PARASITOLOGY FOR MEDICAL AND CLINICAL LABORATORY PROFESSIONALS

John W. Ridley, Ph.D.

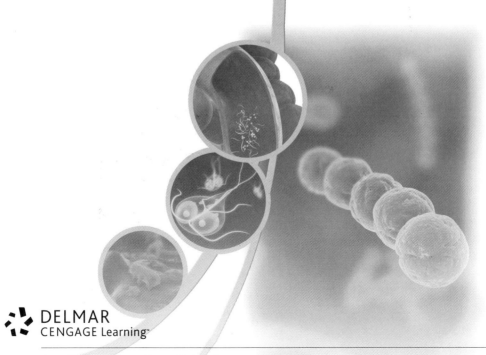

DELMAR
CENGAGE Learning

Australia • Brazil • Japan • Korea • Mexico • Singapore • Spain • United Kingdom • United States

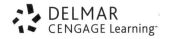

**Parasitology for Medical and Clinical
Laboratory Professionals**

John W. Ridley

Vice President, Editorial, Career Education &
Training Solutions: Dave Garza

Director of Learning Solutions:
Matthew Kane

Senior Acquisitions Editor: Sherry Dickinson

Managing Editor: Marah Bellegarde

Product Manager: Natalie Pashoukos

Editorial Assistant: Anthony Souza

Vice President, Marketing, Career Education &
Training Solutions: Jennifer Ann Baker

Marketing Director: Wendy Mapstone

Senior Marketing Manager: Kristin McNary

Marketing Coordinator: Erica Ropitzky

Production Director: Carolyn Miller

Production Manager: Andrew Crouth

Content Project Management:
PreMediaGlobal

Senior Art Director: David Arsenault

For product information and technology assistance, contact us at
Cengage Learning Customer & Sales Support, 1-800-354-9706

For permission to use material from this text or product,
submit all requests online at **cengage.com/permissions**
Further permissions questions can be emailed to
permissionrequest@cengage.com

Library of Congress Control Number: 2011920100

ISBN-13: 978-1-4354-4816-2

ISBN-10: 1-4354-4816-2

Delmar
5 Maxwell Drive
Clifton Park, NY 12065-2919
USA

Cengage Learning products are represented in Canada by
Nelson Education, Ltd.

For your course and learning solutions, visit **delmar.cengage.com**

Visit our corporate website at **cengage.com**

Printed in the United States of America
1 2 3 4 5 6 7 15 14 13 12 11

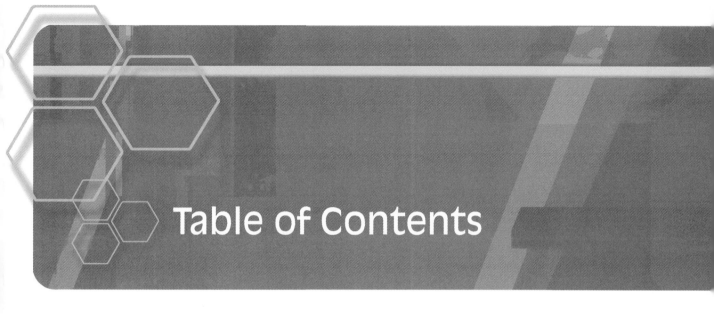

Table of Contents

NOTE: For the purpose of providing a logical sequence in presenting the parasites, and to offer discussions of parasites that infect the human body, this book is organized by body site and the type of tissue in which the various parasites are found. This relieves the beginning student of the task of trying to remember the body site where the ovum (egg) or the adult parasite being discussed is typically found. In areas of the body where numerous organisms are found, such as in the gastrointestinal tract, the organisms will be classified as to their respective morphological characteristics.

CHAPTER 3
PROTOZOAL MICROORGANISMS AS
INTESTINAL PARASITES   35

Preface

Parasitology for Medical and Clinical Laboratory Professionals is written in part to provide a beginning course as an important component of the general and holistic training of laboratory technicians and technologists. With the homogenous society that is reflected today even in remote and sparsely populated regions of the country, the well-trained and educated laboratory worker must be alert to the possibility that a parasite may be the root cause of a patient's illness. Or a parasitic infection may be a result of immunological changes through chronic disease or treatment with antibiotics. It is not out of the realm of possibility that a routine complete blood count may provide the startling discovery by the laboratory worker that a patient has a parasite typically found in the blood. The complete education of a laboratory professional provides an expert, a resource to the physician, who is able to take into consideration a number of possibilities that might not be suspected during a physical examination.

This book, entitled *Parasitology for Medical and Clinical Laboratory Professionals,* provides the background and rationale for the elements involved in teaching a section of microbiology that includes microorganisms as well as organisms that may be viewed by the naked eye. Parasites may range form one-celled organisms, some of which are similar to bacteria, to others that are multicellular agents and may also be arthropods (insects) or arachnids (mites). Some parasites must be transported and transmitted to a host by mollusks and insects, which are called vectors. Parasites may be identified by finding various stages of their unique life cycles, or they may produce eggs that hatch organisms that infect organs and

tissues of the body. It is a textbook focused on providing a foundation for understanding parasitology and the relationships of certain clinical findings with a parasitic infection. Blood counts with microscopic observations of intracellular parasites, anemia associated with parasitic infections, and increases in certain white blood cells, as well as the presence of blood antibodies, may all be utilized to provide a diagnosis of parasitic infection.

INTENDED AUDIENCE

Parasitology for Medical and Clinical Laboratory Professionals is designed to provide the primary knowledge and tools to all the medical or clinical laboratory workers, at the technician or technologist level. With the continuing progression toward more complex and technologically advanced laboratory medicine, the basics, such as staining of and identifying parasites, will continue to be of importance, in both the developed world and the lesser developed regions of the earth. Continuing progression of diseases that adversely affect the immune system, such as HIV infections, will most likely increase the number of cases of parasitic infection, as well as new diseases just being discovered or yet to be discovered.

WHY THIS BOOK WAS WRITTEN

This book was written to provide a broad scope of general knowledge related to the tremendous impact of parasitic infection on human health and the quality of life in societies throughout the world. This book is also intended to alert the laboratory worker, regardless of professional level, as to the possibility of endemic areas developing within the more developed countries, due to the prevalence of world travel. It can also be used as a resource for any medical professional for consultation when familiarizing oneself with or exploring topics of human parasitology. Modes of transmission due to contaminated soil, water, and food sources require that the health care professional be familiar with conditions that contribute to contraction of parasitic infections.

The common perception is that only certain areas of the world suffer from large-scale parasitic infections, and that there are only a limited number of the various species that are capable of infecting humans. This is far from the truth, as more than 300 species of helminths have been recorded as the causative organism for these infections. Parasitologists and pathologists have knowledge of the most common parasites that inhabit the digestive tract along with associated organs of digestion such as the liver. However, the laboratory professional is the medical worker who would most likely come into routine contact with specimens such as blood and feces or sputum that may contain eggs of parasites or the actual organism. Therefore, it is mandatory that when performing parasitological procedures, the health care professional become familiar with the most common organisms that affect humans. No less important than this knowledge is the fact that proper collection, transport, and treatment of specimens in order to find evidence that a parasitic infection is present are mandatory to effectively provide accurate results.

The numbers of parasitic organisms found in nature, and those that may become parasitic, are staggering. Even algae, though non-parasitic, has been found to produce epidemic diarrhea. Exotic parasites enter this country on a daily basis, and cause little or no signs or symptoms in their hosts, but become a problem when spread in this country. Zoonotic infections, or those that result from transmission by a vector, such as nematode parasites of animals, accidentally infect humans around the world. Fortunately, many of these show few signs in their human hosts, and eventually die in the tissues of the infected persons. But it is possible that some of these will adapt and will become "new" sources of infections in the years ahead. And to further complicate the situation, nonparasitic entities also morphologically resemble parasites and are confused with parasites.

ORGANIZATION OF THE TEXTBOOK

A topical overview is presented in the early portions of this book to acquaint the student of laboratory medicine to the background and history of the early knowledge of parasites and the growing body of knowledge in diagnosing and handling of parasitic infections. An emphasis is placed on the morphological characteristics of the most common parasites encountered in the clinical laboratory today. The epidemiology of parasitic infections and conditions that give rise to these medical diseases is stressed early in the textbook.

Microorganisms as causative intestinal parasites are classified as five different groups, those of flagellates, ciliates, amoebae, coccidia, and microsporidia. Tissue protozoa are numerous and include blood and other tissues. These protozoa are mostly intracellular but may border on being extracellular as some do not invade the cytoplasm. Several chapters are devoted to the "worms" of the intestinal tract, and include nematodes (roundworms), cestodes (tapeworms), and trematodes (flukes). Tissue parasites, which invade muscle and nerve tissues, are also important causative agents in diseases of humans. Mites and lice are also scourges of mankind, infecting the skin and hair of those infected. Life cycles, identification, and treatment of these various infestations are systematically covered in this book.

It is not sufficient to only be able to identify parasites from their basic structures. In order to control potential epidemics of parasitic infections, it is necessary to be knowledgeable of the hosts and intermediate hosts for stages of these organisms. Vectors are necessary for some of the parasitic organisms to be transmitted to humans. These stages are important to be able to identify, in order to properly prepare specimens and to determine the presence of an infection by parasites. In addition, it is often necessary to gather as much information as possible concerning a patient's recent travel history, food preferences or routine diet, outdoor activities that may expose the person to infection, and to unusual environmental exposure.

Procedures for Identifying Parasitic Organisms

Direct identification involves direct visual observation of a parasite from a properly prepared and frequently stained preparation. The eggs of the more common human parasites are easily visualized, particularly those of intestinal parasites known as worms. The protozoal types are more difficult to distinguish from tissue and blood cells for identification purposes. It might be noted that some parasites of domestic animals may resemble those of humans, with only subtle differences. Indirect identification would most often be a serological test, using the serum from a patient's blood, and testing for the production of antibodies that are stimulated by a particular organism. Serological tests for many parasites are not currently available, but perhaps more indirect and definitive tests will eventually be developed.

Prevalence of Parasitic Infections

A number of organisms that were not originally considered as being parasites may be a result of a parasitic infection, where alterations have occurred in the gastrointestinal system. Certain yeasts may grow as a result of dysbiosis, a condition resulting from a disorder of the normal flora in the intestines. Although fungi, yeasts, and molds are not strictly a human parasite, there are similarities between the two groups. Candida, a common yeast, often occurs in both pathogenic bacterial and parasitic infections. Parasitic infections appear to be more prevalent than most health care professionals would think in this country. Outpatients at a gastroenterology clinic in Elmhurst, New York, were diagnosed with parasites at a rate of 74 percent in one 2002 report and a total of 20 percent of this group also yielded positive findings for other pathogens (Farr). In the same report, public health laboratories reported that 15.6 percent of specimens examined contained at least one parasite. At the Great Smokies Diagnostic Laboratory, almost 30 percent of specimens examined were positive for a parasite (Farr, 2002). It is possible that the rate is much higher, as it required a great deal of diligence to properly collect, prepare, and examine specimens to determine parasitic infections.

Laboratory Tests for Identification of Parasites and Their Ova

Body fluids and tissues are often specific for certain parasitic organisms. Therefore, the proper specimen and the properly timed and performed specimen collection are of the utmost importance. Most important pathogens are found either in the blood or in the stool, although other anatomic sites are of significance. A properly collected and preserved stool specimen is examined by use of the microscope for detecting parasites and their eggs if appropriate. Some microorganisms are found in the bloodstream and of course require proper collection and treatment of blood smears for examination to determine infections of certain intracellular parasites. Serological tests for antibodies formed by the body against specific parasites are available for a few parasitic organisms at this time.

Quality Assurance

The purpose of a quality assurance program is to provide assurance that accurate and reproducible results are produced, from collection and transport of the sample and the initial handling of the specimen. These steps require that other health care professionals who provide direct patient care will adhere to correct practices to insure the best results possible. In addition, the technical worker, usually a laboratory professional, is enabled to troubleshoot and correct any problem areas in the analysis of the samples and the reporting of accurate results. Quality assurance for parasitology is somewhat different than some of the automated procedures in the laboratory, and requires a great deal of critical thinking, attention to details, and even making assumptions at times. Factors affecting the quality of results include environmental conditions, training and competence of practitioners, and availability of adequate supplies and operable equipment.

Quality control is but a component of a good quality assurance program, and prepared slides are available for laboratory workers to stain and to examine for known parasitic organisms. Adequate performance includes preparation and staining, as well as identifying parasitic organisms. Serological testing for antigens and indirect tests for the presence of antibodies may also be done on control specimens to determine effectiveness and competence of the procedures and the testing personnel.

A common belief of many is that the quality of laboratory results solely depends upon the particular laboratory performing an analysis. However, this includes the analytical portion of quality assurance, but no less important are a number of pre-analytical and post-analytical factors which influence the quality of the results obtained by the laboratory and its professionals.

The principle of "GIGO"—"Garbage in Garbage Out" applies to pre- and post-analytical processes, leading to quality results. Some of the important factors influencing quality are listed here:

1. **Specimen**

   This is the single most important factor. Selection of the right sample, proper collection the correct sample (may be timed), adequate quantity, proper transportation with a preservative if required, to the laboratory and processing of the sample before testing, are crucial pre-analytic efforts.

2. **Personnel**

   The quality of the laboratory results generated is directly proportional to the education and training of the laboratory professional. The staff should be monitored for commitment and motivation by supervisory personnel who can do a gread deal in setting a climate that demands accuracy and zealous performance.

3. **Environmental factors**

   Factors that impact accurate processing and analysis include inadequate lighting, workspace or ventilation, and other unsafe conditions may influence laboratory results.

4. **Analytical factors**

   The quality of reagents, chemicals, glassware, stains, culture media, reagent grade water supply, and use of standard procedures and reliable equipment all influence laboratory results. The failure to adequately examine the specimen by surveying a sufficient number of microscope fields can lead to false negative results.

5. **Post-analytical factors**

   Transcription errors, incomplete reports, and improper interpretation can adversely influence the laboratory results. These are perhaps the most easily managed category of error, as a supervisor may approve the results before they are disseminated by using a standardized set of factors to ensure that the report is complete and accurate.

Safety in the Laboratory and Specimen Contact

Safety is the responsibility of everyone in the laboratory. Duties when performing parasitology procedures often require counseling of patients as to the proper collection and transport of specimens, as well as requiring the laboratory professionals to handle fresh specimens. Safety in the area of parasitology also includes handling of specimens and disposal of specimens after processing. The proper manner in which to dispose of specimens is the responsibility of the student, the instructor, and the health care workers who may come into contact with the various specimens. Handling of chemicals such as stains and concentrating fluid, as well as formalin used for preserving samples, also pose a hazard to the laboratory worker. In addition, it is easy for the laboratory worker to contract a parasitic infection unless protective equipment is used, personal hygiene is observed, and specimens are properly handled and discarded.

FEATURES

Each chapter opens with a list of learning objectives and key terms that highlight important topics and terminology throughout the text. Microscopic Diagnostic Features (MDF) throughout the book consist of standardized lists of distinguishing characteristics of microscopic parasites for easy identification by students. The features provided that enable identification and differentiation of various species of parasites include a number of characteristics. These include the specimen type, stage of the organism that most readily lends itself to quick identification, as well as size and shape of the organism and its nucleus(i) along with other features including the appearance of the cytoplasm and the type of motility, if present. The MDF is especially useful when differentiating between organisms with similar morphology, some of which may be nonpathogenic and would then require no treatment. The initial narrative and images provided for each parasitic organism that precede the MDF will provide clues as to the identification of the parasite in question.

Chapters conclude with Case Studies and Study Questions to further test students' comprehension of the material presented throughout the text. Diagnoses to the case studies can be found in the instructor's manual that accompanies the text.

HOW TO USE THIS BOOK

It is important to know the history of the study of parasites and some of the misconceptions associated with them. It is equally important to understand the widespread nature of parasites and the ecological niches they occupy, and the steps in the life cycles of each species. The vectors, and control of them, will do a great deal to eliminate the impact of the scourge of parasitic infections, if not to eliminate some of them entirely, as is being pursued for the guinea worm. The first 11 chapters are written to provide a good background of information related to the origins of parasites and the damages they may cause. Each major group of parasites described in this book is based on body sites that certain organisms predominantly infect. Most major genera and species are presented in the first 11 chapters, and Chapter 12 is designed to present the methodology for recovering parasitic organisms from body wastes and secretions, and identifying them. Complete procedures for concentrating organisms, removing debris, and proper preparation of slides for microscopic evaluation are presented in Chapter 12.

ANCILLARY MATERIALS

The Instructor's Manual includes answers to all of the review questions from the text as well as suggested answers to the case studies. A midterm and final exam have been provided in the manual, as well as the answers to both exams. The manual opens with sample course syllabus and also includes a sample schedule for a one-semester, 15-week course.

ABOUT THE AUTHOR

John W. Ridley received a B.S. in zoology and a master's of education at the University of Georgia. A Ph.D. in health and human services, with an emphasis in psychology, and becoming a registered nurse in 1992 completed his formal education, but not his practical education. During his tenure as a full-time student, he worked in a hospital laboratory as a laboratory technician, educated and trained during the Vietnam conflict in basic medical laboratory procedures at Brooke Army Medical Center, Ft. Sam Houston, Texas. The U.S. Army did not require that laboratory technicians be registered during this period, but the author was qualified by education and experience and did sit for the ASCP registry examination soon after entering the civilian sector. Experiences that have influenced the writing of this book stemmed from military stints as a combat medic and experiences related to civilians and soldiers who contracted a host of parasites.

Many of the military service member victims suffered from multiple infections that robbed them of their strength and vitality. Basic field tests commonly used to quickly identify potential parasitic infections formed the basics of the author's initial exposure to the effects of parasitic infections. Basic pictures used for comparison gave clues for identification of the most common ova (eggs) and parasites, but the inability to have any control over proper collection of specimens and expert consultation left much to be desired. But it was easy to see that many rudimentary laboratory procedures were extremely vital to the welfare of the troops, and this whetted a desire to learn more. The field procedures included many diagnostic tests that were performed outside a building, sometimes in a tent, and with little equipment. But these initial and basic tests were often as or more important than those without medical facilities than those performed in modern labs, providing quick diagnoses and treatment.

Upon entering the teaching profession in 1992, the author found his niche, with 15 years of experience as an ASCP-registered medical technologist in both hospitals and starting a small private commercial laboratory. After a few years of educating students by teaching academic science courses as well as starting two MLT/CLT programs, Dr. Ridley determined that any student for any health care program needed certain basic core knowledge in a variety of areas prior to entering or concurrent with the beginning of the medical laboratory program. It was this belief that led to the writing of this book. His wide experience as a medical technologist and with the added skills from the nursing arena and human services subjects lend a unique blend in the composition and writing style for this book.

REVIEWERS

Tobi L. Camilli BS, ASCP(M)
Adjunct Professor
University of New Mexico, Gallup Branch
Gallup, NM

Mildred K. Fuller, Ph.D., MT(ASCP)
CLS Interim Vice Provost/Dean–Undergraduate and
    Graduate Studies
Norfolk State University
Norfolk, VA

Barbara Wenger, MS, MT(ASCP)
Allied Health Distance Education Coordinator
Manhattan Area Technical College
Manhattan, KS

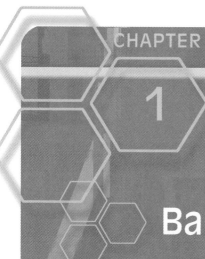

Background of Parasitology

LEARNING OBJECTIVES

Upon completion of this chapter, the learner will be expected to:

- Relate the meaning of the term *parasite*
- Define an organism that qualifies as a parasite
- Describe the importance of hosts in the life cycles of parasites
- Discuss the probable evolution of parasites that infect humans
- List major vectors of parasites and the role they play in causing epidemics
- Define the steps leading to the recovery and identification of most parasites

KEY TERMS

Accidental host

Acquired Immunodeficiency
  Syndrome (AIDS)

Arthropods

Clade

Commensalism

Congenital

Coproliths

Definitive host

Diagnostic stages

Ectoparasites

Endemic

Eukaryotic

Fleas

Guinea worm

Helminthes

Host

Human Immunodeficiency
  Virus (HIV)

Infective stage

Infestation

Intermediate host

Kleptoparasitism

Lice

Malaria

Metazoan

Mites

Mutualism

Nematode

Opportunistic

Parasitism

Pathogenic

Phylogenetically

Prions

Protozoa

Reservoir host

Symbiosis

Syndrome

Zoonoses

INTRODUCTION

Parasitology is a diverse and dynamic field that is still evolving as new technology emerges for earlier and more specific diagnosis and treatment of an infection or infection of parasites. The economic toll for parasitosis around the world is staggering, as it impacts human productivity as well as agricultural pursuits of the various areas of the world. A blurring of the distinction of what is considered a parasite exists, and the list includes bacteriology, virology, and mycology (fungi, yeasts, and molds). Parasites are those organisms that use animal and plant species as a host, and some have more than one host, and sometimes includes intermediate hosts that are necessary for continued reproduction and survival of the various parasites.

The parasites found in specific areas may depend upon one specific host or one set of environmental factors that are present in that locale, and are unable to survive in other areas of the world. Therefore, there are endemic areas of the world which are the only geographical regions where certain parasites exist. Some free-living parasites do not require a host in order to survive, but it is believed that parasites and the parasites that require a host greatly outnumber the numbers of free-living species. Parasitism comprises an ecological relationship between two individuals of different species where the parasite's environment is another living organism.

A diverse group of scientists, including ecologists, molecular biologists, immunologists, and biologists, provide a source of information regarding fundamental biological principles of parasitology. The complex relationships involving parasites and hosts aid the students in a variety of medical professions in understanding the interrelationship of a variety of scientific endeavors. The importance of parasites and the human diseases they cause have been known to humans for perhaps thousands of years as archaeological evidence points to this fact. Hundreds of millions of people suffer from malaria and each year over one million human deaths are caused by this parasitic disease. It should be remembered that at one time malaria was somewhat rampant even in the United States. Many species of parasitic worms, blood flukes, tapeworms, hookworms, and ectoparasites such as fleas and lice range from being an annoyance to humans to vector-borne diseases such as bubonic plague and typhus have contributed to large numbers of deaths. Mosquitoes transmit malaria, yellow fever, encephalitis, other viral diseases, and several species of filarial worms.

Ticks as vectors carry a number of new and emerging diseases such as Lyme disease that are widely viewed as significant to human health.

The field of public health is closely allied with medical parasitology and expands to a global distribution of parasites that offers challenges in the control of conditions, vectors, and parasites. Public health practitioners are employed on a local basis as well as by state and national agencies. International agencies such as the World Health Organization, private industry, private philanthropic and charitable organizations, and military campaigns are organized to coordinate efforts to control parasitism. Educational facilities also use field exercises around the world to increase the body of knowledge necessary to combat parasitic infections and to train workers and educators in areas where parasites are endemic. It is also important that parasitologists work in agricultural pursuits as malnutrition also contributes to the increase in parasitic infections.

Description of the Meaning of the Word *Parasite*

To understand the word *parasite*, breaking down the word into its parts will go a long way in aiding the learner as he or she goes about the task of learning to identify and to report parasitic infections. The word prefix –*para* has several meanings. For the purposes of this book, the following meanings would be appropriate. *Par*, meaning "equal" or "occurring as a pair" would be the meaning in many cases. In a study of parasitology, however, the prefix would encompass the words meaning "near," "beside," "past," "beyond," or "alongside," same as the prefix for the word *parallel*, indicating two organisms living in tandem with each other. When the word suffix –*ology*, meaning "study," is added to the term *para–*, the almost exact meaning of the entire word *parasitology*, would be a "study of those living closely to each other."

Parasitism is the term used for an existing condition where there is an infection by one or more species of organisms classified as parasite(s). A general statement relating to the classification of parasites is that the parasitic organism cannot live separate from the host as the organism in or upon which the parasite lives or exists. Body sites where the parasite survives will be discussed later in this section. Another useful term employed when discussing parasitism is that of symbiosis, which means "living together." Symbiosis is a phenomenon where two or more organisms that differ phylogenetically (term indicating a genetically different lineage) exist over a substantial period of time, although they are completely unrelated. This relationship may be stopped upon the death of one of the organisms, either the parasite or the host.

A number of additional terms are used to describe a parasitic relationship. Symbiosis encompasses **commensalism**, which literally means "eating at the same table," where two organisms co-exist in the same space while one organism benefits but neither helps nor harms the other. The term **mutualism** refers to a condition in which both species derive benefit from the interaction. In the true parasitic **infestation** of humans, the relationship of the organisms is referred to as "parasitism." In this type of relationship, one organism, which is a parasite, is generally the smaller of the two in size. The parasite derives a benefit from the relationship and the other, known as the host, is harmed in some way. Other forms of "social parasitism" exist, such as kleptoparasitism and "cheating parasitism," which include relationships between the parasite and the host that are characterized by a less close association between the parasite and a host, however.

What Are Parasites?

Parasites are organisms that are dependent upon a particular species of host the species and may be seen either macroscopically (by the naked eye) or with the aid of a microscope (microscopically). A parasite depends upon the host for its nutrients, and the true parasites obtain their nutrients at the expense of the host. This category of parasite is normally the one which causes **pathogenic** infections of humans. Other relationships found in nature are called *commensual relationships*, where the host and the parasite live in harmony with each other and neither is harmed by the living arrangements and do not cause human parasitosis. A third relationship between a host and the parasite is called *mutualism*, meaning that the host and the parasite both benefit from a relationship with each other. Some parasites of humans cause little or no physical harm, whereas others cause severe disease and death.

The term used for parasites that cause obvious harm is that of *pathogenic*, which is also ascribed to other microorganisms such as viruses and bacteria. Another important term used in parasitology is *opportunistic*, indicating that the parasite infects those with underlying diseases that predispose them to contract these parasitic infections. Classification of parasites is done by

both the anatomical sites in which they are found, and their basic anatomy. For example, **ectoparasites** (such as lice) live on the body, whereas other parasites including blood and intestinal parasites live in the body. Descriptive morphology includes the term *worms* (Figure 1-1), which includes several morphological types: **protozoa** (one-celled organisms) and **arthropods** (jointed legs), which also includes either insects and spiders or associated arachnids, many of which are non-parasitic. Some parasitic relationships exist that do not entail an organism living off the nutrients from another living organism. An example of this relationship is a lichen, a fungus which grows on dead wood, a condition that is beneficial in nature for breaking down organic wastes.

Pathogenicity of Parasites

Individual factors greatly affect the outcome for a parasitic infection or infestation. The parasite's size and location of infection, as well as the actual immune response

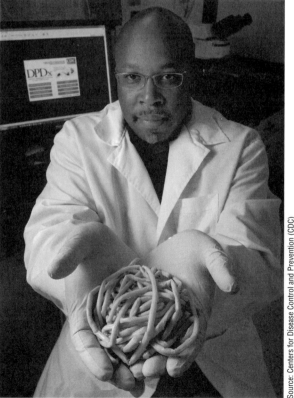

Source: Centers for Disease Control and Prevention (CDC)

FIGURE 1-1 An example of worms as parasites is that of *Ascaris lumbricoides*

the organism stimulates, may either result in physical damage to the host or destruction of the parasite. Or, the infection may result in an absence of symptoms or be only mildly symptomatic. The physical condition of the host and other underlying chronic medical conditions will greatly affect the outcomes of the disease. Some parasites may cause bleeding, irritation of tissues, produce toxins that cause severe reactions, or even obstruct blood vessels or tubular organs of the body. Anemia, organ failure or dysfunction and accompanying bacterial infections and jaundice from destruction of blood or of liver damage may result from significant infections by parasites.

Some parasitic infections are known to have occurred as a congenital condition, which means the fetus was infected while in the uterus of the mother. Infections may occur from direct contact with an infected person, poor food hygiene resulting in the ingestion of the organism or its eggs, by vector transmission, or through dirty water (Figure 1-2). Some organisms, such as the hookworm, may penetrate healthy skin and enter the body.

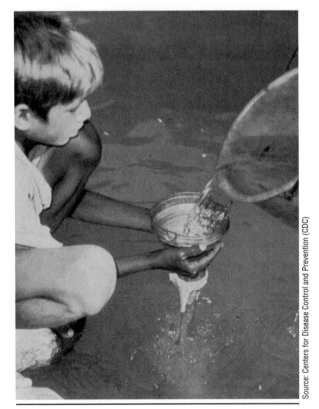

Source: Centers for Disease Control and Prevention (CDC)

FIGURE 1-2 Collecting water using strainer to remove vectors for parasites

Other parasites are contracted from living in close proximity with animals which may be the hosts or reservoirs for a large variety of virulent parasites responsible for tremendous human suffering around the world.

IDENTIFICATION OF PARASITES

Along with the morphology and characteristics of the parasitic organism, the eggs of certain parasites are used to identify a variety of parasites, although this is sometimes problematic in that the eggs of more than one species may appear to be essentially the same. Other identifying characteristics include the type of host the organism infects, and sometimes this is used as a common name; that is, Latin terms for the genus and species of the host. Geographic distribution is another important factor, but this is becoming less significant due to worldwide travel and wholesale immigration. Specific climates are often required for propagation of a species in some cases, accounting for some geographic distribution patterns along with the presence of hosts in the immediate surroundings that are suitable as a site in which the parasite can survive and reproduce. Some parasites require vectors to spread the organism to other individual hosts, so this is also a factor in the patterns of distribution. In some cases, certain stages of a parasite's life cycle require a particular species of animal or insect in which to undergo some of the reproductive phases.

HOSTS REQUIRED IN PARASITIC INFECTIONS

The selection of a host by the parasite and its vectors is an important factor in identifying parasites. Most animal species, including humans, are subject to specific parasitic infections by fulfilling at least some of the requirements of the particular parasite in its life cycle. But some parasites, when the conditions are right, may survive in an entirely different species of host than it ordinarily would and some may be found in a variety of species. Some species of potential hosts are naturally immune to certain parasites and this is sometimes true for humans. For example, humans may not contract some of the parasitic infections to which their pets are subject, such as heart worms in dogs. But some investigators have reported rare cases of *Difilaria immitis* the causative organism for heartworm infections in humans, mostly as pulmonary invasions and often by a single worm.

Those individuals who are in good health and practice good hygiene and food preparation safety are less likely to become infected that those who are not careful in their lifestyles and sanitation practices. It has been documented that parasitic infections on a widespread basis occur more frequently in poor and impoverished regions with a low level of sanitation. Parasites also stimulate an immune response when the body produces antibodies against an invasive organism in the same way as with bacterial and viral infections. In many cases, an indirect identification of an organism may be possible by testing for specific antibodies to known organisms.

Three important terms are used in the subject of host descriptions. The main host is called the *definitive host*, and is the organism in which the adult form of the parasite is found. This is a sexually mature form of the parasitic organism. Some parasites require more than one level of host in order to complete a life cycle, which includes maturation and reproduction. An intermediate host involves a life cycle where a species of host that differs from that of the definitive host is necessary for competion of the developmental stages of a parasite. An example of this relationship is a widespread type of parasite such as the malarial organism, *Plasmodium vivax*. The intermediate host is the human, where asexual or larval forms of the parasite are found, and the definitive host is a species of mosquito where the parasites undergo sexual reproduction.

Reservoir Host

A reservoir host is an organism in which the parasite is harbored until it is transmitted to the main or primary host. The reservoir host may not be harmed extensively or at all while harboring the parasites and is linked to connected populations or environments where a given organism can permanently reside until it is transmitted to a defined target population as a pathogen. Multiple reservoir hosts might exist, and confirmation of the destruction of a reservoir occurs when the target population is free of disease and the parasite has been eliminated. If diseases in the target population are controlled, the presence of a reservoir for the causative organism may never be determined. Practical approaches in identifying reservoirs require field work for identification and effective control of the reservoir hosts.

Reservoir hosts may harbor infectious agents that can infect more than one host species (target population). Zoonoses are infections that are common in animals and may also infect humans. These diseases may comprise well over half the bacterial and parasitic infections suffered by humans and the causative organisms number into the hundreds of species. Many livestock pathogens and those that infect domestic carnivores such as dogs and cats may affect multiple host species, including humans (Haydon, Cleaveland, Taylor and Laurenson, 2002).

Accidental Host

Another term sometimes heard when a parasitic infection is experienced is that of accidental host. This refers to the infection of an animal or human with a parasite or other organism not normally found in the host. Vectors are also involved in the transmission of many parasites, and may be either biological, such as a mosquito or tick, or mechanical, where the parasites are transmitted by food products or by flies that walk on infected wastes and then pass the parasites from one area to another. Humans may become "accidental" hosts when human infection is not required for propagation and continued survival of the infectious agent found in nature. Most emerging or "new" infectious diseases are zoonotic (animal origin). These zoonotic disease agents may be viruses, bacteria, multicellular parasites or prions, the agent associated with "mad cow disease."

TRANSMISSION OF PARASITIC INFECTIONS

The parasitic life cycle is vital in the transmission of parasitic infections. Some parasites spend their entire life cycles in one host, whereas others require more than one host at different developmental stages. Some are parasitic only during periods of development by becoming *free-living* at certain stages. Many parasites also require certain environmental conditions for themselves and their hosts, so many parasites are found in the warmer climates of the world where there is a greater diversity of animal life. Knowledge of the life cycle for suspect organisms is necessary for interrupting the life cycle and thereby minimizing the number of infections, as well as knowing the correct specimen type required for identifying the particular parasite.

The ways humans are infected (modes of transmission) are numerous and often complex. Humans may even infect animals with their own diseases, such as tuberculosis. Animals in which an infectious agent can reproduce with no ill effect on the animal are known as *reservoirs*. Humans come into contact, either directly or

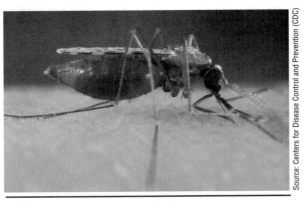

Source: Centers for Disease Control and Prevention (CDC)

FIGURE 1-3 Anopheles mosquito, an effective vector of malaria

indirectly, and transmission then occurs with humans as accidental hosts. The arrival of previously unknown zoonotic diseases may correspond with climatic and ecological changes with a resultant movement of pathogens due to the availability of vectors such as mosquitoes (Figure 1-3) and animals that are hosts to pathogens. The spread of diseases may also be facilitated by genetic changes, and adaptation in the pathogens themselves may occur. Changing human behaviors and the inhabiting of areas formerly void of population centers are also contributing factors. It is the author's opinion that the AIDS-causing organism HIV may have infected humans as an accidental host while the reservoir for the organism could be certain species of monkeys and other simians found in tropical areas of the world.

Stages in the parasitic life cycle are important in the transmission of a parasitic organism. A parasite has two stages in its life cycle: the *infective stage* and the *diagnostic stage*. The infective stage is more important in learning the modes of transmission and how to prevent it, and the diagnostic stage is often crucial in properly identifying the organism. Intestinal parasites most often occupy only one stage, a combination diagnostic-infective stage, making identification somewhat simpler.

DIAGNOSIS OF PARASITIC INFECTION

An infestation or infection by parasites in an individual is often difficult to determine, as symptoms may be vague and testing is only partially sensitive in most cases for finding evidence of parasite infection. The term *infestation* usually refers to an ectoparasite, which includes **mites**, lice, and **fleas**, for the most part. The term *infection* refers primarily to parasites that reside within the body of the victim or host. Identification by indirect methodology includes some tests that are based on serological tests, where antibodies produced by an infected person are tested against known organisms (antigens). These methods of diagnosis are becoming more readily available today and may be more sensitive than the current and traditional methods that require a visual and direct identification of pathogens. An advantage of the indirect tests based on the presence of antibodies against an organism is that they may provide positive results and therefore specific identification of the species when only small fragments of antigens, as only parts of the parasite itself, may be present.

However, there are other organisms that require a relationship in which they are required to feed upon a host and are not considered strictly as parasites of the organism they infect. For instance, some multiple parasites feed off the blood of the animal before detaching themselves. Examples of organisms requiring a host upon which to feed in order to maintain life but not themselves classified as parasites are multiple. One of the examples of this type of relationship that benefits only one partner in the process includes the mosquito, which finds nourishment in the blood of warm-blooded mammals such as humans or birds. The mosquito itself is not a parasite, although parasites such as those that cause the disease of **malaria** as well as a few other significant organisms may be transmitted through bites by the mosquito. Other examples of this relationship will be discussed later in this text.

The most predominant type of parasitism in the field of medical parasitology is one in which the term *parasite* is most often used for a **eukaryotic**, pathogenic organism. A eukaryotic organism is one in which the nucleus is quite organized and is contained within a nuclear membrane. Normally, protozoan (unicellular) and **metazoan** (multicellular) infectious agents are classified as parasites, whereas bacteria and viruses are not as they have no organized nucleus. But they do require a host in or on which to live as do the "true" parasites. Interestingly, fungi are not discussed in textbooks of medical parasitology, even though they are eukaryotic and require tissue, either plant or animal depending upon the species, upon which to grow and reproduce. Another topic open for discussion is the blurring of the distinction between parasitology and tropical medicine, the latter of which includes chiefly bacteria and viruses. Often one will find that all of these studies are conveniently researched by the same organization, such as the World Health Organization, at the same time and in the same location. There will be other references to these practices in this book.

HISTORY OF PARASITES AFFECTING HUMANS

Intestinal parasites most likely have inhabited the gastrointestinal tract of humans since the early beginnings of human habitation of the planet earth. Although it is a rhetorical question, was there a reservoir for the parasites before they infected man? Did they originate early in the history of mankind as part of the normal intestinal organisms that aid in digestion? Or did they possibly function as an aid for stimulating immunity against pathogenic organisms such as some normal bacterial flora now do? A plausible explanation is the possibility that parasites adapted to life in humans after they originated in other animals, with the animal being the reservoir from which humans contracted the organism by eating the meat of the animals or living in close proximity to them. And because intestinal parasites that are similar to those found as pathogens in humans are also found in domesticated dogs and cats as well as in other wild animals, these domesticated animals may have been the original source of parasitic infection (Figure 1-4). And although they differ only slightly for the most part in speciation, these parasites might have specialized for an existence in either man or lower animals from a common obscure origin.

Impact on Human Health by Parasites

Parasites occupy an important position in the history of humans, and are an important part of morbidity and mortality, particularly in the less developed parts of the world. Concurrently with other diseases, medical practitioners are becoming more aware of the possibility of parasitic infections that occur along with, or as a result of, other disease states because a number of parasite species are opportunistic. Anyone who has travelled to a foreign country with poor sanitary conditions for food and human wastes should be evaluated for a parasitic infection, particularly if abdominal bloating or other signs and symptoms arise (Figure 1-5). In addition, migration from those countries where parasites are **endemic** have brought to the shores of the United States and the entire Western world a growing number of heretofore foreign pathogens which have found friendly reservoirs and hosts. Many persons are aware that a health history now almost always questions the patient as to travel within a period of time which might yield clues as to certain infections endemic in some areas of the world. Prior to the United States becoming more advanced and prosperous, humans lived in close proximity with, and had daily contact with, farm animals, so the impact of parasitic infections was much greater in the early history of the United States than it is today.

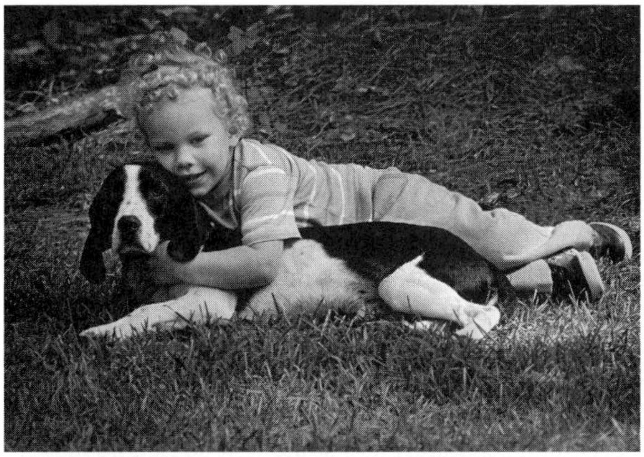

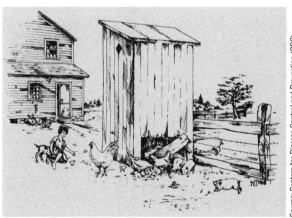

FIGURE 1-4 Dogs may have been a source for original parasite infection in man

Source: Centers for Disease Control and Prevention (CDC)

FIGURE 1-5 Human wastes and unsanitary conditions lead to infections

Source: Centers for Disease Control and Prevention (CDC)

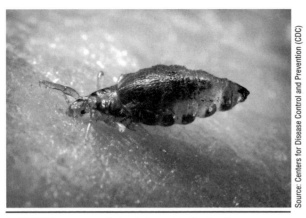

FIGURE 1-6 Female body louse, *Pediculus humanus* var. *corporis*, as it was obtaining a blood-meal from a human host

Although intestinal parasites have received the most attention in modern years, historically the first to receive any attention were those that infected or infested the skin of humans. These ectoparasites were readily visible or at least required immediate attention, due to the discomfort they caused to those infected. The rise of this order of skin parasite or ectoparasite may be used as an example of the manner in which these and other parasites and infectious diseases may travel around the globe. According to current theories on the origins of parasites found to infest the skin of man, it appears that body lice reached the American continents even before early explorers such as the Vikings, who reportedly were the first to reach the North American continent (Figure 1-6). Later, European explorers and possibly the rest of the civilized world, reputedly infected the Native Americans—the North Americans commonly call Indians—along with the Aztecs and Incas. The latter were two indigenous populations that inhabited what is sometimes called the *New World* on both the North and the South American continents. The beginnings of the Aztecs and Indians are even more obscure that those Native American "Indians" we believe had Mongol origins and may have crossed the Behring ice straits between Asia and the western portion of North America.

TRANSFER OF PARASITES FROM ONE AREA OF THE WORLD TO ANOTHER

At any rate, it is believed that the advent of louse infestations predated the Columbian era. This section of the book will use ectoparasites to explain the possibilities for spreading organisms about the world. Just as some larger mammals and other animals are indigenous to one area but eventually are found in a larger geographic region, the spread can best be explained by the example of an ectoparasite, the louse. These organisms are basically the same around the world, but have differing DNA patterns for various populations of lice, with a history of infecting humans since early history.

It was reported in the *New York Times* (2/7, A16, Wilford) that two independent studies detailed in *The Journal of Infectious Diseases* yielded "well-preserved louse DNA" from a pair of Peruvian mummies, remains of two persons who died more than one thousand years ago. This led researchers to the assumption "that lice had accompanied their human hosts in the original peopling of the Americas, possibly as long as 15,000 years ago." This is the length of time that it is commonly believed than man may have inhabited the two American continents. Just as in the example of the louse, certain intestinal parasites are practically the same in diverse parts of the world. But similar parasitic organisms may have different methods of transmission of infection to humans, based on geographic and environmental conditions.

Spread of an Ectoparasite

The example of body lice and the spread of several strains throughout the world provides clues as to how other species of parasites may have spread and evolved. Three strains of lice invade and inhabit the epidermal tissue of humans and are commonly called *clades*. The term clade is not specific for any particular species, but refers to a group of organisms that have specific genetic material as a distinct species or strain of a species (some species have more than on strain, i.e., common influenza). This term is dependent somewhat on the anatomical location and particularly the geographic sites where they are found. Some clade A–type lice are found almost everywhere humans, birds, and others live. Clade B–type lice are most common in North America and Europe, indicating that they were transported from one region to another through migrations between continents. Lice from the clade C type are seldom found, as they are quite rare. Some research seems to support that clade B–type lice developed separately and somewhat simultaneously in North and South America, with cross-infections between humans and native fauna found on these continents.

So the best and probably most valid theory is that European settlers brought clade A to the American continents, where they contracted infections of clade B and returned the favor by transporting them to Europe where that continent developed a ready pool of organisms which tended to infect the entire continent. Later study, however, from medical reports from both continents indicated that clade A was possibly also distributed along with B across the Americas hundreds of years before the first Europeans arrived, perhaps by the Vikings and possibly by some Middle Eastern peoples (some evidence exists that Egyptians and others may have crossed the stormy Atlantic in reed ships centuries before the Vikings). The presence of these lice supports a theory that visitors from Europe and other parts of the civilized world came to the New World many years before Columbus. Or, it is reasonable that clade B was prevalent in the early nomads who may have crossed the ice of the Behring Straits thousands of years before the Norsemen came to what they called "Vinland."

Spread of Intestinal Helminths and Protozoa

During the relatively short history of humans on earth, the species has acquired a substantial number of organisms labeled as parasites. Approximately 300 different species of wormlike organisms, termed as helminthes, exist. These species encompass the flatworm, at least half of which are parasites, and includes the tapeworm, an extremely important intestinal parasite of humans. A widely varied form of life, flatworms are also found as marine life and these species are not known to be parasitic. But the species that are parasitic are second only to malaria in exacting a toll on human health.

Currently, more than seventy identified species of protozoa are characterized by appearing as one-celled (unicellular) organisms. Some of these are free-living or inhabitants of the environment and include some of the most important parasitic pathogens of man that are found in the kingdom Protista. This kingdom includes protozoa, uni- and multicellular algae, and slime molds. Ironically, rare occurrences of apparent algal infections among humans have been mentioned. Many of these protozoa are rare and accidental parasites, but humans still harbor a number of relatively common species from which a small percentage cause

some of the most celebrated and dangerous parasitic infections in the world. Therefore, this small number that cause serious disease have received the most attention and are targets of worldwide organizations such as the WHO (World Health Organization) that has focused on eliminating them.

Because many of these parasitic diseases occur mainly in the tropics, the field of parasitology has tended to overlap with that of tropical medicine, and it is difficult to separate the two branches as they are inextricably intertwined. In the early part of human civilization, activities necessary for survival may have occurred concurrently with the presence of reservoirs of parasites seeking to find a suitable animal host such as the human to inhabit. It might have been necessary to seek new territory to avoid some of the plagues afflicting mankind and may have actually changed the history of mankind where pockets of dense population have occurred. This would be particularly true where bodies of water necessary for the growth of mosquito larvae to provide efficient vectors exist. Such environments often led to dense populations of the adult mosquito species (Figure 1-7). The Anopheles mosquito is one of the vectors that is capable of transmitting both malaria, a protozoan, and filariasis, a nematode (round worms and thread worms), and the *Aedes* species of mosquito is chiefly responsible for inflicting dengue and yellow fever, diseases which are caused by viruses among large groups of victims.

Although the branch of health care called tropical medicine deals mainly with pathogenic strains of bacteria, it is inevitable that the coexistence of bacteria,

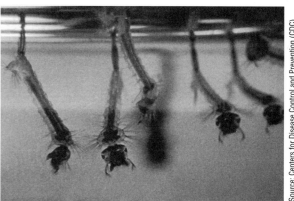

Source: Centers for Disease Control and Prevention (CDC)

FIGURE 1-7 Photograph of mosquito larvae taken during a 1972 study of disease carriers and pests of migrant labor camps

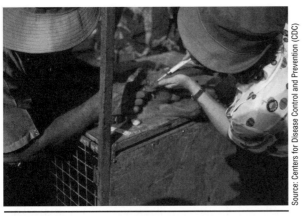

Source: Centers for Disease Control and Prevention (CDC)

FIGURE 1-8   Extracting a blood sample from a green monkey

certain strains of virulent viruses, and numerous parasites would be found that are concurrently surviving. All of these would require surveillance and eradication efforts, lending itself to prevention of all of these categories of infectious agents of humans. So our understanding of parasites and parasitic infections cannot be separated from our knowledge of the history of humans and their spread across virtually the entire globe. In particular, the spread and present distribution of many parasites throughout the world has largely been the result of human activities that includes migration and exposure to animals used for food such as the green monkey of Africa, which may be the source of HIV infections in humans (Figure 1-8). The advent of HIV infections leading to AIDS has added a new chapter to the history of parasitology. Those persons who are immunocompromised by an HIV infection as well as by some of the other infectious diseases that impact the immune status are in some manner with a more diverse collection of animals vulnerable to a host of viral, bacterial, and parasitic organisms to which these persons may fall victim.

EARLIEST EVIDENCE OF PARASITIC INFECTIONS IN MAN

As described earlier, the development and subsequent civilization of humans and the advent of parasitic infections appear to have occurred simultaneously. Due to the knowledge gained from the Human Genome Project, where almost all of the genes contained in the human body have been mapped, scientists are now able to learn more about the origins of diseases affecting the human race than was previously possible. And in a similar fashion, historical evidence of organisms that infected the body and the environment are also able to be studied based on findings within the body of mummies and preserved tissue samples and excrement from humans and other animals.

Physical findings exist as records from tens of thousands of years ago apparently exist, where *Homo sapiens* remains have been found in eastern Africa. Eventually these peoples spread throughout the world, moving somewhat in waves, perhaps based on food supplies or disease in certain areas or for other unknown reasons. It is commonly believed by some that about 15,000 years ago, at the end of the Ice Age, humans had migrated to and had sparsely populated virtually the entire world, taking some parasites with them from their previous dwelling sites and becoming infected by others along the way. The human groups of this period may have diversified their holdings of parasites by retaining those that they seemed to have inherited from their primitive ancestors and then picking up others along the way from other animal groups or from the new environments in which they found themselves.

The greater the dimensions of the geographic areas to which human ancestors moved resulted ultimately in contact with a more diverse collection of animals, insects, and plants, along with an increasingly agricultural environment. These migratory patterns left their mark on the humans who had changed their environment through exposure to a panoply of parasites and other one-celled organisms that are related to parasites but cannot truly be called parasites. These souvenirs remained with the groups as they organized into farms and cities and no longer operated as small nomadic groups with little contact from other groups of humans. These cities and settlements, where populations grew denser, were conducive to the facilitation and the transmission of infections between humans.

A somewhat global trade practice began, but, unlike today, it often took years for products of one area to reach another where they might pass through several regions which later became identified as countries. The opening of these trade routes resulted in a much wider dissemination of parasitic infections as well as other species of microorganisms. Groups of people who might have had genetic protection against some diseases were quite vulnerable to others, and those with some natural protection would be similar to what is called "carriers" today.

Then, as civilization advanced, the slave trade most likely began before recorded history and in biblical times. This resulted in indigenous populations that might have been subjugated during war before being transported to unfamiliar areas of the world but living in close proximity to a genetically different population. Around 1500, the Spaniards sometimes enslaved groups of Native Americans as the first in the New World to be enslaved. Then shortly thereafter, African slaves who might have been captured by other tribes and were sold into slavery were transported to the New World, which included the Caribbean islands, from the Old World. More recently the spread of the Human Immunodeficiency Virus (HIV), and the development of AIDS (Acquired Immunodeficiency Syndrome) from HIV infections, most likely originated on the African continent. This disease serves to initiate immunodepression associated with these conditions and has spread to the rest of the world in great numbers.

This condition predisposes the person suffering from AIDS to becoming infected with a variety of opportunistic parasitic organisms. It has been proposed and not disproven that this ravaging disease originated in the green monkeys of Africa, as these animals were widely hunted for food, often resulting in contact with the animal's blood and body fluids. It should be kept in mind that the origins of the disease are still in dispute, and has led to various theories over the years since the advent of the disease. The syndrome (group of symptoms) of AIDS has resulted in the establishment of a number of new opportunistic parasitic infections that cover the entire globe.

Archaeological Evidence of Parasitic Infections

The past history going back for centuries, and bolstered by archaeological specimens and written records, has confirmed that parasitic infections have a history of infecting humans for as long as any sort of record of humans is available. Much of this information predates written history, with the finding of archaeological specimens that are more ancient than written records. But several thousand years BC, work by ancient Egyptian physicians and then later Greek physicians who wrote of parasitic infections, were recorded. One of the significant areas of the study of parasitology today is that of archaeologists who study the evolution of humans and who have documented the

fact that some of the most important parasites we find today, the helminth worms along with their ova and the protozoa, can now be found in ancient preserved stool specimens, lending verification to what was previously only educated guesses or theory.

The presence of helminth eggs and protozoan cysts have been found in preserved stools called coproliths, a term that literally means "fecal stones" or remnants of the products of bowel elimination that are stone-like. These fecal samples have become fossilized or desiccated (dried) as they are hundreds and even thousands of years in age. These bits of hardened feces often contained naturally preserved bodies of parasites that had infested the gastrointestinal tract of these ancient peoples. Springing from these studies is a new branch of science called *paleoparasitology*. This helps to extend the knowledge base that previously had been more theory than fact. It is possible that less evolved versions of some parasites seen today may be found in preserved remains of animals and humans and the excrement of each. Examples of some of these discoveries will be discussed later. So vast is the field of human parasitology, and with this new and far-reaching evidence and the discoveries made to date from the past, the amount of data will no doubt grow dramatically in the future.

Written documents related to parasitic infection in ancient Egypt from several thousand years BC exist. Ancient medicine men were apparently aware of parasitic infections, as described in the Ebers papyrus of 1500 BC discovered at Thebes. Somewhat later, Greek physicians in the years from 800 to 300 BC described symptoms and signs of diseases of various descriptions, some of which might have been caused by parasites. Persons with raging fevers, which might have been difficult to control without the medical technology enjoyed today, were found in various works, including those of the celebrated Hippocrates, author of the Hippocratic Oath still in use in differing versions and whose corporate works are known as the *Corpus Hippocratorum*. Other documentation of apparent parasitic maladies are found in ancient works from physicians as members of civilizations other than Greek and Middle Eastern areas.

Although the medical literature of the Middle Ages is quite scant, there are many references to the malady of being infected by parasitic worms. In some cases, they were considered as the primary cause of certain diseases. However, generally the literature of the period was rife with those who were somewhat ignorant due to stultifying governmental and religious constraints. In Europe, during the Dark and Middle Ages, many retreated into the superstitious beliefs and lack of tolerance by their rulers, instead of continuing the pursuit of knowledge and enlightenment. This period was characterized by strict religious requirements that were mandated by the mostly monarchial governments.

Unlike the periods of the search for knowledge and advancement as found centuries earlier on the Asian continent and the Mediterranean populace, this entrenchment held back medical progress on the European continent during the Middle Ages. But with the advent of the Renaissance period, the augmentation of many cultural accomplishments and scientific advances occurred in a relatively short time. The flurry of activity during this well-documented period eventually led to some of the great discoveries that characterized the end of the nineteenth century and extending into the beginning of the twentieth century. These discoveries were diverse, and included new cultural pursuits, activities by religious organizations, and scientific research. Scientific knowledge expanded to dispel the commonly accepted theory that spontaneous generation occurred in some dirty environments, leading to advances in microbiology.

In the latter part of the nineteenth century, the theory that many diseases were caused by germs, led by Louis Pasteur and others, demonstrated that diseases could be caused by bacteria, and could be prevented by disinfecting areas where medical procedures were performed. The development of a rudimentary microscope by Leeuwenhoek whereby the visualization of bacteria proved the theory that many diseases were caused by living organisms invisible to the naked eye. A technique was also developed to grow colonies of bacteria on nutrient agar in a Petri dish for identification (Figure 1-9). The presence of an organism even smaller than the bacterium was proven in the discovery of viruses by Pierre-Paul Emile Roux, during this time of great achievement and advancement of knowledge. Robert Koch introduced methods of preventing diseases caused by microorganisms, particularly by showing that organisms from an infected site could be grown in animals, producing the disease in them. A number of what are now considered to be medical pioneers made remarkable discoveries in a number of fields. Sometimes working independently, they made mutual findings and then often their ideas fed off each other.

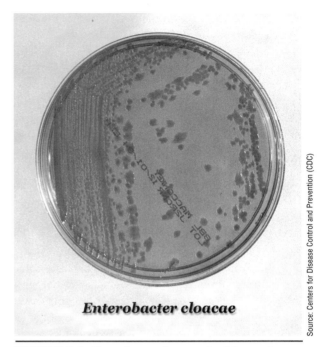

Enterobacter cloacae

Source: Centers for Disease Control and Prevention (CDC)

FIGURE 1-9 *Enterobacter cloacae* colonial growth 24 hours after being inoculated with a specimen sample

Sir Patrick Manson, a London physician, is responsible for discoveries in both tropical medicine and parasitology, close cousins of each other. He emphasized the importance of vectors in the transmission of parasites, and worked with others in discovering that a certain species of mosquito was responsible for harboring and transmitting several of the parasitic organisms that still cause untold suffering and in some cases death in the world. Manson returned to London from the Hong Kong College of Medicine in 1890. He participated in the founding of the School of Tropical Medicine at the Albert Dock Seamen's Hospital in 1899 and later taught there. This school is today known as the London School of Hygiene & Tropical Medicine and is an important training ground for all areas of microbiology, including parasitology.

CLASSIFICATION OF PARASITES

The science of helminthology really took off in earnest during the seventeenth and eighteenth centuries following the reemergence of science and scholarship during the Renaissance period. Carl Linnaeus, known as the father of the classification and naming of living organisms, gave his contribution to science at this time. The term *Linnaean taxonomy* is named for and was devised by Linnaeus and is still largely in use today, although it has changed a great deal since his time. The greatest innovation of Linnaeus, and still the most important aspect of this system, is the general use of binomial nomenclature, the combination of a genus name and a single specific epithet to uniquely identify each species of organism. For example, the human species is uniquely identified by the binomial *Homo sapiens*. No other species of organism can have this dedicated binomial. Prior to the advent of Linnaean taxonomy, animals were classified primarily according to their appendages for locomotion and manner of movement (Niash, 2009).

Because of the importance of and the large size of some helminths, such as the roundworm called *Ascaris* and the tapeworms, it is almost for certain that our earliest ancestors were aware of these common worms. There is some evidence for this assumption based on contemporary studies of primitive tribes in Sarawak and North Borneo, where Dr. Reinhard Hoeppli found that most people are aware of their intestinal roundworms and tapeworms. Hoeppli was best known as a distinguished parasitologist following his service as a German naval physician during the First World War. Some historians have identified references to helminth worms and their diseases in the Bible, but the relevant passages are open to several interpretations. As mentioned previously, the Egyptian medical papyri called the Ebers papyrus, refers to intestinal worms. Again, these records can be validated by the discovery of ossified helminth eggs in mummies dating from 1200 BC.

Also, the Greeks, which again included Hippocrates (460 to 375 BC), knew about the sources of parasitic worms contracted from fishes, domesticated animals, and humans. Following the fall and consequent demise of scientific discovery in the Roman Empire, the focus on medical research and discovery fell to the Arabic physicians. Therefore, some of the names of currently important parasites derive their names from the Arabic influence, including not only the tapeworm but also the **guinea worm**. Many of these discoveries have been recorded in parts of the Arab world, particularly around the Red Sea, for more than a thousand years.

SUMMARY

Parasites have been with animals, including humans, and in some cases plants for the entire history of mankind from the available evidence. Some of the biblical writings of tribulations visited upon humans apparently referred to parasitic infections. Parasites come in many forms, including shapes and sizes, and that impact specific areas of the body and the organs of the body for most species. Parasites can be sufficiently small enough as to require a microscope for identification or as large as helminthes that are capable of growing to several meters in length.

Relationships exist between the parasite and its host, in which the true parasite gains its nourishment from the host. For humans, this strict parasitic relationship is the case in the study of parasites, whereas in nature some parasites and the **host** both benefit from the relationship. In humans, some parasites cause little damage to the host, but some may progress to the point of being fatal to the victim of the infection. Classification of parasites most often depends on the location of the body they infect and their particular type of organism such as amoebae, worms, and insects.

Stages of development of the parasite, and its life cycle, as well as the choice of a host or hosts required for survival and reproduction, are important facets of identification and diagnosis. The main host is called the **definitive host** and in some cases humans are victims as incidental or accidental hosts. For some parasites, a reservoir host is necessary for protecting the parasite until a suitable host, a main host, is available. Basically, a parasite has two life cycle stages: the infective and the **diagnostic stages**. The **infective stage** is the one during which an infection normally occurs, and the diagnostic stage is important for identifying the parasite. Knowledge of the life cycle is important when collecting specimens in order to find the diagnostic stage of development and the likelihood of the highest concentration of parasitic organisms.

The term *infestation* is commonly used for the presence of ectoparasites that parasitize the skin of the body, whereas the term *infection* is used for parasites that colonize the internal organs and body fluids. Identification techniques often include life cycles of parasites and the geographic location where certain organisms are predominantly found. Methodology for collecting and identifying certain parasites that are found inside the tissues of the body (endoparasites) may require different techniques depending upon the body site where they are found. Some of these organisms may require surgical biopsy of tissue specimens for microscopic examination leading to identification of parasites through special staining of the excised tissues. In these cases where surgical techniques are required, knowledge of the life cycle required for isolating the parasites from bodily fluids and wastes may not be necessary for identification as is the case for most intestinal parasites.

Both diet and recent travel are two areas that are extremely important to the investigator of a probable parasitic infection. Both written records and physical evidence of parasitic infections span the ages, with evidence found in mummified remains from thousands of years ago, but today, efforts are being made to completely rid the world of some of the most virulent parasites. The impact of widespread parasitic infections in the endemic pockets of certain infections is still taking a toll on certain groups of peoples, particularly those with a lack of sanitary options. Worldwide organizations are working tirelessly to reduce or eliminate these serious medical problems areas of parasitic infections but it will require years of effort before substantial inroads are achieved in some areas of the world.

STUDY QUESTIONS

1. What mammals may be subject to parasitic infections?

2. Are other species of living or dead organisms subject to attacks by parasites? Think about the answer to this question.

3. What is meant by natural immunity to parasites? Give an example of a type of natural immunity.

4. What are some conditions that may lead to a greater prevalence of parasitic infections in certain groups of people?

5. Define the following terms:
   Reservoir host –
   Definitive host –
   Intermediate host –
   Accidental host –

6. Name several common vectors of parasites.

7. Why is it important in some cases to know the life cycle of a parasite?

8. When are the two stages of a parasite life cycle both important when performing parasitology procedures?

9. Why are the procedures performed prior to identifying the parasite so important?

10. How is it assumed that some parasites that are similar but perhaps not exactly the same in domestic cats and dogs are also found in humans?

11. Describe how ectoparasite such as the louse (species divided into clades or genetic groups) may be used to trace the migration of humans throughout the world.

12. Label the following organisms by the diseases they primarily transmit or cause:
    Anopheles mosquito –
    Nematode –
    Aedes species of mosquito –

13. How was it determined that parasitic infections have been present for thousands of years?

14. What was the invention that greatly facilitated the beginning of proving the existence of microorganisms, including parasites?

15. What is the term for classifying the nomenclature for the order, family, genus, and species of living organisms?

Epidemiology and Conditions Leading to Parasitic Infestations

LEARNING OBJECTIVES

Upon completion of this chapter, the learner will be expected to:

- Describe what is meant by spontaneous generation
- List the three types of parasites as broad classification
- Relate the four pathogenic strains of malaria that infect humans
- Describe an epidemic
- Identify the major vectors that transmit the majority of parasites in the United States
- Define epidemiological surveillance and discuss its importance

KEY TERMS

Acidophilus

Amastigote

Amoebiasis

Ascariasis

Aspergillosis

Asthma

Axoneme

Bronchitis

Cestodiasis

Charcot-Leyden crystals

Chromatin

Chromatoidal bodies

Ciliate

Clonorchiasis

Coccidiomycosis

Contractile vacuoles

Cryptosporidiosis

Cyclosporiasis

Cytoplasm

Cytostome

Dehydration

Dermatitis

Dracunculiasis

Echinococcosis

Edema

Encystation

Eosinophilia

Epidemiology

Excystation

Fibrils

Flagellate

Giardiasis

Glycogen vacuole

Golgi apparatus

Hematoxylin and eosin (H&E)

Histotechnologists

Hydatid (clear) cysts

Infestations

Karyosome

Kinetoplast

Laxative

Leishmaniasis

Liver abscesses

Loiasis

Lymphatic filariasis

Malaria

Microsporidiosis

Myeloproliferative disorders

Onchocerciasis

Opisthorchiasis

Paragonimiasis

Pemphigus

Pica

Pinworms

Pneumocystosis

Pneumonia

Precystic form

Pseudopod

Rhinitis

Schistosomiasis

Strongyloidiasis

Subcutaneous

Toxocariasis

Toxoplasmosis

Trichinosis

Trophozoite

Undulating membrane

Vacuole

Vincent's angina

Volutin

Whipworms

EPIDEMIOLOGY

Humans are hosts to nearly 300 species of parasitic worms and over 70 species of protozoa, some derived from our primate ancestors and some acquired from the animals we have domesticated or come in contact with during our relatively short history on Earth. Acquiring knowledge of parasitic infections extends into antiquity, as evidenced from some of the earlier writings. Descriptions and drawings of parasites and of the effects of parasitic infections are common topics of the earliest writings. This written evidence has largely been confirmed by the finding of parasites in archaeological material obtained from explorations of ancient civilized areas.

The systematic study of parasites began to gain impetus with the rejection of the theory of spontaneous generation and the promulgation of the germ theory. Thereafter, the history of human parasitology proceeded along two lines. First, the discovery of a parasite occurred along with its subsequent association with disease. Second, the recognition of a disease led to the subsequent discovery that it was caused by a parasite. This review is concerned with the major helminth (worm) and protozoan infections of humans. Many exotic-sounding names will be used in the following chapters dealing with classes of parasites. Some of these are as follows (see Table 2-1), and will be discussed individually in most cases.

PATTERNS OF PARASITIC OUTBREAKS

Parasite infections tend to be concentrated within small geographic areas, within families, and within a short distance (in miles) where large numbers of those suffering from parasitic infections reside. Sometimes the overall parasitic infections will encompass large numbers of individuals; however, certain species will be predominant in one area, whereas nearby, another entirely different species of parasite will be the dominant finding. Therefore, by passing the organisms within families and to those who live nearby, the closest condition to an epidemic is created. These individuals may also share certain aspects of life, such as a common water source (Figure 2-1) or fields and gardens fertilized by human waste, which could spread the organisms(s) between groups closely related in their daily routines. There are even differences in the dispersal area of certain parasitic species for those in urban versus rural areas, with the rural areas normally encompassing a smaller area. This is possibly due to less daily contact in the rural areas with a sparser population density than that found in urban environments.

Epidemiological Surveillance

Most epidemiological surveys are performed by governmental agencies and most often are conducted through global organizations of countries, such as the United Nations (UN), the World Health Organization (WHO), and others (Figure 2-2). As shown previously by the limited nature of parasitic epidemiology, studies of human helminth (worm) infections show that there is seldom if ever a wholesale distribution of parasites, but that they are aggregated among given pockets of population. Even in endemic areas, the vast majority of parasitic populations are usually concentrated in only a small representation of the host population. Contracting of the parasites found only in certain areas of the globe is due to a number of factors, including those of an environmental nature. The presence of risk factors among the indigenous population and the presence of reservoirs of infection as well as vectors for transmitting the organisms, if applicable, lead to pockets of infections.

Determination of these small-scale infestations is easily accomplished today due to the availability of global positioning satellites and handheld devices, where specific locales

TABLE 2-1 Examples of Major Organisms Involved in the Following Parasitic Diseases

DISEASE	CAUSATIVE ORGANISM
Amoebiasis	*Entamoeba histolytica; Acanthamoeba sp.; Naegleria fowleri*
Ascariasis	*Ascaris lumbricoides*
Cestodiasis	*Taenia solium; Taenia saginata*
Clonorchiasis	*Clonorchis sinensis*
Cryptosporidiosis	*Cryptosporidium sp.; Isospora belli*
Cyclosporiasis	*Cyclospora cayetanensis*
Dracunculiasis	*Dracunculus meninensis*
Giardiasis	*Giardia lamblia*
Leishmaniasis	*Leishmania sp.*
Loiasis	*Loa loa*
Lymphatic filariasis	*Wuchereria bancrofti*
Malaria	*Plasmodium sp.*
Microsporidiosis	Numerous genera and species
Onchocerciasis	*Onchocerca sp.*
Opisthorchiasis	*Opisthorchis felineus*
Paragonimiasis	*Paragonimus westermani*
Pneumonia	**Pneumocystis carinii (P. jirovecii)*
Schistosomiasis	*Schistosoma mansoni; S. hematobium; S. japonicum*
Strongyloidiasis	*Strongyloides stercoralis*
Toxoplasmosis	*Toxoplasma gondii*
Trichinosis	*Trichinella spiralis*
Trypanosomiasis, African, South American	*Trypanosoma sp.*

Pneumocystis pneumonia (PCP), or pneumocystosis, is a form of **pneumonia chiefly found in those persons afflicted with cancer or HIV infections and caused by the yeast-like fungus Pneumocystis jirovecii. P. carinii is no longer correct for the human variant but is still in common use in many facilities and medical practices.*

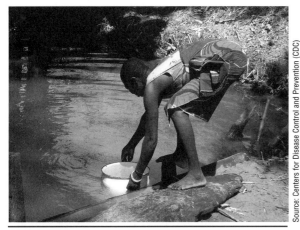

FIGURE 2-1 Gathering water from a local pond, which is used as a source of drinking water

Source: Centers for Disease Control and Prevention (CDC)

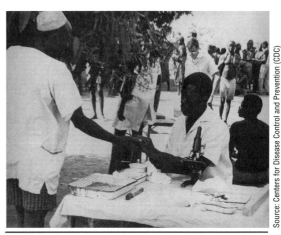

FIGURE 2-2 Epidemiological survey for control of sleeping sickness, measles, yellow fever, and malaria

Source: Centers for Disease Control and Prevention (CDC)

may be determined. Easily transportable field laboratories are now available for working in remote locations, where organisms may be identified microscopically and then preserved for further study. Medical treatment teams from the military services, private charitable organizations, and other governmental agencies often accompany the surveillance teams to provide treatment for residents of the area.

Most areas of the world contain both rural and metropolitan regions that are available for definitive studies related to outbreaks. This information is important academically as well as for scientific study by agencies such as the WHO, divisions of the United Nations, and even U.S. agencies such as the CDC. Certain climactic conditions as well as living conditions contribute to creating an environment for transmission of parasites. Rural dwellers who drink ground water from shallow wells that may have runoff from agricultural sites and animal grazing in the area contribute heavily to the transmission of many parasites. A lifestyle involving contamination of food and water sources, coupled with the lack of availability of health care and sanitation devices and services, are involved in the majority of clusters of parasitic infection.

In order to perform a study in a geographic location, it is necessary to obtain permission from the government agencies and sometimes on a local level, where the indigenous population may be suspicious of strangers in their midst making observations. Meetings are necessary with community members to explain the purpose and manner in which the study will be conducted. Participation is voluntary, and participants must be allowed to withdraw from the study at any time. Most helminth infections may be diagnosed by grossly observing the organism on stool (fecal) specimens, or by finding the eggs (ova) of the organisms by performing certain sedimentary procedures, with the use of ethyl acetate, which has largely replaced the ether and formalin method, to assess the specimens for eggs. Some specimens must be examined as soon as possible, as some features of the eggs may be difficult or impossible to visualize after being passed as much as an hour earlier.

Although parasitic infections do not progress to the proportions by which viral and bacterial infections leading to epidemics and pandemics are characterized, they are, nonetheless, of vital importance. The infestations or infections are usually limited to small groups and are dependent upon the presence of proper conditions for survival and passing of the parasites. The morbidity of the infestations and the mortality as well as the number of worms present in the host (intensity level of infestation) is required for categorization by the WHO. Blood loss in heavy infections and malnutrition associated with heavy infections often prompt treatment by a number of health organizations that operate throughout the world. Parasitic infections of a widespread nature tend to rob the population of vital energy and the will to progress toward a better lifestyle.

SIGNS AND SYMPTOMS OF PARASITIC INFECTIONS

Signs (what you can see) and symptoms (what the patient feels) are many and varied and are dependent upon the type of parasite or parasites with which the victim is infected. People with intestinal parasite infections are usually undernourished and weak, and may be concurrently infected with viruses, fungi, or bacteria. The malnourished state may also lead to certain types of chemical and metal poisoning due to toxins excreted by the organisms. There is no difference in age or gender of those who experience parasitism, as human intestinal parasites can be present with any disease, in any person, and at any age. Parasitic infections may show a broad and confusing array of symptoms, many of which are related to the gastrointestinal tract. The most commonly reported complaints are periods of diarrhea, alternating with periods of constipation. This may be accompanied by bloating and possibly edema, nausea, loss of appetite, and other signs of an irritated bowel (Figure 2-3). Other symptoms not related to the intestinal tract may include night sweats, low tolerance to exercise, intermittent low-grade fevers, recurrent sore throats, low energy, more "allergic"-type reactions, and possibly behavioral changes.

General symptoms and signs will be covered in the sections of this book dealing specifically with the identification of particular organisms. Symptoms of some of the various remaining parasites not described previously may generally cause such clinical signs as anemia, irritation of the gastrointestinal mucosa, and blockage of the organs as common complaints. Cysts that are embedded in tissues of the body and that resemble cancer may also occur with some of these virulent organisms (Figure 2-4). Dehydration from severe diarrhea or anemia related to parasitic infections also provides important diagnostic information to health care teams.

Spirochetes are very tiny bacteria and are spiral-shaped as a group and include both aerobic and anaerobic species. Spirochetes exist as both free-living and parasitic forms, where they multiply in the blood

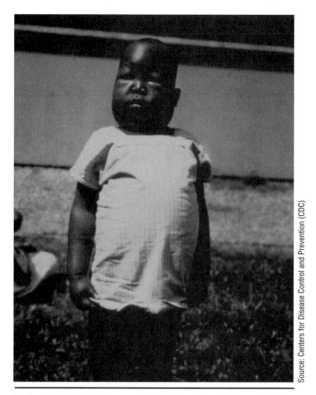

FIGURE 2-3 **Edema exhibited by this African child was brought on by nephrosis associated with malaria**

Source: Centers for Disease Control and Prevention (CDC)

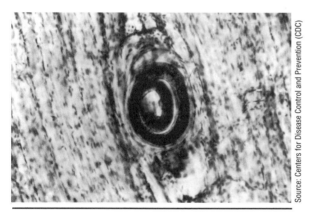

FIGURE 2-4 *Trichinella spiralis* **cyst seen embedded in a muscle tissue specimen**

Source: Centers for Disease Control and Prevention (CDC)

and lymphatic system, and as do parasites, may invade the tissues of the host. The hosts or carriers, sometimes called *vectors*, are usually lice, ticks, fleas, mites, and flying insects, which then transmit the parasites to humans and other mammals. Parasitic spirochetes are responsible for relapsing fever, infectious jaundice, Lyme disease, sores, ulcers, **Vincent's angina** (a disease that causes destruction of the gums), and Wyles disease, a condition resulting from a spirochetal infection, in which the infective organism is spread by insects and **arachnids**.

There are a number of anatomical forms of "worms" that are known to invade the human body. Certain intestinal organisms called *flukes* may cause severe disease of the gastrointestinal tract, bladder, or liver and may also destroy large numbers of blood cells. Some parasitic worms have the ability to fool bodies into thinking they are normal part of the tissue or organ and the immune system will not fight off the intruders. A number of worm-caused infections can cause physical trauma by perforating (burrowing) into the intestines, the circulatory system, the lungs, the liver, or the skin of body (Figure 2-5). They can break down, damage, or block organs of the body by forming clumps as balls or tumors, and sometimes are even mistaken for cancer tumors. A number of species are also able to travel to the brain, heart, and lungs, where they invade the tissues of these vital organs.

Eosinophilia

An important clinical finding that is sometimes discovered in a common blood test is found in the CBC (complete blood count), which includes a count of the percentages of certain white blood cells that might show an increase in a white blood cell called the *eosinophil*. Eosinophils are white blood cells that normally comprise only a small percentage of up to 3 percent of the leukocytes in the blood. The eosinophils have a polymorphic nucleus and pronounced cytoplasmic granules that stain an orange color when an acid stain is used. They increase significantly in many allergic responses and during extremely serious allergic reactions that include bronchoconstriction as often found in **asthma**,

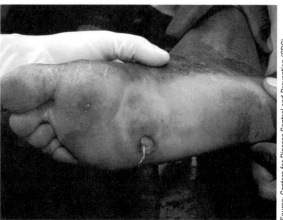

Source: Centers for Disease Control and Prevention (CDC)

FIGURE 2-5 **Subcutaneous emergence of a female Guinea worm**

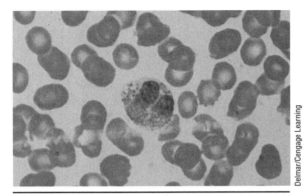

Delmar/Cengage Learning

FIGURE 2-6 Eosinophil, a form of white blood cell present in allergic reactions and parasitic infections

dermatitis, rhinitis, graft rejection, pemphigus (autoimmune skin disease), graft versus host reaction, and certain diseases of the lung (Figure 2-6). But there is an even more dramatic elevation in the numbers of eosinophils for certain parasitic infections and in particular where tissue invasion by parasites has occurred. Although a number of other conditions are known to lead to an increase in eosinophils, an increase for parasitic infections may rise to level where 40 to 50 percent of the white blood cells are eosinophils.

There are also a number of other lesser known illnesses other than parasitic infections and allergies that result in eosinophilia. Reactions to a variety of drugs and food allergies also result in higher levels of eosinophils. Therefore, if a significant rise in the eosinophil count is found, a parasitic infection would be but one of the possibilities for the increase. Substantial increases in the eosinophil count must also be differentiated from malignant disorders such as myeloproliferative disorders. However, elevated levels of eosinophils are also found in a number of parasite infestations that produce an increased eosinophil count. Extreme cases of parasitic infestations may sometimes involve multiple species of organisms infecting a single patient. Some of the kinds of parasites and medical conditions that may elicit a significant increase in eosinophils include:

CONDITIONS LEADING TO PARASITIC INFESTATION

Parasitic infections are more common in areas of the world where sanitation practices are difficult due to lifestyle, availability of water, and detergents for personal cleansing and for preparing food in a manner that will kill any parasites or their ova that may be on the food. Parasites may also result from an underlying larger problem such as in some areas of the country where the patients are largely agrarian. Where most residents of an area drink water from a well, the possibility of contracting a parasitic infection is increased. The symptoms of parasitic infections depend upon what organs of the body are most affected. Specific parasites are able to infest every area and organ of the body, depending upon the species and the medical condition of the patient.

Underlying health conditions may lead to, or exacerbate, an infection by a parasite or parasites. Everyone is at risk and there are many reservoirs in which the parasite may safely reside for considerable periods of time until a more favorable set of conditions, such as a vulnerable victim, becomes available. The human bowel provides the perfect environment for many of the intestinal parasites to flourish, especially if overall health is poor. They can and often do irritate or exacerbate any other health problems already present in the victim. Parasites are responsible for many health problems as some species secrete toxins that affect the body and some steal the vital nutrients from the bodies of those infected. The presence of animals and the conditions they create also contribute to the transmission of parasites to humans, as many different species of animals act as vectors of or are intermediate hosts for important parasites. The relationship between hosts, vectors, and humans is often quite complex for a number of parasite species.

Other medical conditions that may promote parasitic infections occur when excess mucus is formed, and may lead to an imbalance of normally occurring bacteria called *normal intestinal flora*. Chronic constipation where the intestines are infected will also lead to a

Trichinosis	Toxocariasis	Filariasis	Echinococcosis
Aspergillosis*	Coccidiomycosis	Strongyloidiasis	Ascariasis
Shistosomiasis	*Pneumocystis jirovecii*		

Some species of Aspergillus, a fungal disease, like high temperatures with optimum growth at a normal human temperature. It is therefore recognized as a parasite of humans, other mammals, and birds even though it is not among the organisms commonly considered parasites.

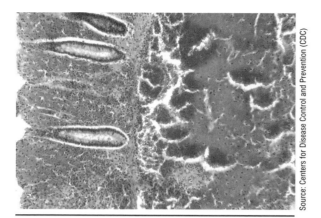

FIGURE 2-7 Human intestine is a perfect environment for intestinal parasites

build-up of toxins in the body that have been released from the metabolism of the parasites (Figure 2-7). The nose is intended for acting as a filter and air conditioner during respiration, by picking up oxygen and exhaling carbon dioxide. By filtering the air with nasal hairs, while warming and moistening the air that is breathed, the interior of the body is able to avoid many of the harmful products found in the atmosphere including pathogens.

Problems associated with the nose may include sinusitis, an inflammation of the sinuses, along with nasal polyps and tumors that may cause restrictions in the nasal passage and further hinder the amount of oxygen inhaled. All of the conditions may be responsible for aiding in the contraction of a parasitic infection. Ironically, parasites often take advantage of certain medical conditions in order to gain a toehold in the body, and then the parasites themselves cause a deterioration of the physical condition of the human body, opening the person to more infections that include bacterial and viral infections.

HOW PARASITES ARE COMMONLY CONTRACTED

Dogs, cats, domestic animals, fowl, and insect vectors such as the mosquito are examples of intermediate hosts, but some parasites, such as *Ascaris lumbricoides*, do not require an intermediate host. Eliminating the source of parasitic infections and improvement of environmental conditions that prevent parasites from reproducing would decrease greatly the numbers of infections that occur. Many physicians even in more advanced countries are not aware of the extent of parasitic infections and the prevalence of parasite infections. Those trained and educated in

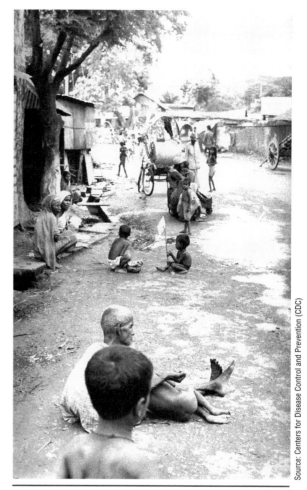

FIGURE 2-8 Crowded and poor living conditions lead to parasitosis

the more advanced areas of the world may not be equipped to recognize the signs and symptoms of parasitic infections they may encounter in the developed countries.

Crowded living conditions, contact with infected persons and infected animals, or exposure to vectors and to unsanitary conditions are the most common conditions leading to the condition of parasitosis (Figure 2-8). With world travel increasing the possibility of bringing parasites to developed countries, the influx of foreign visitors continues to create challenges for health care systems. Routine testing procedures still fall short of being even reasonably accurate and efficient. It is estimated that with traditional testing for parasites, accuracy of recovery and identification of even the most common parasites is perhaps only 20 percent, and is greatly dependent upon the training and diligence practiced by the laboratory personnel conducting the testing. The best way to avoid problems associated with parasite infections is by educating oneself and others to avoid infection and to seek treatment when signs present themselves.

MEDICAL CONDITIONS CREATED BY PARASITIC INFECTIONS

Large numbers of intestinal parasites may even block the intestinal tract or cause hemorrhage if they perforate the intestinal wall. Other extreme medical conditions produced by parasitic infestation are: liver abscesses; appendicitis; peritonitis; hemorrhagic pancreatitis; anorexia (loss of appetite); and anemia and vitamin insufficiency related to poor absorption of digested foods. Hookworm larvae penetrate the skin and are most often contracted through contact with contaminated soil. When hookworms reach adulthood, they may also steal the victim's strength and vitality. Young hookworms have tooth-like structures by which they burrow through the intestinal walls and feed on blood. Symptoms from hookworms are iron deficiency, abdominal pain, loss of appetite, pica (abnormal craving to eat soil), protein deficiency, dry skin and hair, skin irritations, and edema. Advanced cases are characterized by a distended abdomen, stunted growth, delayed puberty, mental dullness, cardiac failure, and death.

Common Organisms That Cause Parasitic Infections

As many or more species of parasites exist than do different mammals and other basic forms of life that can potentially infect humans and other mammals, marine life, plants, and those organisms that dwell in the ground. In addition, many of these may serve as hosts or intermediate hosts, and are capable of infecting humans throughout the world. There are several anatomic categories of parasites have the ability to produce parasitosis in humans, to varying degrees.

CATEGORIES OF PARASITES

The varieties of parasites that inhabit hosts throughout the world are almost endless. The organisms range from single-celled to multicelled organisms that are capable of infecting every living organism in existence. Some cause extensive symptoms, signs, and suffering, whereas others exist at the expense of the host but cause little harm.

Helminthes (worms) and protozoa comprise the basic groups of parasites that infect humans. Another group, ectoparasites that live on the skin and hair, is common but does not cause the extreme medical conditions that the previous two categories do.

Helminths

Helminths, or worms, inhabit most areas of the world and produce a large proportion of the parasitic infections suffered by humans. Two main groups, pinworms and whipworms, are thought to comprise the majority of these infections. The most common "worm" infecting children is pinworms. The organism, *Enterobius vermicularis*, infects a significant number of children annually around the world, including the United States. Symptoms are itching and irritation of the anus or vagina, digestive disorders, insomnia, irritability, or nervousness. Female worms crawl out of the anus and lay up to 15,000 eggs per day. Once exposed to the air, the eggs can survive about two days anywhere in the individual's living environment. On a global basis it is estimated that up to 500 million people may be infected at any given time with pinworms. These worms are white and can grow to about a half inch in length.

The most commonly encountered whipworm, called *Trichuris trichiura*, is also estimated to be the causative agent for up to five hundred million cases throughout the world. Although infections with *T. trichiura* are considered a tropical disease, most cases are found in Asia and to a lesser extent in Africa and South America. The infection rate is low in the United States but may be responsible for several million cases which are found mostly in the rural Southeast. Poor hygiene is responsible for most if not all infections by the whipworm, as food raised in shady and moist soil that has become contaminated with human feces can lead to an increased rate of infection. Mostly children with a high risk of exposure are infected by this parasite. Symptoms of whipworms are bloody stools, pain in the lower abdomen, weight loss, rectal prolapse, nausea, and anemia. Hemorrhage can occur when worms penetrate the intestinal wall and bacterial infections from the normal flora that is found in large numbers in the intestine will usually follow.

Protozoa

The levels of infection are significant and the varieties of parasites that infect humans number into the hundreds.

Causative agents may be the well-known "amoeba," of which several species are quite prevalent. As an introduction to some of the names, which will be discussed at length later in this book, some of the better known parasites will be listed as follows. Of the amoebae that inhabit the human body, a species called *Entamoeba histolytica* is possibly the most common pathogenic amoeba encountered. Another of the amoebae is *Endolimax nana*, which is also found frequently even in the more advanced parts of the world. Several different species of these organisms may infect the human body simultaneously. Another category that includes common parasites is that of the flagellate class that chiefly includes *Giardia lamblia* and *Trichomonas hominis*. In addition to the flagellates *Trichomonas* and *Giardia*, there is another general class called a ciliate, but the most common type of parasitic infestation in some parts of the world are the heminths, which are worms. Other causative agents commonly found world-wide other than worms and protozoa include those of *Blastocystis hominis*, Microsporidium, and Cryptosporidium.

The term *protozoa* refers to single-celled parasites that inhabit various parts of the body, some of which are capable of causing serious damage, whereas others may be scarcely noticed by carriers of the organisms (Figure 2-9). These forms of parasitic organisms include amoebae, protozoa infections, toxoplasmosis, cryptosporidiosis, giardiasis, sarcocystosis, and *Trichomonas vaginalis*. Amoebae are irregularly shaped microorganisms that infect chiefly the end of the smaller intestine and colon. Amebiasis is the most common protozoal infection by a pathogenic species and is caused by the species *Entamoeba histolytica*. It is necessary to identify nonpathogenic protozoa such as *Entaboeba coli*

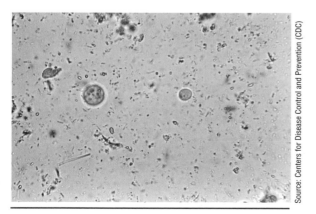

FIGURE 2-9 Cyst of the protozoan parasite, *Entamoeba coli*

Source: Centers for Disease Control and Prevention (CDC)

that are sometimes misidentified or confused with a pathogenic organism such as *Entamoeba histolytica*.

The one-celled amoebae also release an enzyme that causes ulcers or abscesses where they enter the bloodstream. They can eventually reach other organs including the brain or liver. Cryptosporidial infections are usually associated with waterborne outbreaks. Victims of this ailment often experience diarrhea and abdominal pain lasting for about 10 days. The protozoal organism called *Giardia* is the most prevalent intestinal parasite in humans and is found in drinking water throughout the world. Organisms of the genus *Giardia* reside in the smaller intestine and at times in the gallbladder and millions of these organisms will coat the intestinal walls, preventing the absorption of nutrients and later causing illness. Symptoms include mild to moderate abdominal cramps, intestinal gas, light-colored stools, poor absorption of nutrients, weakness, chills, stomach bloating, flatulence, and diarrhea.

Trichomonas vaginalis organisms are a class of pathogens that commonly reside in the vagina of females and the urethra, epididymis, and the prostate gland in males. In women there is sometimes a yellowish discharge accompanied by itching and burning. The organism is almost exclusively transmitted sexually and is quite common in those with multiple sex partners. The female will most commonly become aware of the illness first and it is medically necessary to treat both the male and the female who are in a sexual relationship when one is diagnosed with the infection.

Bloodborne Protozoa

Malaria is the most prevalent and debilitating disease on a world-wide scope and is also caused by a protozoa category of parasite. Malaria is caused by one or perhaps several of the four strains of the genus *Plasmodium*, those of *Plasmodium vivax*, *P. ovale*, *P. malaria*, and *P. falciparum*. These organisms are found in various geographic areas throuhout the world, and the potentially most malignant species is *P. falciparum*. Some of these and in some cases all four strains may be found in one area of the world, particularly in Southeast Asia. As many as half a billion people worldwide may be infected by malaria and about two million people worldwide die annually from malaria. There are a number of organisms that may cause malaria in animals. Several species other than the four known human strains are known to infect animals and birds, but these strains are not yet known to be passed on to people.

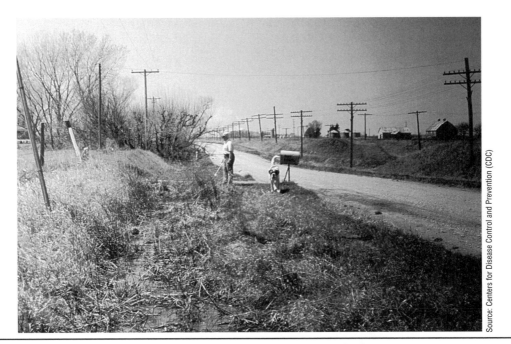

Source: Centers for Disease Control and Prevention (CDC)

FIGURE 2-10 Standing, stagnant water is a perfect breeding place for mosquito larvae

Antimalarial drugs such as chloroquine are often begun prophylactically before traveling to endemic areas. The drug is not always perfectly protective, and insect repellent along with mosquito barriers of fine mesh are used in addition to prophylactic therapy. Malaria cases have also been reduced dramatically by preventing standing water in which mosquitoes breed (Figure 2-10). Many birds, including those in North America, may be infected with various species. This disease is spread to man by a certain species of the Anopheles mosquito, which is infected while taking a blood meal from an infected victim. In rare cases, the organism has been transmitted through blood transfusions. Complex stages of the malaria life cycle that differ according to species occur in both the human host and the mosquito.

Mosquitoes consume both microgametocytes and macrogametocytes. Further development takes place in the mosquito that produces infectious sporozoites that are injected into humans from organisms mixed with the mosquito's saliva. Mosquitoes apparently suffer no ill effects from being infected. Many parasites rob their hosts of vital vitamin and mineral nutrients, the amino acids needed for muscle building, and digestion enzymes. Some sufferers become anemic and are drowsy and fatigued after eating. Many of the parasites release waste products (toxic waste) that are products of their metabolism and that may poison the body. Sometimes these toxins are reabsorbed in the intestines and patients have difficulty ridding their bodies of the toxins that are recycled over and over. The immune system may be overwhelmed as parasites are capable of producing prodigious numbers of offspring on a daily basis. These organisms have hijacked the bodies of humans or animals infected by the parasitic organisms to the detriment of the one infected. The immune system may appear depressed in the presence of infection and this may lead to further damage from bacteria and viruses concomitant with the parasitic infection.

ROUTES OF PARASITIC INFECTION

Parasitic infections occur via three main routes of infection. The organisms listed previously, along with many other species less commonly encountered, are contracted predominantly by drinking contaminated water (Figure 2-11). In the United States, *Giardia lamblia* is extremely prevalent in our water supply, particularly water coming from private wells that are still common

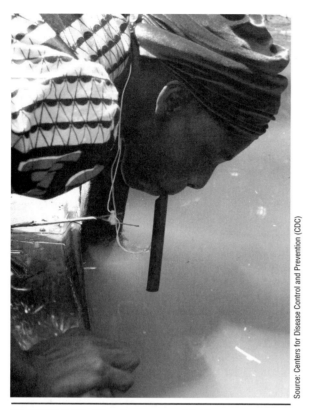

Source: Centers for Disease Control and Prevention (CDC)

FIGURE 2-11 Nigerian woman drinking water directly from a local pond through a pipe filter

DIAGNOSING PARASITIC INFECTION

Diagnosis usually includes a stool examination obtained by routine methods, the aid of a bulk-producing **laxative**, or mechanical removal of the stool specimen from constipated individuals. The test for parasites from the intestine utilizing fecal matter is called the "O&P," indicating that both the ova (eggs) and the parasites may be found. Unfortunately, these procedures lack sensitivity, meaning that they yield a high rate of false negatives. Although the appearance of the parasite eggs is characteristic of the species, it is sometimes a problem in differentiating some species by this method. Also, different labs may have different parameters for determining a parasitic infection.

Stool and Rectal Mucosa Examinations

Although stool examinations are the most common manner of diagnosing intestinal parasite infections, the most reliable but least convenient is that of a rectal mucosal examination to directly find the parasite or eggs (ova) of the parasite. The rectal mucosal surface becomes tender and more delicate, easily bleeding in the quite large expanse of tissue in the region which provides a large amount of mucous secretion. In addition, a rectal mucus swab may be useful for collecting parasites and detecting a parasitic infection by which the mucous membranes are firmly swabbed and the specimen is placed on a slide for staining before a direct identification can be performed. Other lab tests to enhance the diagnosis of a parasitic infection include a sedimentation procedure for concentrating the organisms or the eggs from a fecal specimen where applicable for certain species.

DIRECT TESTING FOR PARASITES

Although the most straightforward way to diagnose parasites is with microscopic examination for either or both ova or more rarely the parasite itself, specific identification is becoming more readily available with direct tests for the antigens (usually proteins) of parasites. Some parasites may be specific to the blood for certain bodily tissues but the most prevalent parasites are found in the human intestine. As with any micro-evaluation of body samples, such as with fecal specimens, this also relies on the laboratory professional's skill and diligence in picking

in many rural areas. Secondly, when travelling to certain parts of the world, the visitor is often exposed to greater amounts of parasites than the body is able to handle. You will often see the people living in these areas who do not become infected or at least show no symptoms, even though sanitary practices related to water sources and food handling are inadequate. Their bodies have developed the immune systems to a point that enables them to avoid becoming inhabited by intestinal parasites by acquired immunity. The third common way to contract infections is exposure to foods from restaurants and street vendors where food handlers may be carriers but show no signs of illness. Even though the human body mounts a strong reaction to parasites upon becoming infected, the disease is not cured unless medication is administered to eliminate the organisms. Sometimes the level of parasites in an infected person may diminish to the point that few symptoms or signs may be visible although transmission of the disease by these persons may still occur.

out the proverbial needle from the haystack. This is true whether looking for and finding filarial (small wormlike organisms), eggs, and protozoa or other manifestations of parasites from blood and other specimens.

When some groups of parasites are suspected, such as *Entamoeba*, roundworm, hookworm, *Strongyloides*, and *Pneumocystis jirovicii*, it is possible to perform tests with sputum specimens to establish that an infection is present. Initially, *P. carinii* (now chiefly reported as *P. jirovicii*) was thought to be the cyst form of a parasite. Some parasites, particularly roundworms, are found in the lungs during part of their life cycle and cause symptoms of bronchitis and even asthma. This cycle of reproduction involves coughing up of the larvae and then they are routinely swallowed with saliva and mucous and continuously repopulate the digestive tract. The cycle is repeated as they reproduce and begin their migration to the lungs again. Even the urine may be a viable specimen for finding some parasites as some organisms identified as blood flukes can be diagnosed through urine sediment examination. Urine samples are used for testing for certain microfilaria and particularly for *Trichomonas vaginalis* infections.

Swabbing the perianal area can often detect pinworms, which are most often found in small children. Pinworms are often discovered when the child complains of itching or is seen to frequently scratch the anal region. Pinworms are most often diagnosed by the peculiarity of their eggs, and they are rarely found with either a purge or other rectal procedures. These organisms come out of the anus at night to lay their eggs, and the eggs are most often found by using a Scotch-tape prep of the perianal area obtained before daylight while the child is still somewhat sleeping. This procedure may also recover eggs of the beef and the pork tapeworms as well as blood flukes. Sometimes scrapings of the perianal area will also reveal amoebae infections. All of the major parasites that invade the human body will be discussed at length, along with methods of identification, in the chapters of this book.

Due to some parasites that imbed themselves in tissues where they prefer to live, detection is often not possible without some sort of invasive procedures. Muscle biopsy can reveal the pork tapeworm or trichinella, the latter which migrates into muscle tissue. Rectal biopsy can reveal flukes, and liver biopsies are used for visceral larva migrans. Hydatid (clear) cysts should have a biopsy (tissue sample surgically excised) to determine the type of tapeworm that inhabits the cyst. Needle biopsy can show heartworms on rare occasions in the lungs of humans (often a single worm of *Difilaria immitis* is found in humans) as well as *Pneumocystis jiroveci*.

Lymph biopsies are used in some cases to detect toxoplasmosis caused by a protozoan called *Toxoplasma gondii*. The realm of parasitology that involves the study of tissue sections is not medically indicated as frequently in the United States as in other countries. Entire textbooks are devoted to studies of tissue parasites and are often included in a specialty called *tropical medicine*. Technologists and technicians do not ordinarily perform these tests, although they may prepare and stain the specimens for microscopic examination, particularly those technical personnel called histotechnologists. These tests are often performed by doctoral scientists and pathologists from stained tissue specimens removed from the body surgically. Although the organism has a complex life cycle, the diagnostic stage is most often made by microscopic examination of tissues stained with hematoxylin and eosin (H&E).

MICROSCOPIC DIAGNOSTIC FEATURE

General Classification	Sporozoan
Organism	*Toxoplasma gondii*
Specimen Required	Tissue biopsy specimen (for direct examination)
Stage	Cyst stage is diagnostic
Size	Tissue cysts in the brain often spheroidal and reach a diameter of 70 μm; intramuscular cysts elongated and may be up to 100 μm long
Shape	Often crescent-shaped
Motility	Gliding movement for invading the host cells
Nucleus(i)	Prominent and most often situated centrally
Cytoplasm	No remarkable characteristics; organelles with envelopes
Other Features	None

Direct testing for the actual infective organisms by testing specimens against known antibodies commercially available are gaining acceptance. The use of antibodies is similar to that of indirect testing with the exception that the patient's antibodies are not used but are obtained from a commercial source. This procedure is still considered direct testing because the antigen, a part of the actual organism, is being tested for. These fragments that are comprised of parts of the organism may be present in stool specimens and will yield a positive result when using this methodology. Three of the parasitic organisms mentioned previously have screening tests that measure the presence of antigens from the parasites by using antibodies formed against the organism. These three are *Giardia lamblia, Cryptosporidium,* and *Entamoeba histolytica* antigen tests. Commercially prepared antibodies against the organisms are used to test for antigens from parasites which might have disintegrated in the intestine.

INDIRECT TESTING FOR PARASITES

Other recent developments provide an immunological profile of the blood that can be used to indicate some but not all parasites that may infect humans. This type of test is quite effective unless the immune system has been greatly diminished by some underlying medical condition, as merely having a parasite infection serves to wreak havoc with the immune system. When a blood test is used, it is possible to determine the presence of antibodies formed against parasitic organisms to confirm the presence of parasitic pathogens such as *Entamoeba; Strongyloides*; blood, liver, and lung flukes; heartworm found most often in dogs; malaria; *Toxoplasma*; microfilaria; and *Trichinella*, as well as others. It is necessary to collect a sample of blood at established intervals, such as every 4 to 6 hours for 72 hours around the clock, because some parasites only come out of the tissue in which they spend most of their time during the middle of the night. A shortcoming of the procedure that determines the presence of antibodies to the various parasites is that it would be impossible to determine if the antibodies were due to a past or a present exposure.

Indirect testing is related to procedures where the evidence of an immune reaction against a parasitic infection exists rather than actually finding the organism itself. The eosinophil count (for a type of white blood cell already mentioned) is most likely increased when tissue invasion occurs, rising to several times the normal percentage of less than the normal range of 1 to 3 percent of the white blood cells. An elevated eosinophil count does not aid in identifying the particular organism with which the victim is infected. It merely shows that there may be a tissue invasion by a parasite. Specific antibodies against some of the more common pathogens are used to identify components of the parasite, and measuring specific antibodies the host has developed is another method for specifically identifying an infecting parasite. Secretory IgA, an immunoglobulin of which antibodies are comprised, may also be measured to determine the ability of the intestinal tract to fight infection in local areas of the body, such as the intestinal tract.

All persons who become infected with a bacterial, viral, or parasitic pathogen should exhibit an immune reaction by forming antibodies that are specific against the infective agent. Parasitic infections also cause the formation of specific antibodies, and although the techniques for testing have evolved fairly recently, the antibodies formed against the particular parasite in some cases may be used as an *indirect* manner of identification of the parasite. An indirect test measures the body's response against the causative organism, and does not require direct evidence of the organism itself where it may be viewed microscopically. Testing for antibodies against parasites is not as well developed as those for viruses.

IDENTIFICATION OF PARASITES AND THEIR OVA IN BODY FLUIDS AND WASTES

This is an area in which laboratory workers perform the vast majority of the diagnoses of parasite infections. It is important to bear in mind that parasites range from unicellular organisms such as amoebae to large "worms" of several feet in length. Therefore, microscopic features of one-celled organisms and identification of the eggs of larger parasite forms may be required to properly identify a parasite. A number of characteristic morphological structures associated with various species of parasites enable definitive identification of the most common varieties of parasites routinely found in infected persons of the developed world. Observation of certain morphological characteristics may be valuable in identifying the genus and sometimes the species of some parasitic organisms known as protozoa (one-celled organisms) as provided in the following chart (Table 2-2). This table

TABLE 2-2 Anatomical Features Contributing to the Identification of Intestinal Parasites

Amastigote	A form of organism such as the genus *Leishmania*, which is a nonflagellated form (flagella are used for movement); promastigote forms become amastigotes when engulfed by macropahges
Axoneme	An intracellular axis through the core of the parasite, dividing it longitudinally; an extension of the axoneme comprises the flagellum or cilium for parasites that contain cilia or flagella
Charcot-Leyden Crystals	Crystallized structures of varying sizes that are found in feces, sputum, and body tissues of those with helminth infestations; originate from eosinophils and are found in allergic infections and parasitic infections
Chromatin	Nuclear components that stain when appropriate staining materials and techniques are employed
Chromatoidal Bodies	Bar-shaped inclusions in the cytoplasm that are stained but are not a part of the nuclear material such as chromatin
Contractile Vacuoles	Organelles (little organs) that pump accumulated fluids from protozoa (unicellular organisms) to regulate internal pressure
Cyst	A stage of a protozoan that is nonmotile and is surrounded by a protective wall; stage that is readily transmitted to new hosts; the trophozoite stage is motile but the organism may be transformed between these two stages (cyst and trophozoite) readily
Cytoplasm	Also called protoplasm; includes all parts of the cell except nuclear material
Cytostome	Mouth-like opening of certain protozoa (the term –*stoma* means "mouth")
Encystation	Process of transformation into a cyst from a trophozoite
Excystation	Process of "hatching" of a cyst, which becomes metacystic trophozoites
Fibrils	Fibers that extend from the axial components of the organisms as flagella; some organisms have fibrils that appear as cellular inclusions that do not extend from the body of the cell
Glycogen vacuole	Glycogen is similar to starch and will stain with a variety of stains; this is a food storage vacuole found in certain amoebae; humans also store glycogen for energy sources
Golgi apparatus	Series of curved and parallel sacs that may package secretory products
Karyosome	A body included in the chromatin of the nucleus that usually stains a darker color than the remainder of the nucleus
Kinetoplast	Small mass that stains darkly and is the base of the flagellum; provides movement to the flagella
Macronucleus	Found in eukaryocytes where the nucleus is organized into one large structure and is surrounded by a nuclear membrane (prokaryocytes, as are most bacteria, lack the organized nucleus surrounded by a nucleus)
Oocyst	Cystic form of a sporozoan (protozoan) that might or might not have a hard, resistant membrane for protection
Precystic form	A trophozoite (motile form) stage often found just before complete encystations
Pseudopod	Means "false foot" and is a temporary extension or protrusion of an amoeba that is used for locomotion and for phagocytosis (surrounding and feeding)
Trophozoite	This is the motile form of many protozoa during which time the organism feeds, multiplies, and grows within the host it has infected; other names for this form are "vegetative" and "trophic" forms

TABLE 2-2 Anatomical Features Contributing to the Identification of Intestinal Parasites (continued)	
Undulating membrane	Occurs in flagellated forms of some organisms such as that of *Trypanosoma*, which has a finlike ridge along the dorsal area of the organism. A flagellum may be buried in this ridge, with the end extending as a flagellum for locomotion; movement of this structure causes the body of the organism to undulate in wave-like movements.
Vacuole	Any of various types of spaces and cavities within the cytoplasm of a protozoan cell; may be used for storage
Vector	Organism that carries and perhaps transports parasites from one host to another; snails, other mollusks, and insects often serve as vectors for parasites as well as viruses and bacteria
Volutin	Chromosomal (chromatoid) substance found in the cytoplasm of certain protozoans, appearing as granules

is designed to provide characteristics to assist in identifying parasites. An extensive glossary of other terms important in the study of parasitology will be found at the end of this book.

Likelihood of Recovering Parasites and Their Ova

Remember this answer to the question, "Will an O&P (stool examination for ova and parasites) detect all parasites?" The answer is an emphatic "No!" Technique, specimen collection, and stage during which the specimen is collected are vital for properly finding and identifying parasitic infections. Only the parasites that live in the gastrointestinal tract and whose eggs are passed through the feces will be diagnosed by a simple stool specimen. And if the organisms are embedded in the tissue, they may not be seen in the stool, but would need a swab from a mucosal membrane to find and identify them by morphology of the eggs or the organism itself. Some parasites are only detectable at certain cycles of the disease, and occur in a form that enables identification during certain cycles, such as the fever cycle for determining the species of protozoan responsible for malaria (remember there are four major species that infect humans). Then there are also other tests specific for parasites such as pinworms or blood parasites that cause malaria as well as a number of other bloodborne organisms. In addition, immunological tests for either antibodies or antigens may be required for identification and proper treatment.

TREATING INFECTION BY PARASITES

After diagnosis of the type of organism present, a drug must be chosen that will be effective in the treatment of a specific parasitic infection. Treatment by drug therapy is directed toward destroying the parasite. For amoebae, the most common drug is Flagyl (metronidazole), which is also used for organisms other than parasites, such as a few select bacteria. Side effects often include nausea, headache, vomiting, insomnia, and vertigo. For giardiasis (infection by *G. lamblia*), the drug commonly used is Atabrine (quinacrine HCl). Side effects often experienced when this drug is prescribed and used are dizziness, headache, vomiting, and diarrhea. Other drugs used for parasitic infections include Humatin (paromomycin), Furoxone (furazolidone), and Yodoxin (iodoquinol). Some treatments utilize a nondrug therapy, which may include an herb known as *Artemesia annus* (par qing), as well as other natural dietary substances. However, the side effects of using *Artemesia* as well as other methods may result in side effects such as gas and bloating. Another commonly used product from plants that grow in specific geographic locations is a seed extract from the citrus fruit (grapefruit), which appears to be an especially effective antiparasite agent.

It often takes a period of three or more months to eradicate an infestation of parasites. This lapse of time between treatment and cure is due to the various life cycles of some parasites, where they may survive while undergoing certain stages of development because they may be shielded from therapeutic treatment by hiding in certain tissues of the body. If treatment is stopped because symptoms have disappeared, a full-blown infection may recur when only a few organisms escaped eradication and begin to multiply. Treatment is tailored for both strengthening the body of the patient and killing the parasite. The residual damage from the infection may require treatment for a period of time following the complete destruction of the parasites.

Dietary Considerations for Victims of Parasitosis

Certain dietary regimens are followed to prevent infection by parasites as preventive practices in some parts of the world. Dietary guidelines include avoiding irritants such as alcohol and caffeine that would give a toehold in the digestive system for some organisms. Lowering the level of sugar and avoiding dairy products and fruit has been found to be potentially beneficial. Fruit is usually considered a "good" food, but in the situation where one is infected by a parasite, it is best to avoid these food groups in the early stages of treatment. Optimally the diet would consist mostly of complex carbohydrates obtained by eating rice and potatoes along with cooked vegetables and lean meats.

But the most important factor in avoiding infection or reinfection would lie in the thorough washing of salad ingredients and by personal hygiene. There are specific cleaners available for greens that do not damage the food or leave an undesirable taste on the plants. This means that the victim of an intestinal parasite infection should probably avoid ordering salads at restaurants until completely recovered from an illness. All water consumed should be filtered; do not drink water straight from the tap! Supportive measures include supplemental bowel flora (acidophilus and bifidus), vitamin A, and folic acid. Normalization of neurological and visceral reflexes by your chiropractor would be beneficial as well.

AVOIDING RISK OF PARASITIC INFECTION

What can be done to prevent a parasitic infection? Avoiding the ingestion of risky foods and water is the best manner to avoid a parasitic infection, especially when in an area where the visitor is unfamiliar with the local foods and drinks, especially during travel to a foreign country. In developing nations even ice in a drink

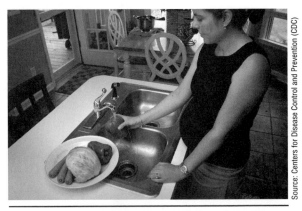

Source: Centers for Disease Control and Prevention (CDC)

FIGURE 2-12 Wash fresh, uncooked produce. Rinse fresh fruits and vegetables in running tap water to remove visible dirt and grime

or a dinner salad (Figure 2-12) may expose the diner to a variety of parasites. Many of the local inhabitants may have learned to live with the organism and will show no symptoms, but may be carriers. So the best manner of prevention is to avoid food and water that is suspected of being contaminated. Even the clearest and coolest mountain stream should be considered a risk, as it may be contaminated with *Giardia lamblia*, particularly if cattle and other animals are upstream.

Most parasites are invisible to the naked eye and you will not be able to smell them or taste them in the water or in food. And if a family member has a parasitic infection, careful hand washing after going to the bathroom is the best way to prevent passing the parasite on to others in the family (Figure 2-13). An infected person

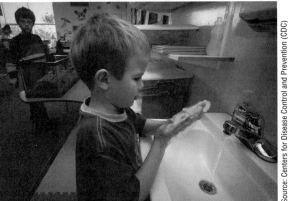

Source: Centers for Disease Control and Prevention (CDC)

FIGURE 2-13 A young child is appropriately washing his hands

should not be allowed to prepare food for others until all symptoms are gone. Remember that parasites are transmitted most often under dirty conditions, and some may even be present in the lungs and could be transmitted through sputum during certain stages of their life cycles, so are easily spread.

OTHER CONSIDERATIONS FOR EFFECTIVE IDENTIFICATION AND TREATMENT FOR PARASITES

Is it necessary to have a fresh stool sample? Yes, the fresher the better, as the morphology of the parasites and even the eggs may be deteriorated in unpreserved stool, which would destroy the identifying characteristics of the parasite and make the infection more difficult to detect. In addition, trophozoites are more easily visualized in fresh samples. Sometimes, if a specimen is impossible to examine while it is fresh, a small amount of formalin-ether (diluted formaldehyde) can be added to preserve the organisms for a period of time. The sample should be viewed microscopically if possible to determine the presence of parasites before preserving the sample for transport to another location for identification. There are a number of other preservatives, including polyvinyl alcohol (PVA), which contains the fixative mercuric chloride. PVA has been considered the "gold standard" for the fixation of ova and parasites in the preparation of permanently stained smears of stool specimens. However, mercuric chloride is potentially hazardous to laboratory personnel and may also present disposal problems.

It is common for the inexperienced student or laboratory worker to mistakenly identify normal cells and other components of the stool as parasites. Small parasitic worms that are thought to be present in a stool sample may be undigested food (cellulose) fibers from vegetables that were recently ingested. Most of the common parasites are much too small to be seen with the naked eye and the fact that solid material from the stool is present compounds the problem of discovery and identification. However, parasites have characteristic external and internal structures that fibers do not have. Only experience will enable the laboratory worker to quickly discount suspect elements that are not parasites such as vegetable cells and fibers.

For the limited number of parasites that have had serological tests developed for determining the presence of antigens that were developed only relatively recently, these tests may be a valuable adjunct to confirm the findings as parasites when suspicious objects are seen microscopically. The antigen tests have been developed for several common parasites including tests for *Giardia*, cryptosporidium, and *E. histolytica*. The antigen tests detect protein structures on the parasite, and they can detect the presence of fragments of the parasite in a stool sample if no intact parasites can be seen. An advantage of this is allowing detection of a specific parasite even if it is not definitely seen in the microscopic O&P examination.

Blood antibody tests may also be ordered to determine if a patient has had previous exposure to a parasite, because specific antibodies may persist throughout life for those with previous infections. These tests may indicate a past or a chronic infection but are not used to detect a current infection. Sometimes it is necessary to obtain a biopsy of the small intestines, where a small amount of tissue is examined for parasitic infestation. Remember that reinfection may occur by repeat exposure or by an incomplete treatment for parasitic infections. It is quite common to become reinfected with a repeat exposure, particularly in cases where a family member has an asymptomatic parasitic infection, such as giardiasis (due to *Giardia lamblia* infection), and continues to shed the organisms and reinfects others until everyone is treated.

A person infected by a parasite should not take an antidiarrhea medicine unless prescribed by the treating physician. This is due to the fact that diarrhea is one of the ways in which the body helps to rid itself of the infection. If the normal activity (peristalsis) of the intestines slows down and prevents the fecal material along with parasites from leaving the body by taking anti-diarrhea medication, the amount of time may be prolonged for a person who is ill and may make the infection become more severe.

SUMMARY

Human parasitic infections are possible when conditions are right. This includes exposure to animals that harbor parasites that may be transmitted to humans. Parasitic infections often are found within isolated and small locations with close quarters, but who share common facilities, land, and water supplies, where human and animal wastes contaminate the land and the produce and other animals that live there.

Travel to certain countries requires exercising caution when buying, preparing, and eating food and drinking the water. For many parasites, specific vectors must be present in order to effectively spread parasites. Surveillance around the world is accomplished through military facilities, private charities, and national health care organizations such as those provided by the United Nations and the WHO, as well as international branches of the Centers for Disease Control and Prevention (CDCP). Conducting epidemiological surveys by these organizations aids greatly in tracking the spread of infections and the treatments that are effective for combating them.

Signs and symptoms are diverse in parasitic infections, and range from very mild to vague symptoms that are suggestive of other illnesses. Symptoms may be similar for many different species of parasite, and are often mistaken for bacterial or viral infections, which are actually found in greater numbers than are those of parasite infections. Pain, bloating, bleeding from a number of sites, allergic reactions with **eosinophilia**, inflammation, and fever are common with parasitic infections, even when the species of parasite is a worm or an amoeba, for instance.

Certain medical conditions and general poor health of individuals actually make them vulnerable for contracting parasitic infections. These organisms are available for transmission anytime a vector is available, or when food is used for transmission of eggs of certain parasites, and may affect almost every organ of the body, from the skin to the urogenital tract, the gastrointestinal tract, blood, muscles, central nervous system tissue, and any other organs or systems of the body, such as the respiratory system. Therefore, there is a parasite to fit almost any geographic location, and any host that is suitable in parts of the life cycle of the particular organism.

In some populations, there are cultural practices that reduce the risk of contracting a parasite. Other methods of avoiding infection include careful cleaning of foods such as those eaten raw in salads. Boiling water for drinking and food preparation in an endemic area, and even not eating ice that is available locally is extremely important in not becoming a victim. Remember that many of the local inhabitants in a country may be carriers and will exhibit no signs of disease, but are still capable of transmitting the parasites to others.

Medications are tailored to the disease with respect to parasite infections. For instance, diarrhea is often the best way to rid the body of pathogens, but unfortunately, may be the best way to transmit the disease to others. So each individual has a responsibility for both him- or herself and others, including the family.

CASE STUDY

1. A 33-year-old man complains to his physician of weight loss and a nonproductive cough that includes a slightly elevated temperature. He privately admits to being homosexual with a number of sex partners. The physician requests a sputum sample and a chest x-ray. The chest x-ray shows numerous infiltrates, suggestive of pneumonia. What organism or organisms would the physician suspect based on the information he has received?

STUDY QUESTIONS

1. What are some reasons for outbreaks of parasites in a given location?

2. What are the percentages for testing procedures and accuracy rates when using current methodology for discovery and identifying of parasites?

3. Describe the symptoms of hookworm infection.

4. List the three major groups or types of parasites.

5. The protozoan that infects the urogenital tract of predominantly females and that is sexually transmitted is that of _____.

6. Why do humans not contract the strains of malaria some birds in North America have?

7. What are two groups of the protozoans called other than amoebae?

8. What is probably the most prevalent parasite found in the United States and what is the source of this infection?

9. What is the most common specimen used to diagnose endoparasites?

10. What is meant by an indirect method for diagnosing a parasitic infection?

11. What condition must be met to perform an indirect test for antibodies against organisms that live inside tissues of the body?

12. Describe the typical test for diagnosing pinworm infections.

13. What are two tissue parasites that may be found in muscular biopsies?

Protozoal Microorganisms as Intestinal Parasites

LEARNING OBJECTIVES

Upon completion of this chapter, the learner will be expected to:

- Describe the life cycle of *Giardia lamblia*
- Differentiate between cyst and trophozoite stages of protozoa
- List steps necessary to perform wet mount on specimen from victim of amoebic dysentery
- Differentiate between fresh cysts of *Entamoeba histolytica* and *Entamoeba coli* or *Endolimax nana* cysts
- Provide the probable origins of infections of *Blastocystis* spp. infections in humans
- Compare the morphology of the various protozoans necessary for identification of each
- Compare morphology of *E. histolytica* with common nonpathogenic amoebae

KEY TERMS

Amoebiasis	Endoplasm	Karyosome
Anaerobic	Endosome	Lugol's iodine
Anoperineal region	Enterocytes	Macrogametes
Binucleate	Febrile	Merozoites
Brightfield microscopy	Fecal-oral route	Microgametes
Charcot-Leyden crystals	Flagellates	Microvilli
Chromatoid bodies	Flatulence	Mitochondrion-like organelles
Ciliates	Fulminant colitis	Multicellular
Colonoscopy	Golgi apparatus	Obligate
Cysts	Gram negative rod	Oocyst
Duodenal fluid	Immunocompromised	Oocytes
Dysentery	Intestinal lumen	Organelles
Ectoplasm	Intracellular	Periodontitis
Empyema	Isosporiasis	Phagocytosis

Pinocytosis   Pseudopodia   Urethritis
Protista   Tenesmus   Vacuoles
Pseudomembranous colitis Trophozoite   Zoonoses

INTRODUCTION

Numerous protozoa live in the gastrointestinal tract of humans and a source of those that cause human infections may come from animals which harbor similar or the same intestinal parasites as humans but that may not be harmful to the animal. It is possible that mutations of animal protozoa and even other classes of parasites may have made it possible for these organisms to inhabit and cause disease in humans. Some protozoa are nonpathogenic, whereas other species may cause only mild discomfort in an episodic manner. A number of medically important single-celled organisms called protozoa may be found that are classified as parasites in humans. These protozoal organisms are found in the phylum of the kingdom called **Protista** and the group includes unicellular and animal-like organisms as opposed to other one-celled free-living organisms such as bacteria that may also be either pathogenic or in some cases helpful. At any rate, both parasites and many species of bacteria may produce serious illnesses.

Intestinal parasites classified as protozoa are most often transmitted by the **fecal-oral route** and are due to poor hygiene and living conditions in many instances. Most exist as a cyst or resistant stage, whereas a few are found only in the **trophozoite** or active stage. The cyst stage with a protective wall offers some protection from adverse conditions and is a resting or dormant stage upon which the cysts become trophozoites upon introduction to the appropriate host. Trophozoites are active in their metabolism and are usually motile, making them easier to identify that cyst stages. These intestinal protozoa often are contracted when a victim is immunocompromised by other disease states such as AIDS and may cause life-threatening diarrhea by causing dehydration and aggravation of existing conditions. In HIV-positive patients and those who have progressed to the chronic disease of AIDS, the patient may have an incompetent immune condition in which the individual has lost the ability of the body to ward off and prevent infection because of a form of immunological dysfunction. The physician must be alert to the underlying causes of new infections based on diseases already present but also to a lifestyle placing the patient at increased risk for contracting infectious diseases.

CLASSIFICATION OF PROTOZOA

Some protozoa are similar under microscopic examination and are easily confused as pathogens when they may actually be nonpathogenic. Morphological and anatomical features are used to differentiate both protozoa and other classes of parasites such as worms that may be differentiated both by the appearance of larvae and adults and by the eggs they produce. Comparison of wet mounts and stained specimens of protozoa that may contain either or both cyst stages and trophozoite stages are helpful.

The taxonomic phylogeny of parasites is complex, and those causing human diseases are no exception. The kingdom Protista includes the phylum Protozoa, which includes a number of species of parasites with which humans become infected. Ordinarily these organisms are loosely divided into three groups and the first set of nomenclature used to differentiate protozoa relates to the type of locomotion, if any, that is present. **Ciliates** use cilia or short hairlike projections to effect movement and belong to the phylum Ciliophora. Basically only one entity of the phylum Ciliophora is described as one that is capable of causing human disease (*Balantidium coli*). **Flagellates** possess longer modified cilia of which there are usually only a few species characterized by this type of ciliate. Amoebae include some of the most pathogenic types of protozoa and most movement is achieved by amoeboid movement where some organisms extend **pseudopodia**, or "false feet," by which they pull themselves along a surface with only minimal movement. These classes of protozoa are presented with representatives of each of the basic types of protozoa that will be presented in the following sections. Table 3-1 depicts the divisions of both pathogenic and nonpathogenic protozoa.

PHYLUM	SUBPHYLUM	ATTRIBUTES	EXAMPLES OF SPECIES
Sarcomastigophora	Sarcodina (amoebae)	Single-celled Motility by pseudopodia Cysts and trophozoite forms Asexual reproduction	*Acanthamoeba* sp. *Endolimax nana* *Entamoeba coli* *Entamoeba hartmanni* *Entamoeba histolytica* *Iodamoeba butschlii* *Naegleria fowleri*
	Mastigophora (flagellates)	Single-celled Movement chiefly by flagella Cysts and trophozoites for intestinal organisms Asexual reproduction Blood flagellates may be included	*Chilomastix mesnili* *Dientamoeba fragilis* *Enteromonas hominis* *Giardia lamblia* *Leishmania* species *Trichomonas hominis* *Trichomonas tenax* *Trichomonas vaginalis* *Trypanosoma* species
	Ciliophora (ciliates)	Single-celled Movement chiefly by cilia Cysts and trophozoites stages Asexual reproduction	*Balantidium coli*
Apicomplexa	Coccidia	Single-celled Inhabit host's cells Life cycle complex and involves insects, mammals other than host Both sexual and asexual reproduction may be involved	*Babesia microti* *Cryptosporidium parvum* *Cyclospora cayetanensis* *Isospora belli* *Plasmodium* species *Pneumocystis carinii (jirovecii)* *Sarcocystis* species *Toxoplasma gondii*

TABLE 3-1 **Classification of Pathogenic and Nonpathogenic Protozoa**

CLASSIFICATION OF CILIATES

A number of important parasites with which humans become infected are found in the class formerly called Ciliata but now are classified as Ciliophora, a phylum of the kingdom Protista; the term *Ciliata* is still widely used. The phylum Ciliophora includes both unicellular and multicellular (colonial, or colony-forming) organisms that possess cilia for locomotion. Some are free-living forms found in the environment and some are parasitic species that will be discussed individually in the following sections of this book (*Balantidium coli*, found next, is one prime example). The cilia these organisms use for locomotion are essentially a sort of flagella that are smaller, thinner, and more hairlike than the longer flagella possessed by some species. These cilia may cover the entire periphery of the membrane of the organism as in the case of *B. coli*.

BALANTIDIUM COLI

The organism called *Balantidium coli* is considered to be the only ciliate found in humans that is pathogenic and is also the largest protozoan parasite found in humans. This organism is of the genus of ciliated protozoa that may be found in a number of hosts generally responsible for infecting humans.

Morphology

This organism called *B. coli* is rather large and is covered peripherally on the entire circumference of the cell by short cilia. The trophozoite stage may vary in size from 30 to 120 μm by 30 to 80 μm, and some larger versions may reach a size of 90 to 120 μm by 60 to 80 μm. The trophozoite is tapered at the anterior portion with an attached cytostome. Two nuclei are visible, with a large kidney bean–shaped macronucleus and a small nucleus called the *micronucleus*. The cyst form is elliptical in shape and measures from 45 to 65 μm. Food **vacuoles** are visible in the cytoplasm and a small opening at the posterior of the organism is used for waste elimination.

Symptoms

In some cases, infection with *B. coli* may result in few or no symptoms. Balantidiasis due to infection with *B. coli* causes generalized symptoms and signs including chronic and recurrent diarrhea, abdominal pain and cramping, vomiting, weakness, and weight loss.

Life Cycle

The ciliate called *Balantidium coli* is chiefly contracted from contaminated water and food, particularly where contact with animals occurs. The cyst is the infective form of *Balantidium coli*, as is the case for most protozoans (Figure 3-1), and the host is infected by ingestion of the infective cysts through water and food. In the cyst form, protozoans are characterized by a thick protective membranous wall that makes them impervious to unfavorable environmental conditions. Excystation (hatching from cyst) occurs in the small intestine and

reproduction occurs by binary fission. Cysts may form in the lumen of the colon for infecting other hosts. The trophozoite form of a protozoan is a stage where the organism is motile and is able to feed during this phase of development (Figure 3-2). The trophozoite is unable to infect a human or other animal but is able to reproduce by division in the host and is capable of causing damage to tissue in the infected individual.

Source: Centers for Disease Control and Prevention (CDC)

FIGURE 3-1 A cyst form of *Balantidium coli*

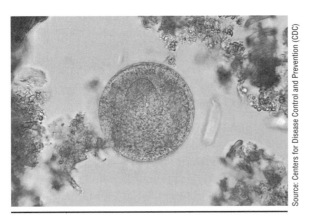

MICROSCOPIC DIAGNOSTIC FEATURE

General Classification	Protozoan, Ciliated
Organism	*Balantidium coli*
Specimen Required	Stool specimen
Stage	Cyst or trophozoite
Size	Cyst = 45–75 μm; trophozoite (two ranges; 45 × 60 μm × 30–40 μm and 90–120 μm × 60–80 μm)
Shape	Oval
Motility	Cilia in rotary motion for trophozoites
Nucleus(i)	2 (kidney bean–shaped and a smaller, round micronucleus)
Cytoplasm	Food vacuoles
Other Features	One of larger protozoa; periphery completely covered by short cilia

Balantidium coli

Trophozoite   Cyst

Delmar/Cengage Learning

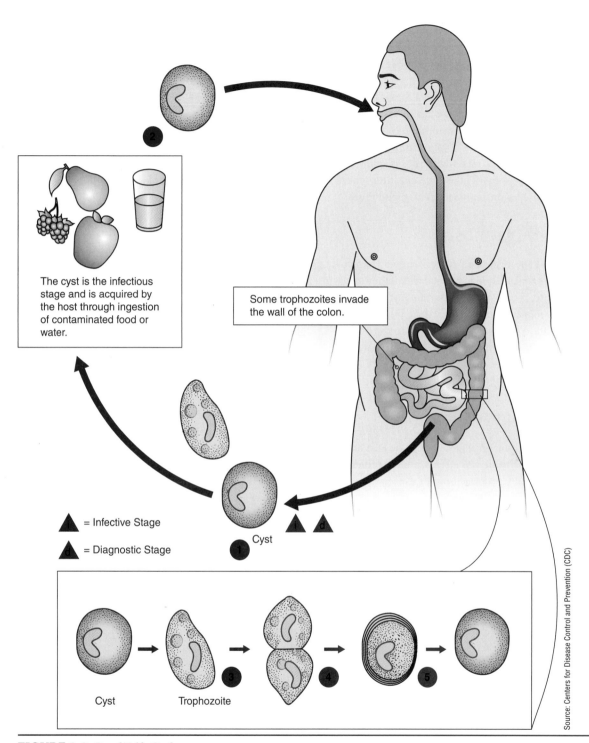

The cyst is the infectious stage and is acquired by the host through ingestion of contaminated food or water.

Some trophozoites invade the wall of the colon.

▲ i = Infective Stage

▲ d = Diagnostic Stage

Cyst

Cyst   Trophozoite

FIGURE 3-2 *B. coli* Life Cycle

Disease Transmission

The infection most frequently occurs in areas where certain animals that harbor the organism come in contact with humans. The parasite *B. coli* is commonly an infection found in a wide group of mammals that includes monkeys and pigs. In areas where pigs are handled by humans on a daily basis, the infection rate has been documented to be as high as 25 percent or more of the general population. This organism is thought to be primarily contracted from pigs which appear to be the natural host for *B. coli* along with perhaps a few other species of animals, and humans become infected through contact with these animals. But there has also been some evidence of human-to-human transmission of the infection, which might allow for the 25 percent rate of infection in areas where close contact with pigs is common. The organism affects primarily the large intestine, where it is known to cause lesions in the mucosal membranes.

Laboratory Diagnosis

A wet mount of the organism *B. coli*, viewed microscopically, reveals cilia that may be seen where they affect rotary motion of the parasite. A permanent slide of a stained fecal specimen or material obtained by sigmoidoscopic examination (endoscope inserted into the bowel) enables identification by the large size and surrounding cilia in the trophozoite stage. In the cyst stage, the two wall layers are ciliated but are difficult to visualize.

Treatment and Prevention

Consistency in performing personal hygiene and managing sanitary conditions are effective in preventing infection with *B. coli*. Caution should be exercised when handling monkeys or working with them in zoos and in research laboratories where these animals may be utilized, although it has been theorized that there may be a cyst stage that is implicated in fecal-oral transmission. But pigs and the raising and processing of them lead to the greatest number of infections. Antibiotics including metronidazole, iodoquinol, and tetracycline should be effective in resolving the infection.

PATHOGENIC FLAGELLATES OF THE UROGENITAL AND INTESTINAL SYSTEMS

Another major group of parasites with medical importance that inhabit the intestinal tract are the flagellates. These organisms have a rather simple life cycle, and at least three of the following four species do not have a cyst stage but only a trophozoite stage, during which unlike many protozoa they are infective. These are *Dientamoeba fragilis, Trichomonas vaginalis, Trichomonas tenax,* and *Trichomonas hominis,* although there are others that may be found in both cystic and trophozoitic forms. Also remember that these organisms may be characterized by exhibiting an undulating membrane, as previously listed in Table 2-1.

DIENTAMOEBA FRAGILIS

The organism *Dientamoeba fragilis* does not have external flagella that are prominent as do other flagellates. It is considered a flagellate because it retains flagellar characteristics which could be considered vestigial morphology where the flagellae have been lost. *D. fragilis* is considered to be more akin to the trichomonad, a true flagellated organism, due to the type of motility it is capable of exhibiting. Although the organism primarily moves in amoeboid fashion by extending pseudopodia with somewhat serrated (sharp-toothed) edges, *D. fragilis* also frequently exhibits active motility resembling that of other flagellates. Therefore it has been suggested that *D. fragilis* is an amoeba of flagellate ancestry, as the nuclear structure of the organism is more similar to that of flagellated trichomonads than to other species of *Entamoeba*. As mentioned previously, there arguably appears to be no cyst stage that provides protection for the organism against the environment, so the trophozoite does not survive for long outside the body, preventing easy transmission directly from one host to another (see "Life Cycle").

Morphology

D. fragilis is a single-celled parasite that infects the gastrointestinal tract of humans. In the binucleate form of the organism there is a spindle structure located between the two nuclei, which stems from certain polar configurations adjacent to a nucleus. A complex Golgi apparatus, a parallel series of flattened saclike structures, is seen best with an electron microscope.

Symptoms

The *Dientamoeba fragilis* organism, not always considered a pathogen, was originally considered to be an amoeba rather than a flagellate (Figure 3-3). However, gastrointestinal symptoms of pain, diarrhea, and tenderness are present in conjunction with the finding of this organism in the stool. Some persons may exhibit mild diarrhea, abdominal pain, and flatulence, as well as nausea and fatigue, whereas others may experience rather

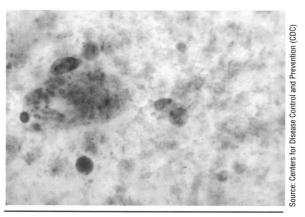

FIGURE 3-3 Trichrome stain of *Dientamoeba fragilis*, an amoebic parasite

Source: Centers for Disease Control and Prevention (CDC)

intense diarrhea accompanied with blood or mucus, abdominal pain, and anal pruritis (a tingling itch or burning sensation).

Dientamoeba fragilis Infection
(Dientamoeba fragilis)

Life Cycle

The *Dientamoeba fragilis* life cycle is simple because it is only characterized primarily by the trophozoite stage, as does the trichomonad group, although it is theorized that there may be a cyst stage that is not readily visible but that is implicated in fecal-oral transmission (Figure 3-4). It is thought that *Dientamoeba* is transmitted along with the eggs of other parasites such as intestinal worms, and especially simultaneously with that of the pinworm, *Enterobius vermicularis*. Because this organism does not appear to have a cystic stage, the beginning medical scientist upon seeing the non-motile forms with a circular outline, will often mistake them most commonly for the cysts of *E. histolytica*.

Dientamoeba fragilis organisms reproduce by cellular division called *binary fission* (simple longitudinal division) and move by pseudopodia (false feet), a mode of locomotion similar to many amoebae. Humans are

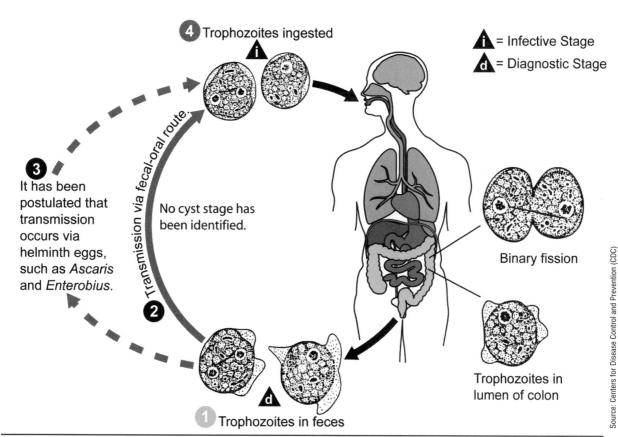

FIGURE 3-4 *Dientamoeba fragilis* life cycle

Source: Centers for Disease Control and Prevention (CDC)

apparently infected by the trophozoite or active stage of metabolism in the life cycle of *D. fragilis*. The organism obtains nutrition by **phagocytosis**, as it extends the pseudopodia and envelopes its prey, which it then proceeds to break down into simple nutrient materials. The cytoplasm most often contains numerous food vacuoles with ingested debris that may include bacteria. The conclusion whereby *D. fragilis* was classified as a nonpathogen was based on its insatiable appetite for the normal bacteria found in the gut rather than the intestinal and other tissues of its host. Waste materials are eliminated from the cell through digestive vacuoles by exocytosis.

Disease Transmission by *D. fragilis*

Although *Dientamoeba fragilis* was originally identified in 1918, the single-celled parasite that is frequently found in the gastrointestinal tract of some humans and particularly in pigs and gorillas and as stated previously was initially thought to be nonpathogenic and therefore received little medical attention. Infection by *D. fragilis* results in intestinal upset in some people but in others it does not appear to cause any distress. It is an important cause of traveler's diarrhea and chronic diarrhea, and infections with the parasite have been thought to result in a failure to thrive in children. A definitively established life cycle for this parasite has not yet been completely described but due to the fact that only trophozoite stage has been found in infected persons would lead to the assumption that a cyst stage must be present in some stage of the development of the organism. Like most other intestinal parasites, *D. fragilis* is most likely transmitted by a fecal-oral transmission resulting from close contact with animals.

Laboratory Diagnosis

Trophozoites of *D. fragilis* characteristically have two nuclei (binucleated), hence the di- (meaning two) prefix to the genus name (Figure 3-5). However, the rest of the genus name indicates that it is an enteric amoeba and not that it is related to intestinal parasites of the genus *Entamoeba*. The term *fragile* in its name refers to the fact that the trophozoite stages are fragile and do not survive long in the stool after leaving the body of the human host. Because they reproduce by binary fission, there are no complex stages for reproduction as are seen in other species of parasites. But the life cycle of this parasite has not

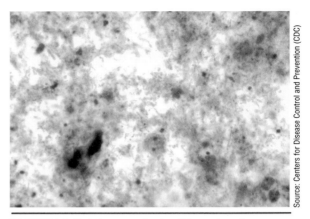

FIGURE 3-5 *Dientamoeba fragilis* trophozoite, binucleated, stained with iron-hematoxylin

Source: Centers for Disease Control and Prevention (CDC)

yet been completely determined, and some suppositions have been made based on clinical data.

Currently, because an environmentally resistant cyst stage has not been identified in *D. fragilis*, the trophozoite is the only stage found in stools of infected individuals. Unlike some other parasitic protozoa that form cysts, *D. fragilis* organisms as trophozoites are quite fragile and cannot live for long periods of time outside the intestinal system. Like other intestinal parasites, *D. fragilis* is most likely, from outward appearance, transmitted by the fecal-oral route. And because there is no known cyst form, transmission through eggs of pinworms (*Enterobius* sp.) and helminth eggs (e.g., *Ascaris*), which operate as vectors for the organism, has been strongly suggested.

D. fragilis is difficult to visualize, even when a special stain called "trichrome" is used, as it is quite small and is obscured by fecal material and bacteria ordinarily found in stool specimens. The trophozoite is only 5 to 12 µm, which may be slightly smaller than most red blood cells. Usually two nuclei exist and the cytoplasm has 4 to 8 granules separate from each other in the **karyosome**; it is composed of irregular clumps of chromatin material. The organism has a single flagellum, characteristic of the subphylum Mastigophora, which is an organism that is not visible when using **brightfield microscopy**.

Treatment and Prevention

Treatment of the symptoms may be required where some experience irritation of the intestinal mucosa. This disease, called dientamoebiasis, may also be associated with

MICROSCOPIC DIAGNOSTIC FEATURE

General Classification	Amoeba
Organism	*Dientamoeba fragilis*
Specimen Required	Stool specimen
Stage	Trophozoite only
Size	5–12 µm
Shape	Irregular and amoeboid
Motility	Nondirectional; contains what is thought to be vestiges of flagella and related to the *Trichomonas* organism
Nucleus(i)	2 (Approximately 50–80% of organisms have 2 nuclei); no peripheral chromatin; and nuclei composed of 5–8 discrete granules
Cytoplasm	Indistinct appearance in stained specimen
Other Features	Organism may be found in eggs of *Enterobius vermicularis*; does not survive for long following excretion

Dientamoeba fragilis

Trophozoite stage

Delmar/Cengage Learning

symptoms of abdominal pain, diarrhea, weight loss, and fever that require treatment other than metronidazole. It was found that by treating the organism as a pathogen, symptoms concurrently subsided. Only a few symptoms may occur in some who are infected and only a small percentage of these show any overt symptoms or signs.

TRICHOMONAS VAGINALIS

T. vaginalis is a protozoan with flagella that is capable of surviving in an **anaerobic** (without oxygen) environment. It is the most common pathogenic protozoan infection of humans in industrialized countries and infection rates between men and women are the same. Women often show symptoms, whereas men do not. The World Health Organization (WHO) estimates that there is a worldwide infection rate of 180 million new cases annually.

The organism *T. vaginalis* is one of the most frequently sexually transmitted organisms with many millions of cases reported each year. In most states and in many countries, it is required that physicians and other health care practitioners report sexually transmitted diseases (STDs) but this is not always the case. Therefore, the rate may be much higher than that reported and there are significant numbers of cases that go undiagnosed. This organism is found in the urogenital tracts of both males and females, and humans are the only hosts at this time (Figure 3-6). This infection is also concurrent with the presence of other sexually transmitted diseases, most often with gonorrhea. As listed previously, this organism has no cyst stage and is vulnerable to drying out and not surviving to be transmitted to others when found in body fluids outside the body, but a few cases have been known to be transmitted by nonsexual means.

Morphology

In females, the diagnosis is generally made by finding the trophozoite in either the urine or in vaginal discharge. Men may also produce the trophozoites in urine specimens and in prostatic secretions. The organisms have four anterior flagella and the cell membrane undulates in those that are highly motile. Dead or dying trophozoites are more problematic for visual diagnosis and may be identified as white blood cells. Therefore, the specimen should be read microscopically as quickly as possible upon collection of the specimen, as the vitality of the organism diminishes rapidly in the open air and light. A stained

Trichomoniasis
(Trichomonas vaginalis)

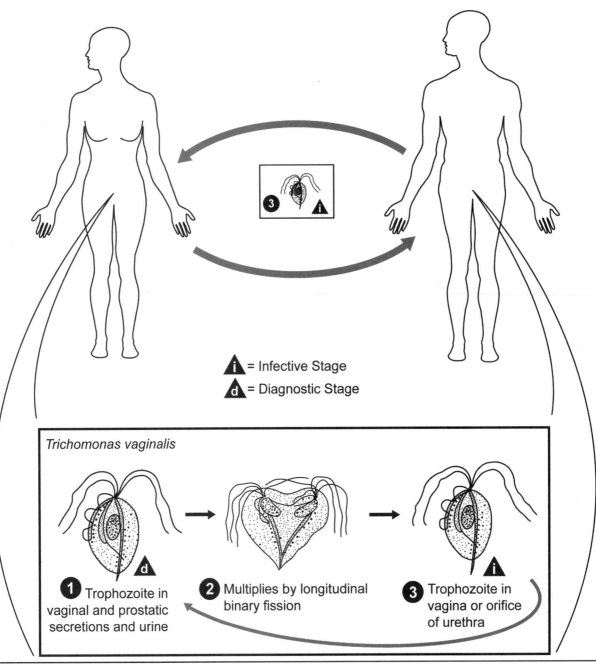

= Infective Stage

= Diagnostic Stage

Trichomonas vaginalis

1 Trophozoite in vaginal and prostatic secretions and urine

2 Multiplies by longitudinal binary fission

3 Trophozoite in vagina or orifice of urethra

Source: Centers for Disease Control and Prevention (CDC)

FIGURE 3-6 *Trichomonas vaginalis* infection routes

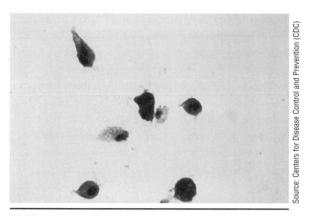

Source: Centers for Disease Control and Prevention (CDC)

FIGURE 3-7 *Trichomonas vaginalis* stained with Giemsa dye

specimen will yield a pear-shaped cell with an axostyle, a centrally located line extending throughout the length of the organism (Figure 3-7). One nucleus is generally visible at the anterior end, and the organism is generally 5 to 19 μm. This is also within the range of white blood cells, so it is easy to miss a *T. vaginalis* infection when the specimen is more than a few minutes old and where white cells are also present. Another important group of pathogenic flagellates are those found chiefly in the blood and tissues, and will be discussed in a later section.

Symptoms

The infected individual may suffer itching, burning, and considerable irritation of the surrounding tissues of the vaginal mucosa, and in some cases produce a foul-smelling and yellowish discharge with lesions. Men may be asymptomatic or suffer from prostate and upper urogenital tenderness and even swelling.

Life Cycle

The trophozoite stage, again the only one found in infections with *T. vaginalis*, is motile and somewhat easy to distinguish in urine samples and in vaginal secretions. However, they can be confused with white blood cells, especially if the organisms are sluggish due to temperature, light, and other adverse environmental conditions. Due to the difficulty of maintaining viability of *Trichomonas* organisms for microscopic examination and perhaps culture, a routine universal transport medium may be indicated, and a number of these are available commercially. Fifty percent of infected women are asymptomatic even

MICROSCOPIC DIAGNOSTIC FEATURE

General Classification	Flagellate
Organism	*Trichomonas vaginalis*
Specimen Required	Urine, vaginal and prostatic secretions
Stage	Trophozoites most easily distinguishable
Size	8–23 μm in length and 5–12 μm in width
Shape	Pear-shaped trophozoite
Motility	Nondirectional but sometimes vigorous in fresh specimens
Nucleus(i)	1, somewhat centrally located
Cytoplasm	Evenly distributed chromatin with granules near axostyle
Other Features	Prominent axostyle with 4–6 flagella and undulating membrane

T. vaginalis

Trophozoite

Delmar/Cengage Learning

though large numbers of organisms are present in the vaginal discharges. Men are usually asymptomatic and serve as carriers, but may develop a milky discharge and a nonspecific urethritis.

Disease Transmission

Symptoms range from mild to none at all. Women in particular may be asymptomatic but are capable of transmitting the organism to others. The condition is quite contagious and both partners in a sexual relationship should be treated, as reinfection may occur on a regular basis when one partner is asymptomatic.

Laboratory Diagnosis

The diagnosis of infection by *T. vaginalis* is accomplished by direct observation of motile trophozoites. Because the organisms may be mistaken for white blood cells, the sample should be immediately examined upon receipt of the sample. All body fluids, including urine, vaginal discharges, or urethral secretions, should not be allowed to cool before examination occurs. A liquid microbiological media is sometimes used to culture the organism and permanent stained slides are possible but yield a number of false positive and false negative results. Some serological tests are available but are not widely used.

Treatment and Prevention

The medication of choice is metronidazole. Prevention is accomplished by the avoidance of unprotected sex with partners whose history is not known. Prompt treatment and diagnosis of men who are asymptomatic and who may readily transmit the organism is important.

NONPATHOGENIC FLAGELLATES OF THE DIGESTIVE SYSTEM (*T. HOMINIS, T. TENAX*)

It is important to distinguish pathogenic from nonpathogenic flagellates. Perhaps the most common of these nonpathogenic organisms is that of *Trichomonas hominis*. *T. hominis* is small and is usually not found or identified from stool specimens due to the concentration of bacteria and undigested materials in the fecal specimen. *T. hominis* is found as a trophozoite and has no known cyst stage associated with its life cycle. *T. hominis* exhibits an undulating membrane as does *T. vaginalis*. Differentiating between the two nonpathogenic species, *Trichomonas tenax*, which is found in the human mouth, and *T. hominis*, which is found in the intestine, may be necessary in some cases but both are considered harmless commensal parasites. Rare cases of pulmonary trichomoniasis have been documented medically and a few cases of trichomonal empyema (inflammation with body fluids often found between the pleura) have been reported.

Only *T. tenax* will be covered here, as it may be necessary to differentiate between *T. vaginalis* and *T. tenax*.

TRICHOMONAS TENAX

T. tenax is primarily found in the mouth and for this reason it may be necessary to determine the presence of and identification of the organism. The *T. tenax* organism is considered a harmless commensal and is frequently found in the tartar (plaque) that has hardened around the teeth.

Morphology

The trophozoite of *T. tenax* is similar to other trichomonads, particularly when compared with *T. hominis*, with the exception that it is more slender. This organism ranges in size from 5 to 11 µm in length and 7 to 10 µm in width. *T. tenax* has five flagella from the anterior end, with four extending to the anterior portion of the organism and one to the posterior. An undulating membrane runs the length of the trophozoite as does *T. hominis*. Stained specimens will yield a pear-shaped cell with an axostyle, a centrally located line extending virtually throughout the length of the organism. One nucleus is generally visible at the anterior end, and the size is the general range for the smaller white blood cells, so it is easy to miss *T. tenax* as easily as *T. vaginalis*, especially for an older specimen where the motility has decreased.

Symptoms

T. tenax may find crevices in the gingiva, the gum tissue that surrounds the neck of the teeth. Generalized inflammation may occur and is most prevalent in smokers and those with poor dental hygiene. The condition is predominantly asymptomatic, however.

Life Cycle

T. tenax is considered a commensal, living harmless in the mouth, particularly those with pyorrhea (pus-associated inflammation) and those with poor oral hygiene, especially in smokers. The trophozoite stage of *T. tenax* is simple as are the other trichomonads. Reproduction is by simple longitudinal binary fission.

Disease Transmission

The mode or modes for transmission has not been firmly established. It is theorized that exchange of oral secretions by oral to oral contact such as in kissing is a possible route for infection. Contaminated dishes and perhaps contaminated food may be another possible means for the organism to become introduced to the oral tissues.

Laboratory Diagnosis

The diagnosis of infection by *T. tenax* is accomplished by direct observation of motile trophozoites in wet preps, hanging drop suspensions, and surgically obtained gum scrapings. The disease is often accompanied with other pathogenic bacteria as opportunistic organisms when dental hygiene is poor or absent. The organism may also be cultured in the same manner used for *T. vaginalis*, but this is not a common practice.

Treatment and Prevention

This parasite is generally considered to be a nonpathogenic organism. Therefore, no medication is generally prescribed for the condition. Treatment includes deep dental cleaning by periodontal specialists and oral prophylaxis (preventive measures) on a regular basis.

DIFFERENTIATING THE ORGANISM(S) *TRICHOMONAS HOMINIS* AND *CHILOMASTIX MESNILI*

It is absolutely necessary to differentiate between *T. hominis* and *C. mesnili*. For this reason, these two organisms will be discussed together in this section in order to provide a convenient comparison. A wide variety of protozoa inhabit the intestinal tract of humans, most of which are transmitted by the fecal-oral route through ingestion of food or water contaminated with cyst forms of flagellates. *T. hominis* and *Chilomastix mesnili*, which are the two flagellates that are encountered most frequently, are used as comparison for the more pathogenic organisms. The flagellates belong to the Magistophora and possess more than one flagellum. Beating these flagella enable them to move. Unlike amoebae, flagellates can swim which enables them to invade tissues quickly and to find environments more conducive to survival. Flagellates may be found in the reproductive tract, alimentary canal, tissue sites, and also the blood stream.

Morphology

Both *T. hominis* and *C. mesnili* are found as trophozoites only, although this point is somewhat argumental. Both are found in the intestine and are excreted in the feces, but are often missed during microscopic examination. The *C. mesnili* parasite is also found widely in chimpanzees, orangutans, monkeys, and pigs. Although transmission occurs chiefly through eating and drinking, areas where monkeys and other simians are common, provides a ready source for infection of humans and is possibly directly transferred between the species.

T. hominis is identified in a similar method as that for *T. vaginalis*. *T. hominis* trophozoites are seldom identified microscopically in the urine except in fecally contaminated specimens. The axostyle and an oval nucleus are similar to that of the *T. vaginalis* organism. It too has an undulating membrane attached along the length of the costa or ribs of the organism, and contains four flagella as a feature common with that of the pathogenic *T. vaginalis* and is attached to the anterior portion of the organism.

Symptoms

This organism, known as *T. hominis,* is found particularly in warm climates and most often an asymptomatic condition is common with this infection. The organism may cause diarrhea even though it is considered to be nonpathogenic.

Life Cycle

T. hominis, like the other trichomonads, reproduce simply by longitudinal binary fission. These active trophozoites feed on bacteria primarily in the cecal portion of the intestine, but encystation is not known to occur.

Disease Transmission

These two intestinal organisms, *T. hominis* and *C. mesnili*, are considered to be nonpathogenic flagellates that must be distinguished from pathogenic flagellates. It is often quite common for *T. hominis* to be found in the urine of females due to the close proximity of the anus and the urethra. It is poorly defined as to the transmission but is generally conceded to gain entrance to the human bowel by fecal-oral means. An infection by *C. mesnili* results in a lack of symptoms and the parasite is more prevalent in tropical climates with warm and humid weather. Transmission occurs by ingesting infective cysts from food and water where poor sanitary conditions are found (*C. mesnili* cysts and trophozoites are similar in appearance).

Laboratory Diagnosis

The identification of *C. mesnili* and *T. hominis* are performed by microscopic examination. Both stained and unstained specimens should be prepared for study. The *C. mesnili* organism is slightly larger than that of *T. hominis*. *C. mesnili* has a pear-shaped appearance and the nucleus is surrounded by fibrils that curl around the cytostome, often seen near the nucleus, giving a characteristic shepherd's crook appearance. In the opinion of most parasitologists and medical professions, neither the flagellates *T. hominis* nor *C. mesnili* are considered pathogenic, but they are included for comparison as they may be found and cause confusion as to their respective identities. The nucleus, cytostome, and curved fibrils are readily visible on a stained smear. The trophozoites of *C. mesnili* are also pear-shaped and measure from 6 to 24 μm in length and 4 to 8 μm wide. The single nucleus usually has a prominent karyosome, whereas the anterior flagella are difficult to see.

Treatment and Prevention

No treatment is indicated for either *C. mesnili* or *T. hominis*. Because both are transmitted in a similar fashion and both are considered to be nonpathogenic, overall hygiene suffices to prevent the majority of infections by the two organisms.

GIARDIA LAMBLIA

Giardiasis in humans is caused by the infection of the small intestine by a single-celled flagellate called *Giardia lamblia*. Giardiasis occurs worldwide and may infect up to a third of the population in developing countries. The organism is also found in other mammals, which serves to make the disease difficult to eradicate. The Centers for Disease Control and Prevention (CDCP) estimates as many as 2.5 million people annually are infected in the Unites States alone.

Giardia infections are frequently referred to as giardiasis, and is the most common of all intestinal flagellates. This organism is often found in the upper areas of the small intestine, and is commonly found in isolated areas throughout the world. Because *Giardia* is likely the most common organism isolated from human stool specimens, it is likely that van Leeuwenhoek observed the organism in stool specimens after developing the first known microscope, but he never published any description or drawings of the organism. The first known description of *G. lamblia* occurred in the stool of a pediatric patient in 1859. *Giardia* infections do not lead to invasive damage to the gastrointestinal tract as is true of some other pathogens, and the patient may be asymptomatic, but is able to transmit the organism by the fecal-oral route.

Morphology

Both trophozoites and cysts may be found in the stool sample, with cysts found most often in formed stools and trophozoites in liquid or loose stools. Cysts are the most diagnostic stage found in a laboratory sample, perhaps because most stools are formed that reach the laboratory for examination are formed.

Trophozoites of *G. lamblia* are either oval or pear-shaped and range from 9 to 21 μm in length and 5 to 15 μm in width. The trophozoite form of this organism has been likened to a "monkey face" with two nuclei as eyes that contain central karyosomes which lack peripheral chromatin. The trophozoite stage is bilaterally symmetrical with an axostyle evenly dividing the cell down the middle. Two curved structures, called *median bodies*, lie parallel to each other and perhaps contribute to the metabolism of the parasite. These morphological features cross the axoneme at slight angles, giving the appearance of a smiling mouth. Four lateral flagella along with two caudal and two lateral flagella extend from the central spine or plane of the parasite. Three of these pairs are attached to the dorsal surface and one pair with a ventral origin. Some of these flagella, a total of eight, may not be readily visible microscopically.

The most infective stage, the *G. lamblia* cyst, is oval and ranges from 8 to 17 μm by 7 to 10 μm. The karyosomes may be less concentric than those of the trophozoites, and in the mature cyst, four median bodies are present. Longitudinal fibers are visible and four nuclei are seen in the cyst form of *G. lamblia*. There may be a clear zone between the cytoplasm and the cell wall, unlike that of the trophozoite.

Symptoms

Some victims of an infection by *G. lamblia* may suffer from either an acute or chronic diarrhea accompanied by severe intestinal discomfort. Following an incubation period of 2 to 3 weeks after exposure to the organism, water and smelly diarrhea, abdominal cramps, flatulence, and anorexia, sometimes accompanied by nausea, may occur. Vitamin deficiencies, particularly the fat-soluble vitamins A, D, E and K, along with folic acid, may create a number of health problems. Weight loss and malabsorption syndrome as well as steatorrhea (fatty stools) may occur.

Life Cycle

The cyst form of *Giardia lamblia* is the stage that causes infection when ingested from sources such as water and food as well as several other means. The cyst is broken down by the acid in the stomach, where the trophozoite emerges from the cyst wall in the duodenum. The cyst is broken down within a few minutes of exposure to the acidic environment of the stomach and the flagella become active quickly. Within a half hour or so, the trophozoite stage of the *Giardia lamblia* organism will undergo cytokinesis, which restores the binucleate morphology of the organism and results in two binucleated trophozoites through fission. Note that *G. lamblia* is also known as *G. intestinalis* and *G. duodenalis*. This rapid replication makes it possible to experience a heavy infection only days following an initial infection. The trophozoite obtains necessary nutrition from the intestinal lumen (tube opening) by a process called pinocytosis, where an organism or a cell absorbs nutrients and fluids from tissue. *Giardia* is sometimes stained to visualize structures

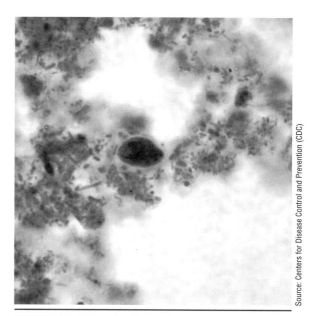

Source: Centers for Disease Control and Prevention (CDC)

FIGURE 3-8 A stained *Giardia intestinalis* protozoa cyst

of the organisms (Figure 3-8) but the wet mount is the most common method of identification.

Disease Transmission

The intestinal flagellate called *G. lamblia* is the most pathogenic intestinal flagellate known. This organism is familiar around the world and is the most common intestinal parasite in the United States. It is found commonly in humans but is also found in other mammals, particularly water-dwelling animals of ponds, lakes, and streams where the water is contaminated by a variety of animals. City water systems may also harbor this parasite because it is impervious to chlorine and only filtering will remove the organisms, which is not readily practiced in water treatment plants. Contaminated foods are also implicated, such as raw vegetables and through oral-anal sexual practices.

Laboratory Diagnosis

The trophozoite stage of *G. lamblia* is the most commonly found stage and is described as a characteristic pear or teardrop shape. These trophozoites are highly motile and move in a twisting and erratic manner, similar to that of a falling leaf. These flagella will be more apparent following a review of images of trophozoites

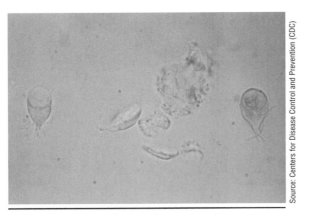

Source: Centers for Disease Control and Prevention (CDC)

FIGURE 3-9 *Giardia lamblia* trophozoites on a wet mount; can be found in the small intestine of an infected host

presented in this section. One other important anatomical feature of *G. lamblia* is an adhesive disc which is difficult to visualize as an organelle (small organ) on the ventral side of the organism.

Sometimes identification of *G. lamblia* is necessary by obtaining a biopsy of the small intestine or from the examination of **duodenal fluid**. Another method requires the patient to swallow a gelatin capsule attached by a nylon string, the end of which is taped to the patient's cheek. After 4 to 8 hours the capsule is withdrawn and the bile-stained mucous on the end of the string where the capsule is attached is microscopically examined by either a wet mount (Figure 3-9) or by permanent staining. A wet mount is merely a drop of water or saline in which the specimen is mixed, after which a cover slip is placed over the mixture and the specimen is examined microscopically.

Treatment and Prevention

Children in daycare centers and in those from rural areas who drink water from streams and contaminated wells are frequently afforded the greatest opportunity for infection along with male homosexual contacts. Domestic cats are also a source of giardiasis where close contact enables the transmission of the organism to humans. A sanitary lifestyle for both the body and for food eaten as well as a safe water source would prevent most of the infections contracted worldwide. The common practice of using human waste as fertilizer, found in several parts of the world, is probably the most causative factor in the transmission of this disease.

MICROSCOPIC DIAGNOSTIC FEATURE

General Classification	Flagellate
Organism	*Giardia lamblia*
Specimen Required	Stool specimen
Stage	Trophozoites and cysts, with cyst stage being the most diagnostic
Size	Trophozoite—9–21 × 5–15 μm; Cysts—8–17 × 7–10 μm
Shape	Pear-shaped trophozoites; oval and somewhat elongated cysts
Motility	Characteristic "falling leaf" motility on wet mount
Nucleus(i)	2 for trophozoites and up to 4 for cysts
Cytoplasm	Unremarkable
Other Features	4 pairs of refractile flagella

Giardia lamblia

Trophozoite   Cyst

Delmar/Cengage Learning

ENTERIC AMOEBAE

Intestinal **amoebiasis** is a potentially serious infection, although trophozoites may inhabit the intestines for years without causing damage or symptoms, during which time the person infected is an asymptomatic carrier. The majority in whom amoebal infections exist will fall into this group and they may spend most of their lives unaware of the infection. But some who are infected will develop amoebic colitis or **fulminant colitis** in which overt symptoms will be found. The organism chiefly responsible for amoebiasis is that of *Entamoeba histolytica*. Another similar amoeboid organism, *Entaboeba dispar* is considered nonpathogenic, although it inhabits the colon of many people. These two organisms are found worldwide, especially in tropical countries and in those with low sanitation standards. As many as 50 million new cases of amoebiasis appear per year in the world, which result in the death of possibly up to 100,000 people annually.

ENTAMOEBA HISTOLYTICA

In cases where amoebic **dysentery** is suspected, a fresh fecal sample is necessary. If a rectal ulcer is present, a swab from either the stool or the site of the ulcer should be examined with the use of a microscope, via a wet mount. A fresh stool while still warm should be examined quickly in order to see the colorless and motile trophozoites. Motility increasingly disappears as a specimen cools and when this happens the parasites are difficult to recognize. It is important to distinguish these organisms from motile macrophages that may also be in the site as an immune reaction. The motile form of the trophozoite has one nucleus but in a fresh specimen, the colorless nucleus is barely discernible if at all. However, staining the specimen gives moderate visibility of the nucleus. **Lugol's iodine** is frequently used and the stain kills the parasite almost immediately, upon which the motility consequently disappears.

Stained *Entamoeba histolytica* trophozoites have a transparent outer border (**ectoplasm**) and an opaque inner border (**endoplasm**). The border between endoplasm and ectoplasm is not distinct in *Entamoeba coli*. This is a physical feature that allows differentiation between *E. histolytica* and *E. coli*. The trophozoite of *E. histolytica* measures 20 to 40 μm and may contain red blood cells (unlike other amoebae). The last detail is pathognomonic (diagnostic) for pathogenic *Entamoeba histolytica* but is not always present. Ribosomes can be arranged in characteristically shaped elongate bars with rounded ends that are called *chromatoid bodies*.

Differentiation Between *E. histolytica* and Harmless Amoebae

The intestines often yield several species of harmless commensal (living together as nonparasitic) amoebae. The organisms that are often observed but that are considered nonpathogenic are described in this section. It is necessary to compare organisms as a technique to enable a laboratory worker to differentiate by comparison between those amoebae that are known to be pathogenic and those that are somewhat debatable as to their pathogenicity. Differentiation of the *Entamoeba histolytica* organism and other nonpathogenic amoebae is extremely important to rule out other causative factors of intestinal problems that might lead to unnecessary therapy (Table 3-2). These nonpathogens and the designation as a pathogen or nonpathogen is arguable even among experts, and often confuse both experienced and inexperienced personnel who are performing diagnostic testing of stool samples.

Morphology

Amoebic colitis is the term for generalized inflammation of the colon and is often used to describe an inflammation of the large intestine, which includes the colon, cecum, and the rectum.

TABLE 3-2 Common Nonpathogenic Amoebal Parasites Encountered	
PARASITE	**PATHOGENICITY**
Entamoeba hartmanni	Debated among professionals
Entamoeba coli	Nonpathogenic
Entamoeba polecki	Most often considered as nonpathogenic
Endolimax nana	Nonpathogenic
Iodamoebic butschlii	Nonpathogenic

Entamoeba histolytica is the most pathogenic of the intestinal amoeba that plagues humans. Trophozoites of *E. histolytica* can sometimes remain in the intestinal lumen (tubelike opening) for years without causing any damage and in this case the patients who are asymptomatic are carriers who can potentially transmit the organisms to others. The majority (90 percent) of patients fall into this group. Asymptomatic carriers are defined as those who are infected by a given organism but report no symptoms and show no signs of the condition of amoebiasis. Disease states in these persons can most often be detected by fecal analyses. The procedure may also reveal cysts of nonpathogenic *E. dispar*, which for unknown reasons is not invasive or as potentially harmful as those of the pathogenic *E. histolytica* (Figure 3-10), which possesses four nuclei. The nuclei are not always visible at various levels within the organism so it is necessary to focus up and down at several levels with the microscope in order to see all the nuclei present. It is also important to differentiate cysts of *Entamoeba coli* that are larger than *E. histolytica* and have eight nuclei (Figure 3-11) from other parasitic organisms, as the *Entamoeba coli* organism is also not pathogenic but may lead to difficulty in the identification of *E. histolytica*.

Symptoms

In amoebic colitis the incubation period varies greatly. During some period of the infection the *E. histolytica* organisms may begin to invade the tissues of the intestinal mucosa and produce ulcerations of the mucus membranes of the colon, resulting in the breaking down of the tissues in the gastrointestinal (GI) tract. Clinical signs often include abdominal pain, diarrhea with blood in the stool specimen, and some patients may be moderately febrile, while appearing to be in good health. If the rectum is affected there may be a condition called tenesmus, which means painful cramps in the anal region. Perianal ulcers may occur by direct spread of organisms from rectal amoebiasis (Figure 3-12). The ulcers develop rapidly and are often quite painful. After suffering from amoebic colitis there may be persistent intestinal problems, the origins of which are not clearly understood.

Life Cycle

Enteric amoebae all have a similar life cycle but an invasive stage that involves organs outside the intestine is seen with *E. histolytica* but not with the others, at least to any great extent. The mature cysts are ingested and passed

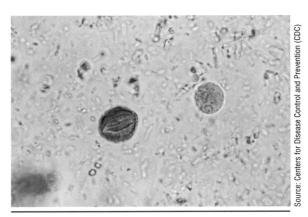

FIGURE 3-10 *Entamoeba histolytica* cysts that when mature, will reveal four nuclei

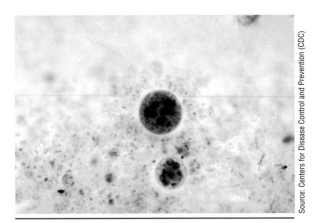

FIGURE 3-11 *Entamoeba coli* (larger) and *Entamoeba histolytica* (smaller) cysts

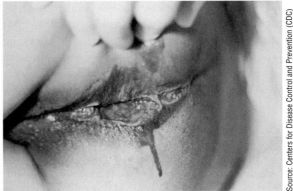

FIGURE 3-12 Amebiasis patient presented with tissue destruction, and granulation of the perianal and anoperineal region due to an *Entamoeba histolytica* infection

Source: Centers for Disease Control and Prevention (CDC)

into the small intestine where excystation ("hatching") takes place. The "freed" cyst then develops into a trophozoite form and proceeds to multiply through binary fission in the lumen (tubelike opening of the colon). Trophozoites may then initiate a process called *encystations*, and immature cysts are excreted where fecal contamination begins the infective cycle that would impact other animals. Both immature and mature cysts are found in the feces along with trophozoites, a stage that is most prevalent in watery stools. Some trophozoites may invade the colon's wall where they multiply and pass into the vascular system to infect organs outside the colon.

Disease Transmission

E. histolytica is one of the most important and most widely distributed human protozoans to infect humans. *E. dispar* is considered by some medical practitioners a nonpathogenic strain of *E. histolytica*. Food and water contaminated with amoebic cyst and sexual intercourse involving anal penetration are the sources of most cases of amebiasis. Asymptomatic carriers, particularly food handlers, may transmit the disease to significant numbers of victims. The incubation period before symptoms arise may range from several days to several months. Symptomatic patients often have diarrhea and abdominal pain. With the progression of the infection leading to dysentery, blood may be contained in the feces. Ulcers sometimes occur in the appendix and all parts of the colon. Symptoms may mimic ulcerative colitis and diverticulitis, leading to erroneous diagnoses. When *E. histolytica* trophozoites pass through the colon walls and enter the circulatory system, the development of abscesses may occur in diverse tissues and organs of the body, including the liver and the brain or lungs.

Fulminant colitis due to amoebal infection is a condition indicated by a severe and sudden onset. This condition is characterized by high fever and intestinal bleeding and sometimes perforation of the colon. The transfer of intestinal contents would release a variety of bacterial organisms into the peritoneum that would result in the patient becoming seriously ill. This condition will often be manifested by a distended abdomen and a form of intestinal paralysis where peristalsis is halted. A fulminant course may occur when patients are misdiagnosed as suffering from Crohn's disease or ulcerative colitis in which the patient is treated with steroids. Another condition that occurs in rare cases is a condition called *amoeboma* in which a mass may occur, resulting in a diagnosis of colon cancer. Countless trophozoites are found in the infected tissues of the intestines but cysts are never found in these conditions.

Laboratory Diagnosis

It may be difficult, both for the beginning student of parasitology as well as for an experienced laboratory technician or technologist, to identify trophozoites of amoebae. Features of single organisms, including observation of stained specimens for nuclei and the overall cytoplasmic appearance, cannot often be made without examining a representative number of organisms before arriving at a conclusion. Several different features and several different individual organisms must be examined before a presumptive identification may be made. Cyst forms of amoebae are usually less variable and can be more easily identified under normal conditions. Certain features that are peculiar to only one species may be helpful. In addition, other findings such as Charcot-Leyden crystals for disintegrated white blood cells called eosinophils may provide clues that parasites may be present.

Features that distinguish the differences between trophozoite and cyst stages of intestinal amoebae are used by experienced parasitologists to aid in identifying the various organisms. Remember, there are even cases where some parasitic organisms do not exhibit both stages of development, and this is also used as a valuable piece of information for finding and identifying some of these organisms. In addition, a great many artifacts may appear as parasites, but on further examination will turn out to be harmless elements or artifacts from the diet and from the environment. The following table, Table 3-3, will identify features of both cyst and trophozoite stages of amoebae found in the intestine. Descriptions of the features for differentiation are used comparatively.

In active dysentery, no cysts of *E. histolytica* are found in the feces but if there is little diarrhea that could quickly result in the organisms being quickly expelled, the parasites have time to encyst in the tissues of the digestive system. Since excretion of the parasites is intermittent, it is best to carry out three different stool analyses before deciding upon a negative result. Sometimes it is easier to reveal the parasites in a stool obtained by means of a purgative medication or a laxative. Other tests for identification of *Entamoeba histolytica* antigen in the feces have been developed, but further evaluation may be needed in order to determine the validity of these tests. These tests may, however, permit

TABLE 3-3 Comparison of Trophozoites and Cysts

	TROPHOZOITES	CYSTS
Motility	Rapid or sluggish motility	Not applicable
Cytoplasmic Appearance	Finely or coarsely granular, vacuolated	Not applicable
Cytoplasmic Inclusions	RBCs, bacteria, or yeasts	Not applicable
Nucleus or Nuclei	Number present	Number present
Karyosome	Location and size	Location and size
Peripheral Chromatin	Present or absent	Present or absent
Chromatoid Bodies	Present or absent	Present or absent
Glycogen Vacuole	Present or absent	Present or absent
Size	Same importance with both stages	Same importance with both stages
Shape		Shapes vary

swift differentiation between *E. histolytica* and the non-pathogenic *E. dispar*.

Treatment and Prevention

Parasites in the tissues (intestinal wall) can be treated with metronidazole or tinidazole. The dose of metronidazole (Flagyl) is also the treatment for certain bacterial infections, as well as for certain amebic parasites. These drugs are rapidly absorbed in the proximal intestine. For this reason they are not very effective in combating the parasites in the distal intestinal lumen (tubelike opening) near the anus. These amebic parasites are best treated with diloxanide furoate, which kills amoebae upon contact. However, parasites that have invaded the tissues are not affected by this drug, as it is difficult for the drug to gain contact with the imbedded parasites. Other contact amoebicides are iodoquinol and paromomycine, which result in a somewhat higher relapse percentage, but this is not always the case.

Humans act as reservoirs for the infectious *E. histolytica*. The cysts for this organism are extremely hardy and can be transmitted by infected water. The cyst stages of the organisms can survive environmental extremes and require both filtration and chemical treatment of water in order to kill or remove the organism. During military operations where water is taken from wells, springs, lakes, and running water, iodine is used to ensure safety when drinking the water from local and untreated sources. Sanitary living conditions are mandatory in order to prevent transmission of this parasitic amoeba.

ENTAMOEBA COLI

It is important to be able to identify *E. coli* (not to be confused with the bacteria *Escherichia coli*), which is nonpathogenic by comparing *E. coli* and *E. histolytica*. The **microscopic diagnostic features** that follow for *E. coli* and *E. histolytica* will be helpful in differentiating between the two organisms, one of which if pathogenic (*E. histolytica*) and the other (*E. coli*) is not.

Morphology

Entamoeba coli is one several nonpathogenic varieties of amoebic parasites, but is medically important not because it is pathogenic, but because it can be confused during the microscopic examination of stained stool specimens with the pathogenic *Entamoeba histolytica*. Differentiation between these two species is typically accomplished by visual examination of the parasitic cysts by use of light microscopy. But new and emerging methods using molecular biology techniques have been developed and are currently on the market, whereas others are currently being developed to provide improved and more rapid. The identification of *E. coli* is not in itself of enough significance to seek treatment as it is considered harmless. But other pathogenic organisms may have been ingested at the same time the patient was infected by this benign species of *Entamoeba* because the route of infection for most species of amoebae is the same.

Entamoeba coli as a nonpathogenic species of *Entamoeba* that frequently exists as a commensal parasite

MICROSCOPIC DIAGNOSTIC FEATURE

General Classification	Amoeba
Organism	*Entamoeba histolytica*
Specimen Required	Stool specimen
Stage	Trophozoites most diagnostic stage
Size	Trophozoite—15–25 × 5–15 μm; Cysts—10–20 μm
Shape	Elongated trophozo-ites and round cysts
Motility	Directional and progressive by pseudopodia
Nucleus(i)	1 for trophozoites and up to 4 for cysts
Cytoplasm	Clear and without ingested particles or vacuoles
Other Features	Tissue invasive; concentric bull's eye karyosome in Chromatoidal bars with rounded terminal ends nucleus (nuclei)

E. histolytica

Trophozoite   Cyst

Delmar/Cengage Learning

in the human gastrointestinal tract. The term *E. coli* is sometimes confused with the bacterium *Escherichia coli*, a **Gram negative rod** that is normal flora in the bowel of humans except for some pathogenic strains that often cause serious illness when contracted. Fresh cysts of *Entamoeba coli* contain what are called *chromatoid bodies* or bars and when they are present they will have sharply pointed and splintered appearances. The cysts are almost perfectly round and contain granular and unevenly distributed peripheral chromatin. The morphology of the *Entamoeba coli* cyst includes a spherical (round) shape and a range in size from 10 to 35 μm but is usually observed in the 15- to 25-μm range. Chromatoid bodies are seen less often in *E. coli* than in *E. histolytica*. When observed, they are usually splinter-like with pointed ends and differ from the chromatoid bodies of *E. histolytica,* which have rounded ends.

Entamoeba coli is one of the larger cysts in intestinal amoebae, containing eight nuclei, but careful focusing at different levels with a light microscope may be necessary to visualize all eight nuclei. Mature *E. coli* cysts usually have 8 nuclei (but it has been reported that sometimes 16 nuclei are present) in completely mature cysts that measure 10 to 35 μm. In addition to at least 8 nuclei, the mature cysts will have a large karyosome (central or eccentric) in each nucleus and an irregular (but sometimes regular) chromatin pattern (Figure 3-13). Immature cysts contain 8 or fewer nuclei and may have one or two large nuclei with a large and easily discernable glycogen vacuole. The nuclei can be enumerated by carefully focusing up and down with the microscope

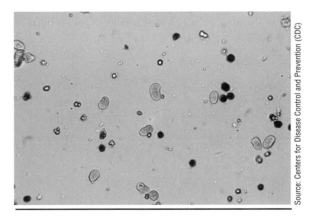

Source: Centers for Disease Control and Prevention (CDC)

FIGURE 3-13 *Entamoeba coli* cysts typically have 8 nuclei

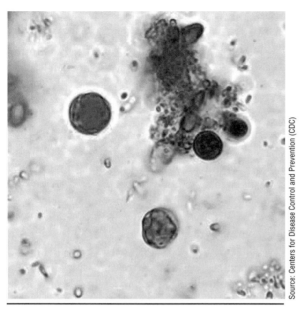

Source: Centers for Disease Control and Prevention (CDC)

FIGURE 3-14 *Endolimax nana* cysts from wet mount with iodine stain

MICROSCOPIC DIAGNOSTIC FEATURE

General Classification	Amoeba
Organism	*Entamoeba coli*
Specimen Required	Stool specimen
Stage	Trophozoites most diagnostic stage
Shape	Elongated trophozoites and round cysts
Size	Trophozoite—5–50 µm; cysts—15–25 µm
Motility	Nondirectional with no progression
Nucleus(i)	1 for trophozoites and up to 8 for cysts; coarse and uneven peripheral chromatin
Cytoplasm	Vacuoles present along with ingested bacteria
Other Features	Chromatoidal bars with splintered terminal ends
	Eccentric karyosome in nucleus of trophozoite

Entamoeba coli

Trophozoite   Cyst

Delmar/Cengage Learning

objective along with adjustment of the condenser. It is important to remember that *E. coli* is the only species of *Entamoeba* with more than four nuclei in the cyst stage.

The trophozoite stage of *E. coli* measures from 15 to 50 µm and the cytoplasm often appears "dirty" due to the coarse granulation as well as ingested bacteria and other fecal debris. A single nucleus is present with peripheral nuclear chromatin that is distributed in clumps. A large eccentric (noncentered) karyosome in the solitary nucleus is characteristic of the trophozoite stage. The motility of the trophozoite is described as sluggish with little progression that is accomplished by blunt pseudopodia.

The nuclei of *E. coli* are best revealed by means of an iodine stain. They have a dark circumference and a dark central point (karyosome). The karyosome of *Entamoeba coli* is not centrally located, but eccentric (off-centered). Staining with an iodine solution (Lugol's) can also detect glycogen bodies or vacuoles (brown) in young cysts. Peripheral chromatin is present in the nuclei of *E. coli* cysts and trophozoites but not in *Endolimax nana* trophozoites (Figure 3-14).

Symptoms

Those infected with *E. coli* are generally asymptomatic because these parasites are not considered pathogenic.

However, it is important to distinguish this organism definitively from those parasites that are pathogenic. *E. coli* may occur simultaneously with another intestinal protozoan.

Life Cycle

E. coli enjoys a similar life cycle as the other amoebae where simple reproduction is accomplished by binary longitudinal fission. However, there is no extra-intestinal stage such as that found with *E. histolytica* where invasion of other tissues occurs.

Disease Transmission

Patients with *E. coli* infections are generally, but not always, asymptomatic. As is the case with many other parasites, transmission is chiefly by ingesting the organism with food and water that are contaminated with amoebic cysts. Cockroaches have also been implicated in transmitting the disease to humans where these insects have contaminated food products.

Laboratory Diagnosis

Diagnosis of the presence of an *E. coli* infection relies on the standard examination of a fresh fecal specimen for ova and parasites for characteristic morphological features and structures. A permanent stained smear is the best means for identifying this organism.

Treatment and Prevention

The nonpathogenic *E. coli* do not require any treatment unless concomitant infection with other organisms occurs. Ensuring cleanliness of food and water that has been purified is necessary to prevent infection. Flies and cockroaches should be prevented from gaining access to foods.

OTHER IMPORTANT AMOEBAL ORGANISMS IN INTESTINAL PARASITOSIS

Although *E. histolytica* is the most important amoeba that is responsible for producing disease of the gastrointestinal tract of humans, there are other species that are pathogenic. An added problem is the ferreting out of organisms that are not pathogenic, and differentiating between them and the important disease-causing parasites. A systematic approach of comparing morphology is helpful in differentiating between the large variety of organisms that might be encountered in stool specimens, and can be a challenge even to experienced medical professionals. The use of table such as Table 3-4 and comparative charts are

TABLE 3-4 Comparison of *E. histolytica* with Common Nonpathogenic Amoebae

E. HISTOLYTICA	E. COLI	E. HARTMANNI	E. DISPAR
Trophozoites	**Trophozoites**	**Trophozoites**	**Trophozoites**
20–40 µm	20–25 µm	8–10 µm	15–20 µm
Motility increased when warm	Sluggish and nondirectional movement	Less progressive motility than *E. dispar*	Progressive movement
Extended pseudopodia	Broad, blunt pseudopodia		Extended pseudopodia
Cysts	**Cysts**	**Cysts**	**Cysts**
8–20 µm	20–25 µm	6–8 µm	12–15 µm
1 to 4 nuclei (4 in mature form)	8 nuclei	4 nuclei	4 nuclei
Squat, oval chromatoid bodies	Pointed chromatoid bodies	Blunt chromatoid bodies	Blunt chromatoid bodies

invaluable when faced with the task of identifying protozoa of the human gastrointestinal tract.

BLASTOCYSTIS HOMINIS

Blastocystis is a single-celled parasite that infects the gastrointestinal tract of humans and other animals. Many different species of the *Blastocystis* genus exist and are prevalent in not only humans but also are found to infect farm animals, birds, various rodents, amphibians, reptiles, fish, and even insects such as cockroaches. This provides for a wide variety of reservoirs from which humans may become infected. The disease known as blastocystosis is often accompanied by symptoms of constipation, diarrhea, and other abdominal distress. These symptoms are also found in a number of other intestinal disorders so the history of exposure to hosts and knowledge of a variety of environmental conditions may be extremely important when attempting a diagnosis.

Morphology

Originally *Blastocystis* was classified as a yeast form because of its appearance as a round, yeast-like glistening image when examined in fresh wet mounts. Initially no amoeboid characteristics were observed such as pseudopodia for locomotion. Later investigation by C. H. Zierdt led to reclassification under the subphylum Sporozoa based on some features of the *Blastocystis* cell that are similar to that of Protista. This decision was based on the presence of an organized nucleus, smooth and rough endoplasmic reticulum, Golgi complex, **mitochondrion**-like organelles, and pseudopodia. Its sensitivity to antiprotozoal drugs and its inability to grow on fungal media further indicated that it was a protozoan (Brumpt, 1912) rather than one of the yeasts. Eventually further revisions were made and more recently the classification of *Blastocystis* was based on modern molecular approaches to classification, through which these studies have shown that *Blastocystis* is neither a yeast nor a protozoan. It has now been placed in a new kingdom known as the *stramenopiles*. Other stramenopiles include brown algae, mildew, diatoms, the organism that caused the Irish potato famine, and the organism responsible for sudden oak death disease.

Considerable diversity appears in the morphological forms in which *Blastocystis* exists, providing for

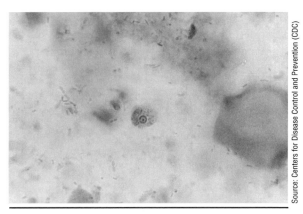

FIGURE 3-15 *Blastocystis hominis* cyst-like forms in wet mounts stained with iodine

Source: Centers for Disease Control and Prevention (CDC)

considerable difficulty in identifying the organism as the causative organism for diarrhea. Four commonly described forms are the vacuolar (otherwise known as central body), granular, amoeboid, and cyst forms, which appear to be mostly dependent upon environmental conditions due to an extreme sensitivity to oxygen levels (Figure 3-15). Whether all four of these forms exist concurrently in the host intestine has not definitely been demonstrated.

This organism is challenging in the preventive steps that must be taken to avoid the diversity and numbers of potential hosts that may transmit the organism and with which almost everyone at some time has had contact. Most species of *Blastocystis* found in mammals and birds are able to cause infection in humans. Along with its challenging nature, even its classification has proved challenging. *Blastocystis* was originally classified as a yeast organism due to its appearance, but later and after further study was reclassified as a protozoan. For many years, scientists believed one species of *Blastocystis* infected humans, whereas different species of *Blastocystis* infected other animals. This led the investigators to call *Blastocystis* found in humans by the term *Blastocystis hominis* (*hominis* for human) and ascribed different species names to *Blastocystis* from other animals, for example *Blastocystis ratti* from rats. Analysis of genetic characteristics of *B. hominis* has proven that the organism does not have a single entity or dedicated single species of *Blastocystis* that infects humans. It is believed that there are perhaps as many as nine distinct "species" of *Blastocystis* (as defined by genetic differences) that can infect humans.

Symptoms

The diagnosis of *Blastocystosis* is arguable because it has not been proven that symptoms associated with the presence of the organism are valid or are a result of the infection. It is argued that many people found to harbor *Blastocystis* might have other infectious organisms responsible for their symptoms. *Blastocystis hominis* organisms are found mostly in asymptomatic people, and only a few persons diagnosed with the infection actually experience any symptoms. Potential symptoms that are common complaints from patients infected by *B. hominis* are watery diarrhea, abdominal pain or cramps, perianal pruritis (itch), and excessive flatulence.

Life Cycle

The life cycle, along with its questionable pathogenicity, appears to not be fully developed. However there are three stages called the *amoebic*, the cyst, and the central body or vacuolated form. The parasite reproduces in the same manner as amoebae, by binary fission, or by sporulation. *B. hominis* feeds on bacteria and detritus of the gastrointestinal tract.

Disease Transmission

A number of investigators do consider *B. hominis* to be at least a possible pathogenic organism. It is assumed that the fecal-oral route of transmission is responsible for infections, although this belief is not supported by any specific characteristics or body of scientific knowledge.

Laboratory Diagnosis

The cyst form is the more recognizable and more recent discovery that has helped in the advancement of understanding the way the infection is transmitted. A permanent stained smear using a stain such as the trichrome stain is most preferred for determining the presence of this organism. Iodine smears, used to identify *B. hominis* organisms, are preliminary procedures for a number of other parasites. As compared to the other three forms, the cyst is generally smaller in size with a thicker cyst wall of several layers. It lacks a large central vacuole and has a few nuclei, although there are small multiple vacuoles and food storage deposits that may be seen. The cyst form is the most resistant form of this parasite and is able to survive in environmental conditions that may not be conducive to life for other organisms due to temperature extremes and drying out because of its thick cyst wall.

When ingested, the organisms appear to be able to survive the high levels of acidic hydrogen chloride in the stomach acid and the other gastric juices such as bile. The cysts are not lysed (destroyed) when placed in distilled water, whereas normal cells may rupture in the low-density water. The cysts have been known to survive successfully at room temperature for up to 19 days, indicating the form's strong resistance (Zaman, Howe, and Ng, 1995; Moe, Singh, Howe, *et al.* 1996).

In another experiment, the cyst form was even able to survive in a liquid culture medium that contained antiprotozoal drugs used for growing bacterial and yeast cultures. This ability to survive such a restricted environment further lends support to the belief that the cyst form of *Blastocystis* is the most resistant of the four forms. The most likely life cycle begins with ingestion of the cyst form. After ingestion, the cyst develops into three other forms which may in turn redevelop into cyst forms. Through human feces, the cyst forms enter the external environment and are transmitted to humans and other animals via the fecal-oral route, repeating the entire cycle.

Treatment and Prevention

Treatment for *Blastocystis* is initiated only when the organism is detected in significant numbers. The agent, metronidazole, that is effective against a variety of parasitic pathogens and some bacteria is the predominant drug used for treatment. Iodoquinol is also sometimes used for treatment when necessary.

ENTAMOEBA HARTMANNI

The *Entamoeba hartmanni* parasite is concentrically round with chromatoid bodies and forms small cysts with four nuclei. It is one of the several parasitic amoebae that may be found in the human intestinal tract but is largely considered to be nonpathogenic, but this is an issue debated among some professionals. *E. hartmanni* is sometimes called a "small-race *E. histolytica.*"

Morphology

Entamoeba hartmanni is sometimes called a "small *E. histolytica*" because these two species share a number

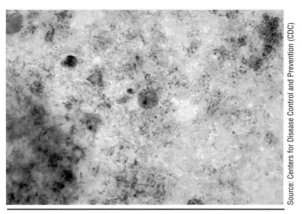

Source: Centers for Disease Control and Prevention (CDC)

FIGURE 3-16 *Entamoeba hartmanni* trophozoite

of morphological characteristics except for the differences in their respective sizes (Figure 3-16). Trophozoites of *E. hartmanni* measure usually 8 to 10 μm (range 5 to 12 μm) and are smaller than those of *E. histolytica* (10 to 60 μm). The trophozoites of *E. hartmanni* have one nucleus (cysts have four nuclei) with fine peripheral chromatin and a small and centrally located karyosome (body included in the chromatin of nucleus that usually stains a darker color than the remainder of the nucleus). The cytoplasm is finely granular. In summary, the trophozoites of *E. hartmanni* strongly resemble the morphology of those of *E. histolytica*, with a small, often centrally located karyosome, fine peripheral chromatin, and finely granular cytoplasm. But the main difference is in their small size: 5 to 12 μm compared to 10 to 60 μm for *E. histolytica*, but it should be noted that there may be some overlap among the smaller size of *E. histolytica*. Trophozoites of *E. hartmanni* also reveal ingestion of such materials as yeasts and other organic materials including bacteria but with no RBC inclusions as a diagnostic feature as is found in *E. histolytica*, and are considered nonpathogenic. When red blood cells are found in *E. histolytica*, this is called a pathognomic (indicative of a disease) condition (CDC).

Symptoms

E. hartmanni is nonpathogenic and no symptoms are usually associated with the presence of the organisms, as infections with the organism result in an asymptomatic condition. The organism is often found when examining microscopic slides of feces for other pathogenic enteric amoebae.

Life Cycle

The life cycle for *E. hartmanni* is the same as for other intestinal amoebae, with reproduction by binary longitudinal fission. Following excystation (when the cyst "hatches" and converts to a trophozoite), the phenomenon of binary fission occurs and trophozoites continue to reproduce in the colon's lumen (tubelike opening).

Disease Transmission

Amoebiasis by *E. hartmanni* as for most other enteric parasites is transmitted by ingestion of food and water containing the cysts of the organism. Again, this organism is not considered a pathogen, even in great numbers.

Laboratory Diagnosis

Diagnosis of the presence of an *E. hartmanni* infection relies on a microscopic examination of a fresh fecal specimen for ova and parasites. A permanent stained smear would provide the best means for identifying this organism. Immature and mature cyst forms as well as trophozoites may be found in the fecal sample.

Treatment and Prevention

The presence of nonpathogenic *E. hartmanni* does not require any treatment. Ensuring cleanliness of food and water that has been purified is necessary to prevent infection. Good personal sanitation practices as well as the availability of clean water and food will usually eliminate infections by *E. hartmanni*.

ENDOLIMAX NANA

Endolimax nana cysts are small, round or oval cysts with two to four nuclei, encompassing a range in size of 6 to 12 μm. The trophozoites of this organism are slow-moving trophozoites (*Limax* is the genus for a slug- or snail-like creature). *Endolimax* is the genus of amoeboid organisms found in the intestines of various animals, including the species *E. nana* found in humans. It causes no known disease and is most significant in medicine as it provides false positives when using other tests for identifying intestinal parasites. It is easy to confuse *E. nana* with the similar species *Entamoeba histolytica*, responsible for amoebic dysentery, and because its presence

MICROSCOPIC DIAGNOSTIC FEATURE

General Classification	Amoeba
Organism	*Entamoeba hartmanni*
Specimen Required	Stool specimen
Stage	Trophozoites most diagnostic stage
Size	4–12 µm for trophozoite and 5–10 µm for cyst stages
Shape	Slightly oval and irregularly shaped trophozoites and oval cysts
Motility	Nondirectional
Nucleus(i)	1 for trophozoites and 4 for cysts
Cytoplasm	Finely granular appearance
Other Features	Large and irregularly shaped, eccentric karyosomes in both
	Confused with *E. histolytica*, except for differences in size stages

E. hartmanni

Trophozoite   Cyst

Delmar/Cengage Learning

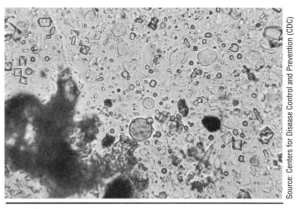

FIGURE 3-17 *Endolimax nana* trophozoite, an amebic parasite

indicates the host has consumed fecal material. The cyst form for *E. nana* contains up to four nuclei, which excyst in the body and become trophozoites (Figure 3-17). *Endolimax nana* nuclei have a large **endosome** somewhat off-center (eccentric), an identification feature that helps in separating *E. nana* from *E. histolytica*, the major causative organism in dysentery. There may be small amounts of visible cytoplasmic chromatin or none at all.

ENTAMOEBA DISPAR

Entamoeba dispar varies in its clinical impact and is a special case among several *Entamoeba* spp. that can result in either a harmless colonization of the intestine or may progress to an invasion of the colon wall and damage to other host tissues such as the liver, lung, and brain (amoebiasis). Often a clinical diagnosis of amoebiasis by *Entamoeba* can be confirmed and usually depends on the visualization of parasites using light microscopy for either a wet smear or a stained smear. *E. coli*, *E. dispar*, *E. histolytica*, and *E. hartmanni* may be differentiated by comparative sizes and minor morphological differences.

Morphology

Same as *E. histolytica*, the *E. dispar* trophozoite ranges from approximately 10 to 60 µm and is indistinguishable from *E. histolytica*. The cytoplasm is finely granular and may contain ingested bacteria. A single nucleus has a consistently arranged nuclear chromatin pattern similar to beads of a necklace. The karyosome is small and is

MICROSCOPIC DIAGNOSTIC FEATURE

General Classification	Amoeba
Organism	*Endolimax nana*
Specimen Required	Stool specimen
Stage	Trophozoites most diagnostic stage
Size	5–12 μm for both trophozoite and cyst stages
Shape	Elongated trophozoites and oval cysts
Motility	Sluggish
Nucleus(i)	1 for trophozoites and 4 for cysts
Cytoplasm	Vacuoles accompanied with granular appearance
Other Features	Large and irregularly shaped karyosomes in both stages

E. nana

Trophozoite   Cyst

Delmar/Cengage Learning

immature cysts but are not likely to be observed in mature cysts. An elongated chromatoid bar has smoothly rounded and blunt ends that sometimes leads to some confusion with *E. histolytica*.

Symptoms

Persons infected with *E. dispar* primarily show no symptoms unless concurrent infections with other organisms are present. But symptomatic patients may suffer from abdominal pain and diarrhea, which may or may not be listed as a cause of infection by *E. dispar* because it is considered nonpathogenic.

Life Cycle

E. dispar is a noninvasive parasite and although it resembles *E. histolytica*, it does not cause disease. The organism reproduces simply by binary longitudinal fission. Excystation occurs primarily in the lower ileum and there the cyst develops into the trophozoite form. Trophozoites continue to multiply in the colon and may become encysted.

Disease Transmission

Amoebiasis is most often achieved by eating contaminated food or drinking water containing the cysts of the various organisms, including *E. dispar*. Transmission of *E. histolytica* and perhaps *E. dispar*, because they are virtually indistinguishable from each other, may be contracted by a sexual route.

Laboratory Diagnosis

The morphological characteristics of *E. histolytica* are compared with the common and so-called non-pathogenic species that cause confusion with identification and differentiation of these various species. *Entamoeba histolytica* and another amoeba, *Entamoeba dispar*, which is about 10 times more common, look the same when seen under a microscope and require extensive investigation to differentiate between the two (see Table 3-4). This table, when used with a properly calibrated micrometer, will enable the medical professional to differentiate between the two species, but a number of organisms must be studied, and average sizes obtained (Figure 3-18).

Actively motile amoebic trophozoites are most commonly found in wet mounts from liquid or soft fecal

centrally located. Motility is demonstrated by directional and progressive movement.

The cyst ranges from 10 to 20 μm and the mature cyst contains four nuclei, whereas the immature cyst contains fewer than four nuclei. The *Entamoeba* genus is characterized by peripheral chromatin organized evenly around the nucleus, and this is not true of any other genus of amoebae. The karyosome is extremely small and centrally located. Glycogen vacuoles may be seen in

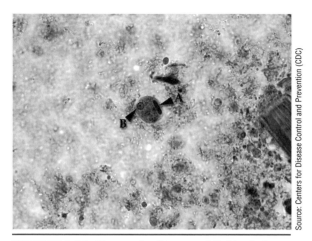

Source: Centers for Disease Control and Prevention (CDC)

FIGURE 3-18 *Entamoeba dispar* and *E. histolytica* appear the same but are not

specimens should be observed. Concentration techniques enhance the recovery rate and the numbers of organisms to be averaged for size, a method of differentiation between *E. dispar* and *E. histolytica,* because there is an overlap in the sizes of both trophozoites and cyst forms for the two species. Serological procedures are available that will definitively differentiate between the two species.

Treatment and Prevention

No treatment is indicated for infections with *E. dispar* but it is vital that a correct identification of the infectious organism be accomplished for differentiation between

E. histolytica and *E. dispar* before a course of treatment or lack of treatment is established. Prevention includes personal hygiene and avoidance of contaminated food and water.

OTHER INTESTINAL AMOEBAE

In addition to the information contained in the Table 3-4, just presented, there are several other non-pathogenic amoebae that have morphology that may require comparison to distinguish them from *E. histolytica*. It should be noted from earlier presentations that *Dientamoeba fragilis,* although grouped with amoebae, is more morphologically similar to flagellates such as *Trichomonas* spp. All three of the organisms presented in the next table have nuclei without a large karyosome and do not possess chromatin. Comparisons for differentiating nonpathogens and eliminating them from consideration are presented in the table (see Table 3-5).

IDENTIFYING MISCELLANEOUS AMOEBOID INFECTIONS

A number of other organisms that may serve to confuse the diagnosis of *E. histolytica* by providing false positive identification are presented here. The basic microscopic procedure using a stained specimen or wet prep is inexpensive and simple but it has several limitations. The procedure does not easily allow for distinguishing between the cysts and trophozoites of the disease-causing

TABLE 3-5 Comparison of Several Common Nonpathogenic Amoebae		
DIENTAMOEBA FRAGILIS	***ENDOLIMAX NANA***	***IODOAMOEBA BUTSCHLII***
Trophozoites	**Trophozoites**	**Trophozoites**
8–10 µm	8–10 µm	12–15 µm
May be binucleated		
Broken (scattered) karyosome		
Cysts	**Cysts**	**Cysts**
No cyst stage	6–8 µm	10–12 µm
	4 nuclei	1 nucleus
		Pronounced glycogen vacuole

species *Entamoeba histolytica*, the nonpathogenic species *Entamoeba dispar*, and other species that occasionally infect humans. Multiple samples often have to be requested and examined as the presence of cysts of the genera for *Entamoeba*, *Iodamoeba*, or *Endolimax* can cause difficulty in making a diagnosis. In sporadic cases of human infection with other species such as *E. moshkovskii* accompanied with both *E. histolytica* and *E. dispar* in young children in Bangladesh (Ali, *et al.*, 2003), the differentiation of the three species in clinical samples by other means becomes of great importance both for diagnosis and for epidemiological studies. Although there is some evidence that following infection with *E. dispar*, pathological changes may occur in some humans (McMillan, *et al.*, 1984), at this point *E. dispar* is still largely considered a nonpathogen.

IODAMOEBA BUTSCHLII

Iodamoeba butschlii organisms present themselves as mononuclear cysts. The most remarkable morphological feature of this organism is a lightly stained and large glycogen supply vacuole. *I. butschlii* is a nonpathogenic amoeba with worldwide distribution and prevalence. Although it can be difficult to differentiate the trophozoites of *I. butschlii* from *Endolimax nana*, this stage of *I. butschlii* is more active than that of *E. nana*.

Morphology

The cysts of *Iodamoeba* are much more distinctive than their trophozoite stage (Figure 3-19). They contain a single nucleus with a large karyosome and inconspicuous peripheral chromatin. Cysts are variable in size but are mostly 5 to 20 μm in diameter and also contain the characteristic and well-defined large glycogen vacuole but no readily discernible chromatoidal bars. The large glycogen vacuole stains a deep reddish-brown with iodine and in permanent stains the vacuole may appear as an unstained intracellular space. In an iodine-stained cyst, the single nucleus is not readily visible, but if discernible, a large karyosome is located eccentrically in the nucleus.

As is the case for other intestinal protozoa, infection occurs via the fecal-oral route. The trophozoites are only slightly larger than the cysts at 10 to 20 μm and their internal structure is similar to that of cysts except that the granular cytoplasm contains many vacuoles. In addition, fecal debris, bacteria, and yeast may be seen in

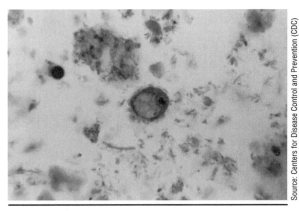

Source: Centers for Disease Control and Prevention (CDC)

FIGURE 3-19 *Iodamoeba buetschlii* cyst, an amoebal parasite

the cytoplasm with a large karyosome that may fill much of the nuclear space within the cytoplasm. No peripheral chromatin may be seen and nonprogressive and slow motility is characteristic of this species.

Symptoms

No symptoms are associated with the presence of this organism. The organism is usually discovered during examinations for other parasites.

Life Cycle

The reproduction of *I. butschlii* is the same as other nonpathogenic amoebae. Longitudinal binary fission is the sole means of reproduction for this organism.

Disease Transmission

Transmission is by the fecal-oral route, as are most of the intestinal amoebae. Personal hygiene and ingestion of foods and water from safe sources will eliminate infections by *I. butschlii*.

Laboratory Diagnosis

Diagnosis is accomplished by the microscopic examination of fecal samples for *I. butschlii*. Wet mounts using solutions of iodine are effective in visualizing *I. butschlii*.

Treatment and Prevention

No treatment is indicated for an infection with *I. butschlii*. Sanitary preparation of food and purification of water is necessary to prevent the infection.

MICROSCOPIC DIAGNOSTIC FEATURE

General Classification	Amoeba
Organism	*Iodamoeba butschlii*
Specimen Required	Stool specimen
Stage	Trophozoites most diagnostic stage
Size	6–20 µm for trophozoite and 6–15 µm for cyst stages
Shape	Irregularly shaped and elongated trophozoites and slightly oval cysts
Motility	Nondirectional
Nucleus(i)	1 for trophozoites and 1 for cysts
Cytoplasm	Sometimes includes ingested bacteria and is vacuolated
Other Features	Large and concentric karyosomes in both stages
	Large defined glycogen vacuole is characteristic of this species

I. butschlii

Trophozoite   Cyst

Delmar/Cengage Learning

DIFFERENTIATING BACTERIAL DYSENTERY FROM AMEBIC DYSENTERY

Dysentery is a disease that is characterized by diarrhea and contains both blood and mucus. The condition may be caused by pathogenic bacteria, viruses, or parasites. Because treatment for the various types of dysentery is quite different, it is necessary to determine the cause of the dysentery prior to initiating treatment. Diagnosis is most often made through clinical signs and stated symptoms expressed by the patient, but dysentery should be confirmed by microscopic examination because diarrhea by any of the three entities listed previously are capable of producing similar signs and symptoms. Bacterial dysentery is diagnosed and the causative organism determined by culture of the bacterial strain on nutrient media, after which an antibiotic sensitivity test will indicate the antibacterial agent that should be most effective in controlling the disease. Viruses may be grown in cell cultures but this procedure is quite time consuming, and may become contaminated. The most common manner of diagnosing a viral infection is by the indirect process of the antibody titer where the body's immune system reacts to the infection and by the presence of clinical signs and symptoms. Parasites, on the other hand, are discovered by examination of blood and body wastes by microscopic evaluation of wet mounts and stained specimens that may also necessitate concentration techniques.

OTHER ASSOCIATED CONDITIONS OF INTESTINAL INFECTIONS

Balantidium coli, a normal parasite of swine as described previously, is a pathogenic ciliate and can cause severe colitis, or irritation of the bowel, and is mentioned for the following reasons. The clinical manifestations are very similar to the intestinal amoebal infections where the diagnosis is most often made by the microscopic examination of stool specimens before treatment is begun. Treatment for *B. coli* infections is with tetracycline, an antibiotic used primarily for bacterial infections. **Pseudomembranous colitis** may mimic parasitic infections, but is an infection of the colon that is often caused by a bacterium called *Clostridium difficile*. The illness is characterized by offensive-smelling diarrhea, fever, and abdominal pain, which are similar to signs and symptoms presented by victims of an intestinal parasitic disease. Therefore, parasitic or bacterial infections should be ruled out by specific lab tests to provide appropriate treatment.

Other intestinal diseases characterized by severe dysentery are Crohn's disease and ulcerative colitis, but both of these conditions are rare in the tropics where parasitosis abounds. Radiological studies and

TABLE 3-6 Differentiation of Bacterial Versus Amebic Dysentery

BACILLARY DYSENTERY	AMEBIC DYSENTERY
Acute onset	Gradual onset
Poor general condition	General condition normal
High fever	Little fever in adults
Severe tenesmus (pain and feelings of needing to empty bowel)	Moderate tenesmus
Dehydration frequent	Little dehydration (adult)
Feces: no forms of bacteria are identified as trophozoites	Feces: trophozoites present
Can be cultured on nutritive media	Unable to culture or grow on media

surgical biopsies are essential for the diagnosis of these conditions.

A standardized approach to empirically differentiating between dysentery caused by bacteria or amebic organisms organisms is shown in Table 3-6.

INTESTINAL AMEBIASIS AND TREATMENT

Infection or colonization of the gastrointestinal system begins in the colon but is capable of spreading to other organs and systems, such as the liver, where lesions are formed. Amebiasis often results from the ingestion of contaminated food and beverages in which mostly cysts of the various organisms are found. The cysts enter the intestines where they release motile trophozoites, and these forms invade the membranes of the colon or spread to the liver though the large vascular system, including the portal vein. Trophozoites divide quickly to form more cysts, which may be excreted in the feces and serve to contaminate water and food that will be ingested by others.

Again, a number of tools are available to diagnose amoebiasis and to prevent damage to the infected patient. The presence of amoebae may be determined by microscopic evaluation of stools, where both cysts and trophozoites may be found, or by serological testing

for antibodies against these amoebae by blood testing. These antibodies will most likely appear by the seventh day of infestation, and an exam called a colonoscopy may be required to obtain tissue samples to differentiate amebic infection from bacterial and other types of intestinal inflammation. In extreme cases a liver abscess may form and produce pain that imitates other diseases and an ultrasound procedure or CT scan may be required to diagnose the involvement of the liver.

ASYMPTOMATIC CARRIERS

Entamoeba dispar is distributed worldwide. Because extremely high numbers of the people in endemic regions of the world may be cyst carriers (e.g., 10 percent), there is little rationale for treating them when they are found by chance in isolated regions with a high infectivity rate. In many cases, perhaps 90 to 95 percent of these people may be chronically infected with this possibly nonpathogenic species of amoebae called *E. dispar*. For service workers, such as food handlers and medical personnel, however, treatment may be indicated with a variety of medications to ensure a reduction in the infective rate of these workers. In regions of high potential for becoming endemic, it may indeed be sensible to treat the patient even though the organism is considered nonpathogenic except in rare cases. This would serve to prevent transmission to the remainder of the uninfected population, creating endemic areas and also to prevent possible development of later cases of invasive amebiasis by *E. dispar*.

NONINTESTINAL AMOEBA

A number of organisms inhabit the mouth but are not found in the intestines. A number of free-living amoebae may occasionally be encountered by humans, usually with little consequences.

ENTAMOEBA GINGIVALIS

In addition to *T. tenax*, *Entamoeba gingivalis* is also a causative agent for gum diseases. *E. gingivalis* is found in the mouth where there is soft tartar between the teeth and in tonsillar fossae and crevices. Sometimes the organism can be recovered from sputum, and specimens from this source must be differentiated from *E. histolytica*. *Entabomeba gingivalis* may be called either *E. gingivalis* or *E. buccalis*. This is a nonpathogenic species of amoeba that inhabits the mouth and is found particularly in periodontal disease and in smokers. *Entamoeba gingivalis* is a protozoan that is renowned as the first amoeba in humans to be described by investigators. It is found only in the mouth between the gingival pockets and near the base of the teeth. *Entamoeba gingivalis* is found in 95 percent of people with periodontitis (gingivitis or inflammatory gum disease) and in 50 percent of people with healthy gums.

Morphology

A cyst form has not been identified, and transmission is believed to occur directly from one person to another by kissing and sharing drinking containers and dining table utensils and dishes. Only the trophozoite form is observed and the organisms range from 10 to 20 µm in diameter. *Entamoeba gingivalis* protozoa have pseudopodia that allow them to move quickly, particularly because they are found only in the trophozoite stage. A round (spheroid) nucleus will be from 2 to 4 µm in diameter and will contain a small central endosome. Numerous food vacuoles are present and cellular materials, blood cells, bacteria, and perhaps other miscellaneous organic materials may have been ingested by the organism.

Symptoms

Most hosts of this organism will be asymptomatic. In some cases severe periodontal conditions, including inflammation and pyorrhea (purulent discharge in periodontal disease) of the gums, iares present. Serious effects of gum disease may lead to loosened teeth accompanied by bleeding, which may eventually lead to loss of teeth if not successfully treated. In addition, periodontal disease is known to lead to cardiac problems.

Life Cycle

Reproduction for *E. gingivitis* is the same as for other amoeboid organisms, through bilateral fission (splitting into two or more parts).

Disease Transmission

Transmission has been linked to kissing people with serious gingivitis, smoking that causes constant and persistent inflammation of the gums, and eating and drinking from equipment contaminated by an individual with an *E. gingivitis* infection.

Laboratory Diagnosis

A cyst form has not been identified at this point, and transmission is believed to occur directly from one person to another by kissing and sharing drinking containers and dining table utensils and dishes. Only the trophozoite form is the sole form observed, and the parasite ranges from 10 to 20 µm in diameter. *Entamoeba gingivalis* protozoa have pseudopodia that allow them to move quickly, as a characteristic typically found in the trophozoite stage. A round (spheroid) nucleus will be from 2 to 4 µm in diameter and will contain a small central endosome. An endosome is a lumen (opening) found in the cytoplasm that serves to differentiate between waste products that are transported into lysosomes for destruction and those materials that can be metabolized by the organism. There are numerous food vacuoles and cellular materials, blood cells, bacteria, and other organic materials that may have been ingested by the organism. A variety of permanent stains are used, such as crystal violet.

Treatment and Prevention

Treatment where symptoms exist is based on good oral care and judicious choices of those whom one kisses. Those at risk or those who have gingivitis should consult with a periodontist (dentist with a specialty practice in diseases of the gums and mouth tissues) where deep cleaning around the roots of the teeth is performed on a regular basis.

COCCIDIA OF THE HUMAN INTESTINE

Several species of sporozoans have recently been found to inhabit the human intestine and that of other mammals. Two of the most prevalent organisms from the subphylum Sporozoa are presented in Table 3-7.

CRYPTOSPORIDIUM PARVUM

Coccidia are classified as members of the subphylum Sporozoa and are nonmotile and obligate intracellular parasites that have complex life cycles of both sexual and asexual states that occur in definitive and intermediate hosts, in that order. Coccidia are found in a number of

TABLE 3-7 Classification of Pathogenic and Nonpathogenic Protozoa

PHYLUM	SUBPHYLUM	ATTRIBUTES	EXAMPLES OF SPECIES
Apicomplexa	Sporozoa	Single-celled and intracellular	*Babesia microti*
		Inhabit host's epithelial cells of the intestine and associated glands	*Cryptosporidium parvum*
			Cyclospora cayetanensis
		Life cycle complex and involves insects, mammals other than host	*Isospora belli*
			Plasmodium species
		Both sexual and asexual reproduction may be involved	*Pneumocystis carinii (jirovecii)*
			Sarcocystis species
			Toxoplasma gondii
	Microspora	Chiefly infects those who are immunodeficient	*Encephalitozoon*
			Enterocytozoon
		Mammal-infecting intracellular parasite	*Microsporidia*
			Nosema
			Pleistophora

animals but are also known to infect humans. The coccidia are a group of organisms of the kingdom Protista. All representatives of this group are intracellular parasites which parasitize the epithelial cells of the intestinal tract. This group includes three species: *Cryptosporidium parvum, Cyclospora cayetanensis,* and *Isospora belli,* of which *C. parvum* and *I. belli* are the most prevalent in the infection of humans (Table 3-7). Note that another important member of the phylum Apicomplexa that infects humans is that of *Toxoplasma gondii*. These intestinal coccidia have been known for the better part of a century as a parasite of dogs, cats, cattle, horses, pigs, and other types of livestock and may also be found in some species of insects. But it was not until the 1980s when severe diseases of the immune system, such as HIV infections, became more prevalent that it became better known as an opportunistic organism.

Morphology

The oocyst of *Cryptosporidium parvum* is small, measuring approximately in a range of 4 to 6 µm and when mature the oocyst contains four sporozoites that may or may not be visible (Figure 3-20). A thick double-layered wall protects the oocyst from environmental stresses and no sporocysts are visible but darkly stained granules may be present.

Symptoms

Symptoms of cryptosporidiosis usually appear within 2 to 10 days, or an average of about a week before symptoms occur, after ingestion of the parasite. Signs and symptoms include watery diarrhea, headache, abdominal cramps, nausea, vomiting, and fever. The respiratory tract may become involved, as well as the gastrointestinal tract. These symptoms sometimes lead to weight loss and dehydration. In healthy individuals, symptoms such as diarrhea are self-limiting and last from one to two weeks, at which time the immune system eliminates the infection. However, in the immunocompromised persons and infants, the infection may continue, progressing to a life-threatening condition.

Life Cycle

Both *C. parvum* and *I. belli* are single-host pathogens, with no intermediate host involved.

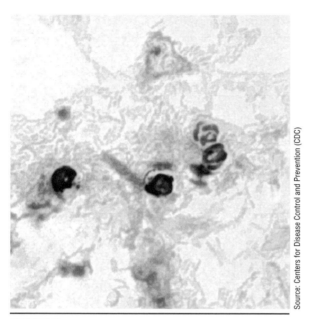

Source: Centers for Disease Control and Prevention (CDC)

FIGURE 3-20 *Cryptosporidium parvum* oocysts (i.e., encapsulated zygotes), which have been stained using the modified acid-fast method

Through fertilization, facilitated by the union of the macrogametes by the microgametes, a zygote is formed, which develops a cell wall and then becomes an oocyst. Ingestion of this oocyst by another host animal starts a new life cycle. These oocysts can survive in the environment for several months until ingested, followed by incubation in the gut of the host for approximately a week. *I. belli* develops only in humans but differs from *C. parvum*, as it is capable of infecting a variety of hosts. However, reproduction for the two organisms is similar except that for *I. belli*, unsporulated oocysts must develop for roughly a week in feces before they reach the infective stage. After oocysts are formed in the cytoplasm of the enterocytes (specialized nutrient-absorbing cells of the small intestine), they are completely developed and are excreted in feces, a form that will infect other hosts.

Disease Transmission

The infective form from animals and humans is the resistant oocyst that is passed in feces. Ingestion of contaminated food and water as well as person-to-person transmission are the main routes of infection. Municipal water systems that become contaminated with fecal material have also been implicated in widespread outbreaks of diarrhea in recent years. Municipal water supplies may sometimes become contaminated with many organisms, including *E. dispar* and other organisms such as *Coccidia*, that are not filtered out in the treatment plants. Standard chlorination levels by water treatment plants do not control this organism and levels of up to 30 times what is normal are necessary in water supplies to destroy the organisms.

In 1993, Milwaukee, Wisconsin, suffered the largest waterborne outbreak most likely in U.S. history. This outbreak of *Cryptosporidium* occurred when one of the water purification plants and the associated water tower became contaminated and treated water showed turbidity levels well above normal. Most of the coccidian infections in man are zoonoses, a term indicating that a distinct possibility of contracting the disease from infectious animals exists. Immunocompetent individuals usually suffer from mild, self-limiting infections that are sometimes not even noticed to an appreciable extent, but for those with an immunocompromised defense system, the symptoms may progress to a much more severe condition.

Laboratory Diagnosis

Examination of fecal samples and biopsy specimens to detect oocysts are the most common laboratory practices for identification. Specialty stains and Sheather's sugar flotation procedure for oocysts that are capable of being seen microscopically, are commonly used. Fluorescent antibody detection methods are now available, as a more sensitive and specific method than microscopic examination.

Treatment and Prevention

A number of antiparasitic agents are ineffective against *C. parvum*, but those who are immunocompetent often are free of symptoms within a short period of time after the appearance of symptoms. Some medications in current use are showing limited success in AIDS victims. Water treatment plants with filtration procedures and sanitary practices could prevent most infections by *C. parvum*, although filtration of water is not a standard practice. Most infections could be eliminated or reduced by the control or elimination of runoff of water from animal pens into water supplies.

ISOSPORA BELLI

Isosporiasis is a human intestinal disease caused by the parasite *Isospora belli*. This organism is found worldwide, especially in tropical and subtropical areas. Infection often occurs in immunocompromised individuals, particularly those who are HIV-infected, and outbreaks have been documented in those who are institutionalized, such as in prisons. The condition has been known since 1915. The coccidian parasite *Isospora belli* infects the mucosal epithelial cells of the small intestine. *I. belli* is less common than two other intestinal coccidia that infect humans, those of Toxoplasma and Cryptosporidium.

Morphology

Isospora is diagnosed most frequently by the study of freshly passed stools. Oocysts are formed by the union of microgametes and macrogametes, resulting in infective oocytes. Morphology of oocysts reveals two sporocysts with each containing four sporozoites. The size of these oocysts vary greatly, measuring an average of 17 to 37 μm.

Symptoms

A self-limiting diarrhea may occur in those who have a healthy immune system, and after a few weeks of incubation, nausea with vomiting, fever, abdominal cramps, loss of appetite, and often watery diarrhea occur. For infants, morbidity and mortality are prevalent as well as in immunocompromised individuals (organism present in many AIDS victims). The respiratory tract may become involved, as well as the gastrointestinal tract.

Life Cycle

The elements of the life cycle of both *C. parvum* and *I. belli* are similar, as both are single-host pathogens with no intermediate host involved. *I. belli* differs from *C. parvum* as it develops only in humans, but reproduction in the two organisms is similar except that for *I. belli*, unsporulated oocysts must develop for roughly a week in feces before they reach the infective stage (Figure 3-21). When infective oocytes are ingested by persons or animals; sporozoites emerge from the oocyst, containing four sporozoites. The sporozoites enter the microvilli of the intestine and develop into trophozoites, an asexual means of reproduction. The trophozoites multiply (schizogony) by forming merozoites that enter other cells and further schizogony occurs, producing microgametes and macrogametes, a form of sexual reproduction. The fusion of these two gametes results in a zygote that develops a cell wall and becomes an oocyst. These oocysts are excreted in feces and for *I. belli*, these oocysts can survive in the environment for several months until ingested and incubated in the gut for about a week. After oocysts develop in the cytoplasm of enterocytes (infected nutrient-absorbing cells of the small intestine), there is no further development until excreted in feces.

Disease Transmission

The resistant oocyst is passed in feces as the infective form from animals and humans. Ingestion of contaminated food and water as well as person-to-person transmission are the main routes of infection. Municipal water systems that become contaminated with fecal material have also been implicated in widespread outbreaks of diarrhea in recent years. Municipal water supplies may sometimes become contaminated with many organisms including *E. dispar* and other organisms such as *Coccidia* that are not filtered out in the treatment plants.

The outbreak in 1993 in Milwaukee, Wisconsin, is a case in point. Such an outbreak of a number of organisms may not be effectively controlled in standard water purification plants. Standard chlorination levels do not control this organism, even at higher levels than normally employed, so additional measures may require implementation such as filtration, or asking the citizens of a community to boil any water used for human consumption. Because most of the coccidian infections in humans are zoonoses, meaning there is a distinct possibility of contracting the disease from infectious animals, measures designed to control runoff of surface water from feeding facilities and where animals are processed for meat may require governmental standards to be implemented and enforced. Most immunocompetent individuals will suffer from mild, self-limiting infections that are sometimes not even noticed. In those who are immunocompromised, the individual's defense system may result in much more serious symptoms and progression to a critical medical condition.

Laboratory Diagnosis

Examination of fecal samples and biopsy specimens to detect oocysts are the most common laboratory practices. Specialty stains and Sheather's sugar flotation procedure

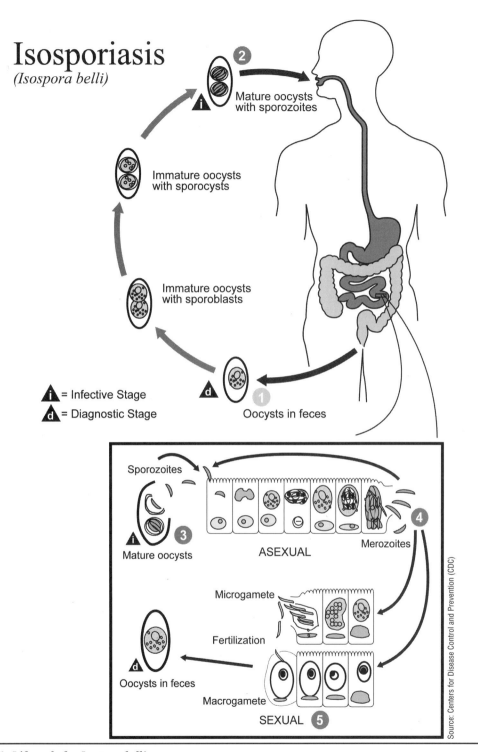

Isosporiasis
(Isospora belli)

2 Mature oocsts with sporozoites

i = Infective Stage

Immature oocysts with sporocysts

Immature oocysts with sporoblasts

d = Diagnostic Stage

1 Oocysts in feces

i = Infective Stage
d = Diagnostic Stage

Sporozoites

3 **i** Mature oocysts

ASEXUAL

4 Merozoites

Microgamete

Fertilization

d Oocysts in feces

Macrogamete

SEXUAL **5**

Source: Centers for Disease Control and Prevention (CDC)

FIGURE 3-21 Life cycle for *Isospora belli*

for oocysts, seen microscopically, are commonly used. Fluorescent antibody detection methods are now available, and are considered more sensitive and specific than microscopic methods.

Treatment and Prevention

A number of antiparasitic agents are ineffective against the organism of *C. parvum*, but those who are immunocompetent often are free of symptoms in a short period of time after symptoms appear. Some medications are showing limited success in AIDS victims. Water treatment plants with filtration procedures and sanitary practices will prevent most infections as well as reduce or eliminate runoff of water from animal pens into water supplies.

MICROSPORIDIA

Spores are oval in shape but are difficult to differentiate from bacteria because they are so small. Identification of spores in feces is actually possible with a modified trichrome stain that will stain spores a red color. Three or more organisms of this class are recognized as possible pathogens of humans and are difficult to differentiate but only recently have been considered as human parasites. Hundreds of species of microsporidian parasites have been isolated from a number of vertebrates, as well as from a variety of crustaceans and insects.

The importance of microsporidia lies in the fact that they are members of the phylum Microspora, are protozoal parasites of animals and insects that are responsible for common diseases of crustaceans and fish, and have been found in most other animal groups, including humans. Microsporidia are obligate, intracellular, spore-forming protozoa known to infect almost any class of animal. These organisms appear to have evolved perhaps hundreds of thousands or even millions of years ago and evidence appears to have been discovered in anthropological samples. As with other similar organisms, those with compromised immune systems are more vulnerable to intestinal infection with *Enterocytozoon bieneusi*. Infection with *E. bieneusi* and the condition is becoming increasingly recognized in patients with AIDS and chronic diarrhea where the prevalence is up to a third of those with these long-term medical conditions affecting the immune system. But there is still argument among professionals over the pathogenic role of *E.bieneusi*. Replication takes place within the host's cells, often in

the duodenum and gallbladder, and the microspiridium spore is the infective stage.

Morphology

The spores are extremely small and vary in size from 1 to 4.5 µm, making them some of the smallest parasites currently known. It is extremely difficult to differentiate between the parasite and a cocci-shaped bacterial cells that are prevalent in stool specimens due to similar size ranges.

Symptoms

Symptoms of sporidiosis are similar to those of cryptosporidiosis. Infants and those who are immunocompromised (prevalent in many AIDS victims) are particularly affected. A self-limiting diarrhea may occur in those who have a healthy immune system, and after a few weeks of incubation, nausea with vomiting, fever, abdominal cramps, loss of appetite, and often watery diarrhea occur. For infants, morbidity and mortality are prevalent as well as in immunocompromised individuals (the organism is present in many AIDS victims). The respiratory tract may become involved, as well as the gastrointestinal tract.

Life Cycle

The life cycle for the various species of microsporidia begins with a spore with thick protective walls to ward off extreme environmental conditions that might harm the organism. A polar tube is used to infect the cells of a host and is characteristic of all microsporidia. A spore that is ingested is stimulated by the gastrointestinal conditions to penetrate the cellular cytoplasm of the host. Sporoplasm is spilled into the host cell and multiplication begins in the cytoplasm of the host's cells. A number of cellular divisions occur by binary fission, resulting in spore production (sporogony).

Disease Transmission

During the process called sporogony the thick cell wall forms to protect against environmental hazards, aiding in the further spread throughout the host. The organisms are excreted in urine and feces where they are able to infect other hosts. Although microsporidiosis is more common in people with weakened immune systems (i.e., immunocompromised), cases do occur less frequently among those with normal immune systems. Microsporidia have the potential to be waterborne because they are released in both feces and urine that may wash into bodies of water. Although the most frequent cause of human microsporidium infection is *Enterocytozoon bieneusi*. Other microsporidia that are well known include: *Encephalitozoon hellem, Encephalitozoon cuniculi, Encephalitozoon intestinalis,* and *Nosema corneum.* Further information may be found on the following Internet site: http://www.dpd.cdc.gov/DPDx/HTML/ImageLibrary/Microsporidiosis_il.htm.

Microsporidia may infect individuals through both the digestive and the respiratory systems. Resistant spores are formed within the host and then are excreted from the body in feces and urine, and perhaps by mucous secretion, but this route has not been fully verified. Therefore, microsporidiosis is predisposed to spread via fecal-oral, urine-oral, and waterborne transmission. Microsporidia spores have been shown to survive for protracted periods of time in water (up to 4 months) and have been detected in surface water (Figure 3-22). The levels of microsporidia spores found in raw sewage correlates well with those of *Cryptosporidium* and *Giardia*.

Microsporidia from contaminated water may infect large segments of the population. Symptoms of individuals infected by microsporidia organisms often range from exhibiting asymptomatic (no symptoms) conditions to bouts of diarrhea, bronchitis, pneumonia, and sinusitis. Microsporidia can also cause bile duct pain and inflammation (pain in the upper-right abdomen).

Laboratory Diagnosis

Microsporidiosis can be diagnosed through examination of stool, urine, or nasal washings. Special fluorescent antibody studies are often needed to detect microsporidia. Thus, species identification is paramount for defining the appropriate treatment before medical intervention begins. These tests for differentiation are not routinely requested by physicians and routine staining procedures

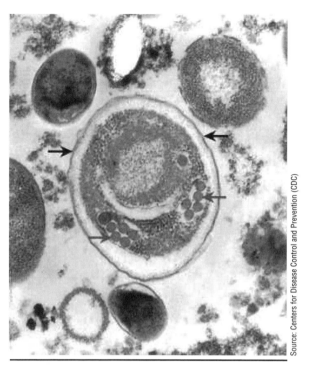

FIGURE 3-22 Microsporidia—electron micrograph of a mature microsporidian spore

with Giemsa or Gram stains are not effective for detecting spores in the presence of bacteria that is normally present in stool specimens and other sources of specimens. But the use of a Giemsa stain is valuable when staining duodenal fluid where both spores and developing stages can be observed.

Treatment and Prevention

Currently no accepted therapies for the microsporidial infections exist, except for perhaps two species. Differentiation between the two major intestinal microsporidia is required for effective treatment of the condition. *E. intestinalis* infections are treated with albendazole, whereas fumagillin has been shown to be effective for eradicating *E. bieneusi*, and *Encephalitozoon intestinalis*, which is treated with albendazole.

SUMMARY

Protozoa are among the most prevalent of parasites, but unfortunately are also among the most difficult to find microscopically. Protozoa are typically spread by the fecal-oral route, meaning that food contaminated by feces may find its way onto the kitchen counter and table, and may result in an infection.

Two major groups of protozoa occur as human pathogens. These are called ciliates and flagellates, and their chief difference lies in their locomotion structures. *Balantidium coli* is an example of a ciliate that is transmitted from monkeys and pigs, for the most part, to human hosts. Primarily pigs, the natural host for *Balantidium coli*, are responsible for the majority of the cases in humans of this disease, but there have been at least a few instances of transmission from human to human. These organisms are quite large and have short hairy cilia surrounding the body, making the organism appear to have a rotary motion.

Four major organisms of the flagellate type have several long hairlike projections that are used by tails for swimming. They also exhibit a phenomenon called an undulating membrane, which makes an organism's exterior morphological structures appear to be rising and falling rhythmically. These organisms are *Trichomonas vaginalis, T. tenax, T. hominis,* and *Dientamoeba fragilis.* At least three of these have no cyst stage, so these organisms have an extremely simple life cycle. *D. fragilis,* originally not considered a pathogen, is now, as symptoms subside upon treatment.

T. vaginalis is a common sexually transmitted organism, and may be found in both males and females. This organism is often confused with white blood cells if movement is not present. *T. tenax,* found in the mouth, and *T. hominis,* found in the intestine, are considered harmless as a parasite of man. *Chilomastix mesnili* is a pear-shaped parasite that like *T. hominis* is considered nonpathogenic.

Infections with *Giardia lamblia* are common throughout the world and are perhaps the most frequently identified intestinal parasite. *G. lamblia* is transmitted mainly through the fecal-oral route and is often found in contaminated well water and streams. Often the infection is accompanied by diarrhea and intestinal pain, but may be asymptomatic. Sanitary life styles will largely prevent infection with *G. lamblia*. Rapid replication that occurs due to the binucleate morphology of *G. lamblia* frequently leads to a heavy infestation only days after infection.

Intestinal amoebae may lead to serious infection, although some cases cause chronic infection with no damage occurring. However, some victims progress to amoebic colitis or fulminant colitis. *Entamoeba histolytica* is pathogenic, and may invade the intestinal walls, whereas *Entamoeba dispar,* as well as *Entamoeba coli,* are considered nonpathogenic. To diagnose *E. histolytica,* a fresh fecal sample or a swab from a rectal ulcer is examined under the microscope. The movements of the motile forms become perceptibly slower as the specimen cools, making it more difficult to identify the parasites. Therefore, careful differentiation is required to distinguish between *E. histolytica* and the other nonpathogenic forms of intestinal amoebae.

Blastocystis hominis was formerly thought to be a yeast, and is prevalent in many animals, birds, and insects, but now is known to be neither a yeast nor a protozoan. Constipation, diarrhea, and abdominal distress are the predominant symptoms and signs of the infections by most strains. Almost all humans and animals have had contact with *Blastocystis* at some point. Four different morphological forms—vacuolar, granular, cyst, and amoeboid—challenge the testing personnel when examining a stool specimen. It is thought that all of these forms may be present in the host simultaneously The cyst forms of this organism are able to survive in harsh environmental conditions due to its thick, multi-layered cyst wall.

Other considerable numbers of amoebae are present in human stools, and are capable of causing pain and other symptoms and signs of distress. Most of these are identified chiefly by size and the numbers of nuclei they possess. Some of these miscellaneous amoebae are harmless when colonizing the intestine, whereas others cause mild to considerable abdominal discomfort. *E. histolytica* is the primary disease-causing species of this sort, and often other species are confused with *E. histolytica*. Another challenge for the microbiologist or parasitologist is that of differentiating between bacterial and amoebic dysentery. Symptoms may be similar, but the treatment is completely different. Diagnosis is mostly made through clinical signs and symptoms, but dysentery must be confirmed by microscopic examination. Other medical conditions must also be ruled out to avoid misdiagnosis and wrongful treatment.

CASE STUDIES

1. A 25-year-old male graduate student from a local university arrived at the emergency department with a sudden onset of fever. Upon arrival, his temperature was 101° F when measured orally and he reported feeling a need to defecate almost constantly. The student most often prepared his own meals or ate at local restaurants and occasionally traveled to a number of Asian countries for research toward his degree. He appeared somewhat thin and pale and somewhat dehydrated. What should the physician consider as the probable type of infection from which the patient is suffering?

2. An anthropology student from a U.S. college was performing field studies of the Mayan ruins in Guatemala, eating and drinking food and beverages from the local farmers and merchants. Shortly before returning from South America, he began to suffer from cramping abdominal pain that worsened during the flight home. Soon after arriving at the campus, the diarrhea showed small amounts of blood and he felt weak and suffered from malaise. At the student health center, the physician ordered a stool culture which revealed no pathogenic bacterial organisms. The laboratory technologist examined a wet mount from a new stool sample and noted round protozoal cysts with finely granular cytoplasm that measured 10 to 20 μm and most of which showed four nuclei with cigar-shaped chromatoidal bars with blunt, rounded, and smooth ends.

3. After summer camp in a rural and wooded area, a group of adolescent students returned home following this two-week trek into the wilderness. On the way home, the driver of the van in which the close friends were riding decided to treat the students to a buffet-type meal at a chain restaurant. All of the children ate a meal similar to each other that included a few items from the same prepared container on the steam table. One day after reaching home, all of the children suffered from camping diarrhea and nausea, accompanied by a moderately elevated temperature. The pediatrician who treated the children considered parasitic involvement, because the children had been to camp and swam in the lake together. Stool examinations were ordered and the microscopic findings reported trophozoites of 30 to 40 μm and cyst forms of approximately 25 μm. The cysts revealed eight nuclei and chromatoidal bars with splintered ends in most of the organisms.

4. A computer software salesperson travels extensively in Asia and parts of Europe. Recently when he returned home from a month of business activities in Southeast Asia, he quickly developed severe diarrhea and intestinal discomfort that worsened over a period of several weeks. His family physician suspected either a bacterial or a parasitic infection, but leaned toward a diagnosis of a parasitic infection because the patient's temperature was not extremely abnormal. A stool specimen sent to the laboratory of the local hospital was negative for the presence of bacterial pathogens but revealed a large protozoan which contained cilia around the entire periphery of each organism. What was the most likely diagnosis for this parasite, and is it nonpathogenic?

5. A 23-year-old sexually active male reported to his physician that he had recently noticed a urethral irritation with slight burning after urination and ejaculation.

(continues)

CASE STUDIES (CONTINUED)

A culture for *Neisseria gonorrhea* and Gram stain from the penis were performed and resulted in negative results. What would be the next most important pathogen that the physician might suspect? What is another important instruction that the physician should give to the patient?

6. A city that is surrounded by farms of mostly cows that produce both milk and beef obtains its water from two lakes into which local streams run. The majority of the population began suffering from watery diarrhea and became dehydrated within a few days of each other, complaining of fever and stomach cramps. The local health department launched an investigation and found that the members of some families suffering from the digestive upset had been out of town during the weekend of the previous two weeks. Family members who had been at home suffered from the ailment. What would be the most important pathogen capable of causing these signs and symptoms that the investigators might suspect? What is another important element the health department should investigate that might have led to the local epidemic?

STUDY QUESTIONS

1. How are most intestinal parasites transmitted?

2. With what organism is *T. hominis* and *C. mesnili*, both nonpathogens, frequently confused?

3. The only ciliate found in humans that is considered to be pathogenic is that of _____.

4. How does the ciliate differ from a flagellate?

5. Flagellates have a simple life cycle. They are infective, unlike many other organisms, in the _____ stage.

6. *T. vaginalis* only has one host. What is it?

7. With what are *T. vaginalis* most often confused?

8. Name two flagellate organisms found in monkeys and simians.

9. What is the most common parasitic organism isolated from the human stool?

10. How is *G. lamblia* able to cause a heavy infection in only a few days?

11. What parasitic infective organism was originally thought to be that of a yeast organism?

Blood (Intracellular) and Other Tissue Protozoa

LEARNING OBJECTIVES

Upon completion of this chapter, the learner will be expected to:

- Describe the life cycle of *Leishmania*
- List the four species of parasite-causing malaria in humans
- Describe the three types of filariasis
- Discuss the transmission of lymphatic filariasis
- Trace the history of dracunculiasi

KEY TERMS

Amastigotes	Elephantiasis	Mucocutaneous
Antihistamines	Encephalitis	Myalgia
Arthralgia	Filariasis	Nagana
Asplenic	Giemsa or Romanowski stain	Nematodes
Asymptomatic carriers	Gundi	Occult filariasis
Babesiosi	Hemiptera	Onchocerciasis
Balkh sore	Hemoflagellates	Oriental sore
Blackflies	Immunodeficient	Promastigotes
Carnivores	Leishmaniasis	Reduviid bug
Caudal	Lyme disease	Ring form
Chagas's disease	Macrophages	Sand gnats
Coccidians	Malaria	Sand flies
Copecod	Merozoites	Schistosomiasis
Corticosteroids	Microfilaria	Seroprevalence
Dracunculiasis	Monocytes	Splenomegaly

Surra
Tabanid flies
Trachoma

Transplacental
Triatomid
Trypanosomiasis

West Nile virus
Wright-Giemsa stain

BABESIOSIS

Organisms of the genus *Babesia* is a parasite that is the causative agent of a somewhat rare disease that occurs most frequently in the New England section of the United States. The infection is most often self-limiting but may become quite severe in asplenic (those without the spleen organ) and elderly whose immune systems are diminished but rarely result in fatalities among the victims. Many different *Babesia* species exist throughout the world and several of these can infect humans. Babesiosis, the disease caused by infection with *Babesia*, is most common in New York (specifically, Long Island), Martha's Vineyard, and Nantucket, but fatalities are rarely recorded in humans. Although more than 100 species of *Babesia* exist across a large geographic span, only a small number of species have been implicated in the majority of diseases known to affect humans. The causative agent of babesiosis varies by species according to geographic regions that support the various parasites.

In the United States, human infections with *Babesia* species are almost exclusively due to *Babesia microti*. The disease is found mostly in the northeastern states, including some offshore islands and coastal areas. Only a few documented cases in the midwestern states as well as in California and Washington State have occurred, leading to speculation that the disease is spreading and may soon be prevalent throughout all areas of the United States. Several cases have been reported in medical literature related to infections acquired from blood transfusions in which the blood donors had lived in or had traveled to an area endemic for the disease. All of these cases have occurred in the United States with the exception of one Canadian patient who received blood from a donor who became infected while in the United States, and a single case reported in Japan. The rate of acquiring *B. microti* from a unit containing red cells from an infected donor has been estimated to be one in several hundred to almost two thousand in endemic areas. Although it is rare to find cases of transmission to fetuses in utero, apparently a few incidences have occurred.

Morphology

The organism may be either a round- or rod-shaped protozoal parasite that is often characterized by a tetrad configuration (Maltese cross). These parasites of the genus *Babesia* are found as intracellular inclusions of the red blood cells and are found in the phylum Apicomplexa (Figure 4-1). Unlike a number of other protozoal organisms, this organism lacks organs for motility such as amoeboid pseudopodia, cilia, or flagella. One species of *Babesia*, called *B. bigemina*, has gained notoriety as the first parasitic disease in which a vector (carrier of the organism) was identified and described. The disease may have been discovered in the late 1880s in diseased cattle herds from Texas, some of which may have been sold to other parts of the country, but most of the general knowledge of human infection has occurred in the past few decades.

Symptoms

After an incubation period of a few weeks (but sometimes after a couple of months), a febrile anemia may occur. The initial symptoms are headache, general malaise with

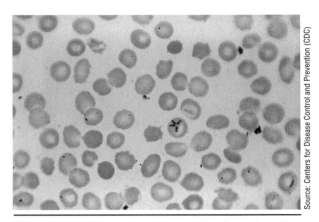

Source: Centers for Disease Control and Prevention (CDC)

FIGURE 4-1 Conventional "tetrad" configuration of these Babesia sp. trophozoites, which resemble *P. falciparum*

fatigue, muscular aches, chills, and fever accompanied by sweating. No periodic episodic fever cycle is found in infections by *Babesia*, as is the case in various species of malaria.

Life Cycle

Babesiosis is similar to malarial infections except for a fever cycle, and some call the disease the "malaria of the northeast." As in malaria, the parasites of the *Babesia* species reproduce inside red blood cells. There they can sometimes be cross-shaped inclusions where four merozoites are asexually budding but are attached together to form a figure similar to that of a Maltese cross. This distortion of the red blood cells results in hemolysis (destruction) of the red blood cells, which produces anemia in a manner similar to that of malaria. Asexual reproduction takes place in human or other mammalian hosts and sexual reproduction occurs in the vector (several species of the ixodid tick). Because the sexual reproductive stage takes place within the tick, this is where the infective sporozoites are formed. The infective stage involving sporozoites are then injected into the host during the blood meal of the tick. These injected organisms spread throughout the circulatory system and invade RBCs (red blood cells) where they undergo asexual reproduction and form intracellular ring forms that approximate those of the *Plasmodium* (malarial) genus. However, gametocytes are not visible in the peripheral blood in the manner they are in malarial infections.

Disease Transmission

Babesia organisms are spread chiefly by the ixodid tick *Ixodes scapularis*, the same vector for Lyme disease, although a number of species are capable of transmitting the *Babesia* organisms. A tick must be embedded for at least 12 hours before transmission takes place, so daily body surveys are necessary to avoid infection. The disease is rarely fatal and is usually resolved without treatment.

Laboratory Diagnosis

Just as in the case of the better-known Lyme disease, the organism for babesiosis, regardless of species, is spread chiefly by deer ticks except for blood transfusions from asymptomatic carriers. The disease requires several weeks to several months of incubation and symptoms of fever, chills, headache, sweats, myalgia, arthralgia, nausea, and vomiting may be so mild as to be ignored in some victims. As in malaria, thick and thin blood films stained with Giemsa or Romanowski stains are used for diagnosis. A polymerase chain reaction is also used for confirmation of the diagnosis.

The parasites of the *Babesia* species must reproduce in red blood cells, and are therefore called obligate organisms. There they can be seen as cross-shaped inclusions where four merozoites are asexually budding but are attached together to form the previously mentioned configuration of a Maltese cross, that results in hemolysis of the red blood cells which produces anemia in a manner similar to that of malaria. Careful scrutiny of multiple blood smears may be required, as *Babesia microti* may be easily overlooked because the organism typically infects fewer than 1 percent of the circulating red blood cells.

MICROSCOPIC DIAGNOSTIC FEATURE

General Classification—Protozoan

Organism	*Babesia microti*
Specimen Required	Blood smear
Stage	Merozoite stage is diagnostic
Size	Ring forms may measure 1.0–5.0 µm
Shape	May appear as ring forms and Maltese cross shapes (tetrads)
Motility	None
Nucleus(i)	Chromatin dot as nucleus
Cytoplasm	Parasites appear as cytoplasmic rings
Other Features	May resemble *P. faciparum*, except for absence of stippling and enlargement of the infected red cells

Treatment and Prevention

Although babesiosis is most often self-limiting in humans, treatment may be necessary to alleviate some of the symptoms by eliminating the parasite. Prevention of the disease is most effective when the tick vectors are controlled in endemic areas by destruction of the habitats of ticks and the use of protective clothing. Insect repellents help to avoid bites from ticks when properly used and body examinations to remove embedded ticks after exposure to ticks will greatly diminish the number of cases of babesiosis.

LEISHMANIASIS (OLD WORLD CUTANEOUS LEISHMANIASIS)

Leishmaniasis is caused by several species of the genus *Leishmania* called hemoflagellates and is transmitted by sand flies, which are often prevalent in desert areas. The disease occurs in various forms in both the Old and New World (the Americas). Upon infection, the parasites infect and multiply in macrophages and are ingested by sand flies when they feed on an infected person. In the gut of the sand fly, the parasites multiply and reach the mouthparts of the insect from which the infective forms are injected into a new host when the sand fly again feeds upon a potential victim (Figure 4-2). The disease leishmaniasis has a number of forms that range from simple cutaneous ulcers to a substantial destruction of cutaneous and subcutaneous tissues in the mucocutaneous forms of the organism. Most often other organs, and in particular the liver, are greatly affected by the visceral form.

From the historical vantage point, it is easiest to consider the Old World forms first. Old World cutaneous leishmaniasis, known as oriental sore, is a disease that has been known for hundreds of years if not longer, and there are descriptions of the conspicuous lesions formed on tablets in the library of King Ashurbanipal from the seventh century, some of which are thought to have been derived from earlier texts from 1500 to 2500 BC (Cox, 2002). Detailed descriptions of oriental sores by Arab physicians in the tenth century described what was (and is) called Balkh sore from northern Afghanistan (Figure 4-3). Later records from various places in the Middle East including Baghdad and Jericho indicate many of the conditions known by local names by which they are still known today (Cox, 2002).

Old World visceral leishmaniasis, or kala-azar, also called black fever, is manifested by fevers and by an enlarged spleen, a condition known as splenomegaly. The visceral type may be caused by *Leishmania donovani*, *L. chagasi*, or *L. infantum*. Cases of cutaneous *Leishmania* have been found in Texas and across the Mexican border in the past few decades, and it is believed that *L. meicana* may be harbored by armadillos. This disease is often confused with other diseases, especially malaria, which is also endemic in the region where leishmaniasis is found. Kala-azar was first noticed in Jessore in India in 1824, where numbers of patients were suffering from fevers. Although it was at first thought to be due to malaria, the disease failed to respond to quinine,

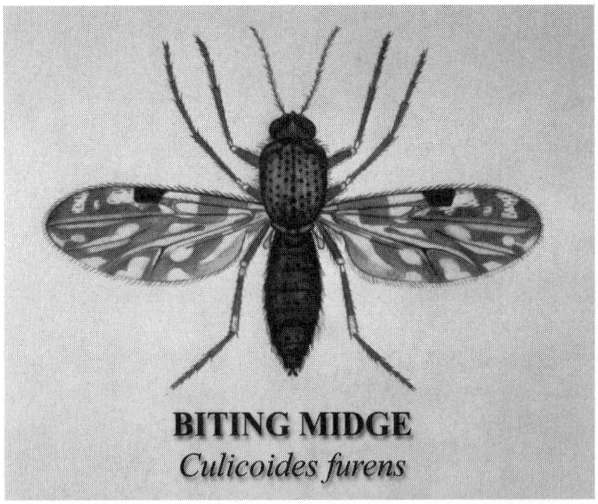

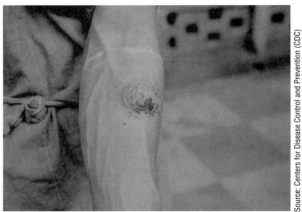

BITING MIDGE
Culicoides furens

Source: Centers for Disease Control and Prevention (CDC)

FIGURE 4-2 Sand fly or biting midge, *Cullicoides furens*

Source: Centers for Disease Control and Prevention (CDC)

FIGURE 4-3 Left arm with a leishmanial lesion

a medication successfully used to prevent malarial infections. In 1862, the disease had spread in a mere 38 years to Burdwan, with infection rates reaching epidemic levels. The disease was thought to be caused by a virulent form of malaria by a number of clinicians, including Ronald Ross. But the cause of the disease remained unknown until the early 1900s, when Leishman and Donovan discovered the parasite, *L. donovani*, lending their names to the infective organism (Cox, 2002).

During the late 1800s, literature in Asia, Europe, and Africa described a number of structures that may or may not have been a species related to *Leishmania*. Some victims had epithelial sores that were labeled as oriental sores by medical practitioners at that time, which could have resulted from any number of organisms that may not have even been a result of intraerythrocytic parasites. Bacterial, viral, and fungal infections may have been the causative agents in at least some of these medical conditions. Credit for the discovery of *Leishmania* is often given to an American, James Homer Wright (Cox, 2002), although there is little doubt that parasites responsible for leishmaniasis were actually seen by David Cunningham in 1885. Cunningham may not have realized what these organisms were. In 1898 a Russian military surgeon, P. F. Borovsky, also discovered similar structural organisms. The discovery of the parasite that causes visceral leishmaniasis, *L. donovani,* is less controversial than those just discussed. It is almost universally accepted that a Scottish army doctor, William Leishman, for whom the organism is named, first definitively identified *L. donovani*. Also, and somewhat concurrently, a professor of physiology at Madras University, Charles Donovan (Cox, 2002), independently discovered the parasite in the spleens of patients with kala-azar. Apparently the discovery by the Russian military surgeon, Borovsky, was unknown to Homer Wright and to Leishman and Donovan, although their discoveries were made during a short period of time.

It was not discovered until 1921 that *Leishmania* was transmitted by a vector. The search leading to the implication of a specific vector was sought for a number of years, before the Sergent brothers, Edouard and Etienne, demonstrated through experimental proof the transmission to humans from sand flies of the genus *Phlebotomus*. However, the actual mode of infection, through the bite of the sand fly, was not finally demonstrated until 1941 (Cox, 2002). The history of Old World leishmaniasis is also extensively described by Garnham, Manson-Bahr, and Wenyon (Cox, 2002).

In the New World, either cutaneous or mucocutaneous leishmaniasis is responsible for causing disfiguring conditions. Evidence of these medical conditions are found in sculptures since the fifth century, and in related writings of Spanish missionaries in the Americas during the sixteenth century. It was originally thought that New World leishmaniasis and Old World leishmaniasis were the same. However, in 1911 Gaspar Vianna found that the parasites in South America differed from those in Africa and India and created a new species, *Leishmania braziliensis*, ostensibly due to the discovery of the diseases in the area of South America. Since then, a number of other species unique to the New World have been described. Following the discovery in 1921 of the sand fly transmission of Old World leishmaniasis, it was assumed that the vectors of *Leishmania* in the New World would also belong to the genus *Phlebotomus* but was later identified as the genus *Lutzomyia*. Over the last two decades, the complex pattern of the life cycle and the transmission of the organism based on the species of both the parasite and the vector, the reservoir host, and the disease has been extensively verified and described by Ralph Lainsonand his colleagues (Cox, 2002).

Morphology

The *Leishmania tropica* complex includes three different species that are similar in many ways but are genetically and therefore serologically different that occupy different geographical regions of the world. The three species are: *Leishmania tropica, Leishmania aethiopica,* and *Leishmania major*. The morphologic forms for these organisms are the amastigote, promastigote, epimastigote, opisthomastigote, and the trypomastigote and they differ significantly in size (Table 4-1).

Symptoms

Tissue destruction occurs as amastigotes are released and invade new macrophage cells. Cutaneous leishmaniasis occurs when a red papular structure develops as a primary lesion that may be 2 centimeters or more in size and is often extremely itchy. Bacterial infections often occur in the primary site due to the breakdown of the skin. "Dry" lesions occur with infections by *L. tropica* and *L. aethiopica* but moist, weeping lesions occur with *L. major*. Lesions heal quickly unless a secondary bacterial infection complicates the condition, but considerable scarring to areas of the body may follow healing of the

TABLE 4-1 Characteristics of Leishmanial Forms

	AMASTIGOTE	PROMASTIGOTE	EPIMASTIGOTE	OPISTHOMAS- TIGOTE	TRYPOMAS- TIGOTE
Size	2–5 µm × 1–3 µm	9–15 µm	9–15 µm	Not available	12–35 µm
Flagella Presence	Reduced or absent	Yes	Yes	Yes	Yes
Shape	Round (oval)	Slender and elongated	Long, slightly wider than promastigotes	Spindle-shaped	Spindle-shaped, C-shapes often seen in blood films

lesions. For victims of leishmaniasis, recovery is based on cellular immunity where macrophages clear the infectious sites of cellular debris and organisms. But those with impaired immunity may progress to a more serious condition called *diffuse cutaneous leishmaniasis*, where nodular lesions occur particularly on the face, arms, and legs. In this case, the lesions are filled with parasites and do not heal as quickly as uncomplicated cases.

Life Cycle

The life cycle of *Leishmania* is no more complex than that of other prominent parasites. The incubation period may range from a few weeks to three years depending on the species. *L. major* has a more rapid onset of symptoms and signs. Two morphologic stages occur in order for the transmission of the disease to take place. A stage called amastigotes occurs in a vertebrate host; after amastigotes, the promastigotes, a developmental and infective stage, occurs only in the insect vector, so both a host and a vector are required in order to transmit the organism (Figure 4-4). As the vector bites the infected host, amastigotes in macrophages (tissue cells that clean up infections and debris) are ingested by the fly or other vector, where the amastigotes undergo changes to become flagellated forms called promastigotes. The promastigotes then multiply rapidly before infecting the proboscis, or biting parts of the vector, which is then transmitted to new victims. Amastigotes often remain in the skin and other tissues through the lymphatic system in the cutaneous forms of the disease. In visceral forms, amastigotes migrate within monocytes, types of protective white blood cells, where the organisms migrate to the spleen, liver, and bone marrow, and then continue to divide and multiply.

Disease Transmission

This disease is transmitted into the skin by sand flies and promastigotes of the three subspecies of *L. tropica* and are ingested by macrophages at the site of the injection of the promastigotes. Inside the macrophages the promastigotes progress into amastigote forms by multiplying greatly. The host cell then ruptures and amastigotes are free to enter uninfected macrophage cells. This continuous cycle of invasion, multiplication, and cell rupture results in the lesions and destruction of tissue.

Laboratory Diagnosis

The presence of amastigotes is the definitive diagnosis for leishmaniasis where aspirates from lesion sites or a biopsy of tissue materials from an active lesion are stained with Wright's or Giemsa stain, or a combination

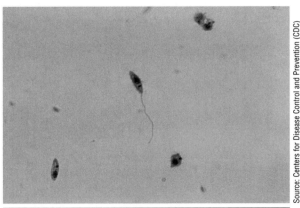

Source: Centers for Disease Control and Prevention (CDC)

FIGURE 4-4 Presence of promastigotes of *Leishmania* sp.

of both. A microscopic examination for evidence of the oval amastigote forms in tissue macrophages are direct evidence of infection. For the various species of *Leishmania*, isoenzyme studies and molecular diagnostic procedures may be utilized. A skin test called the *Montenegro (Leishmania) skin test* is used to screen large numbers of individuals in endemic areas and is a delayed hypersensitivity test similar to that of the PPD for tuberculosis. The Centers for Disease Control and Prevention also has a noncommercial serologic test not in general use that includes an indirect fluorescent antibody assay.

Treatment and Prevention

Antimonial medications are often effective by intramuscular injections for 10 days. Resistant infections may require repeated treatments. Amphotericin B and an antifungal preparation called *ketoconazole* may provide effective treatment if patients suffer from prolonged infections.

Prevention is accomplished through controlling sand fly populations by destroying the vectors and by controlling rodents in endemic areas where the sand flies may also find hosts. In addition, individuals infected with *Leishmania* organisms should be quickly treated to prevent further transmission to other humans from insects that bite the victim and then transmit the organisms to others, leading to a significant and rapid increase in the number of cases of the disease.

LEISHMANIA MEXICANA COMPLEX (NEW WORLD CUTANEOUS LEISHMANIASIS)

New World leishmaniasis is found from southern Texas through Mexico and Central and South America and is disseminated by a number of animal vectors. The species diagnosed in these regions are: *Leishmania Mexicana, Leishmania pifanoi, Leishmania pifanoi, Leishmania amazonensis, Leishmania venezuelensis,* and *Leishmania garnhami.* The treatment and prevention of these strains are similar to the organisms responsible for Old World leishmaniasis. Morphological forms are similar for both Old World and New World leishmaniasis as well as the transmission, pathogenesis, and identification of the two types with a few notable exceptions. The following tables list the basic data for differentiation of each species of the various types of *Leishmania* (see Tables 4-2, 4-3, 4-4).

MALARIA

Malaria is one of the most common infectious diseases in the world, and its history extends into ancient history, no doubt impacting the migration of humans about the world. The disease in humans is caused by four species of the genus *Plasmodium*: *P. falciparum, P. vivax, P. ovale,* and *P. malariae.* Ring-form trophozoites in

TABLE 4-2 Mexican Leishmaniasis Complex—New World

ORGANISM	FORM OF DISEASE	VECTOR	GEOGRAPHICAL REGION	RESERVOIR HOSTS
L. mexicana	Diffuse cutaneous form	Lutzomyia sand fly	Belize, Guatemala, Yucatán Peninsula	Opossums, forest rodents, domestic dogs and cats
L. pifanoi	Diffuse cutaneous form	Lutzomyia sand fly	Amazon River basin, isolated parts—Brazil, Venezuela	Opossums, forest rodents, domestic dogs and cats
L. amazonensis	Both cutaneous and diffuse cutaneous forms	Lutzomyia sand fly	Amazon basin of Brazil	Opossums, forest rodents, domestic dogs and cats
L. venezuelensis	Cutaneous form	Lutzomyia sand fly	Remote forested regions—Venezuela	Opossums, forest rodents, domestic dogs and cats
L. garnhami	Cutaneous form	Lutzomyia sand fly	Venezuelan Andean region	Opossums, forest rodents, domestic dogs and cats

TABLE 4-3 *Leishmania braziliensis* Complex—Mucocutaneous Seishmaniasis

ORGANISM	FORM OF DISEASE	VECTOR	GEOGRAPHI-CAL REGION	RESERVOIR HOSTS
L. braziliensis	Mucocutaneous form around mouth and nose	*Lutzomyia* and *Psychodopygus* sand flies	Rainforests	Animals (zoonoses)
L. panamensis	Mucocutaneous form around mouth and nose	*Lutzomyia* and *Psychodopygus* sand flies	Panama, Colombia	Animals (zoonoses)
L. peruviana	Mucocutaneous form around mouth and nose	*Lutzomyia* and *Psychodopygus* sand flies	Peruvian Andes	Animals (zoonoses)
L. guyamensis	Mucocutaneous form around mouth and nose	*Lutzomyia* and *Psychodopygus* sand flies	Guianas, parts of Brazil and Venezuela	Animals (zoonoses)

TABLE 4-4 *Leishmania donovani* Complex—Visceral Leishmaniasis

Viserotropic—Infects reticuloendothelial cells; infected macrophages are disseminated throughout the body.

ORGANISM	FORM OF DISEASE	VECTOR	GEOGRAPHICAL REGION	*RESERVOIR HOSTS
L. donovani	Diffuse cutaneous form	*Lutzomyia* sand fly	India, Pakistan, Thailand, parts of Africa, Peoples Republic of China	Rodents and dogs
L. infantum	Diffuse cutaneous form	*Lutzomyia* sand fly	Europe, Africa, the Near East, parts of former Soviet Union	Domestic dogs, other canids, porcupines
L. chagasi	Both cutaneous and diffuse cutaneous forms	*Lutzomyia* sand fly	Central and South America	Foxes, domestic dogs and cats

* In India, humans are the only mammalian reservoir.

the red blood cells are sometimes inadvertently found in the blood of asymptomatic patients during routine blood tests (Figure 4-5). Similar parasites are common in monkeys and apes. It is now generally held that malaria arose in our primate ancestors in Africa and evolved with humans, spreading with human migrations first throughout the tropics, subtropics, and temperate regions of the Old World and then to the New World with explorers, missionaries, and slaves. The characteristic periodic fevers of malaria are recorded from every civilized society from China in 2700 BC through the writings of Greek, Roman, Assyrian, Indian, Arabic, and European physicians up to the nineteenth century. The earliest detailed accounts are perhaps from observations by Hippocrates in fifth century BC. The disease was variously believed to be an example of demons afflicting humans, as references to the disease are found in literature from Greece and Italy, and in the areas governed by the Roman Empire.

Certain climactic conditions and the availability of suitable vectors that contribute to the transmission of malaria must be present in order for the disease to be transmitted and to survive and continue to infect individuals. Eventually it became somewhat obvious to scientific investigators that malaria was somewhat endemic in marshy areas, and was not as frequently observed in dry areas with no standing bodies of water. Originally the disease was attributed to the vapors from the marshes, but perhaps there became a gradual realization that in

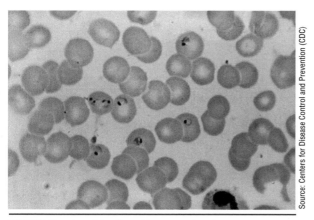

Source: Centers for Disease Control and Prevention (CDC)

FIGURE 4-5 Thin-film Giemsa-stained smear with ring-form of *Plasmodium falciparum* trophozoite

Morphology

Humans are infected by only four species of malaria, although other species are found in other mammals and birds. *Plasmodium vivax* is found in temperate regions and is the most widely distributed and numerous in the cases found worldwide where climactic and geographic features favorable for the breeding of certain species of mosquitoes are found. *P. falciparum* is found in the tropics and subtropics predominantly and is the most serious of the four species affecting humans. *P. malariae* infections are disseminated throughout the tropics and subtropics, whereas *P. ovale* is mostly found in tropical West Africa, South America, and Asia.

Symptoms

Symptoms initially mimic those of minor febrile illnesses accompanied by general malaise, muscle aches with fatigue, headache, abdominal aches, and cycles of fever and chills. Three stages of fever characteristically occur, first with shaking and chills, followed by the second or hot stage where a small amount of sweating occurs and the body's temperature may rise to levels as high as 106°F. After several hours of the hot stage where brain damage may occur, the patient may experience tachycardia (rapid heart rate), cough, head and backache with abdominal pain, vomiting, and diarrhea. The third sweating stage then begins within a few hours as the fever subsides and sleep ensues. Hemolytic anemia is associated with the *P. falciparum* infection due to destruction of infected red blood cells.

Life Cycle

The life cycle is a very complex one that begins when an infected *Anopheles* mosquito injects sporozoites, the infectious stages, into the blood of its host (Figure 4-6). Sporozoites enter and multiply in liver cells, and thousands of daughter forms, merozoites, are released into the blood. These merozoites invade red blood cells, in which another phase of multiplication occurs; this process is repeated indefinitely, causing the symptoms of the disease we call malaria. Some merozoites do not divide but develop into sexual stages, that of male and female gametocytes, which are taken up by another mosquito when it feeds. Then fertilization and zygote formation occur in the mosquito's gut. The zygote develops into an oocyst on the outside of the mosquito's gut, and within the oocyst

seasons where mosquitoes were less prevalent in cold or dry weather and that the transmission rates for malaria diminishes during these drier periods. But it seems that many other inventive explanations arose to rationalize the spread of the disease in terms of the poisons rising from the swamps. The term *miasma,* which meant infectious particles or germs were floating in the air made noxious by the presence of such particles or germs, were freely associated with the incidence of malaria at the time these discoveries were occurring.

Toward the end of the nineteenth century, the germ theory was established that led to the birth of the science called *microbiology.* This basic scientific understanding of invisible life forms that contributed to a number of infectious diseases was embraced and advanced by contributions attributed to a considerable number of medical and scientific pioneers from a number of countries. Malaria exacted such a toll over several thousand years on the human population that it became a primary goal of scientists during the nineteenth century to discover the cause of the disease that was by then threatening many parts of the European empires. Discovery of the origin of the malaria parasite and how it was transmitted are among the most important and historic events in the annals of infectious diseases. In addition to treating the disease that resulted from infection by the *Plasmodium* parasite, control of the vector, a species of mosquito, led to a decrease in malaria in the more developed areas of the world, as is the case in Europe. Malaria still rages in some areas of the world, particularly Southeast Asia and portions of the African continent, despite global efforts to control the impact of this disease on indigenous populations.

Malaria
(Plasmodium spp.)

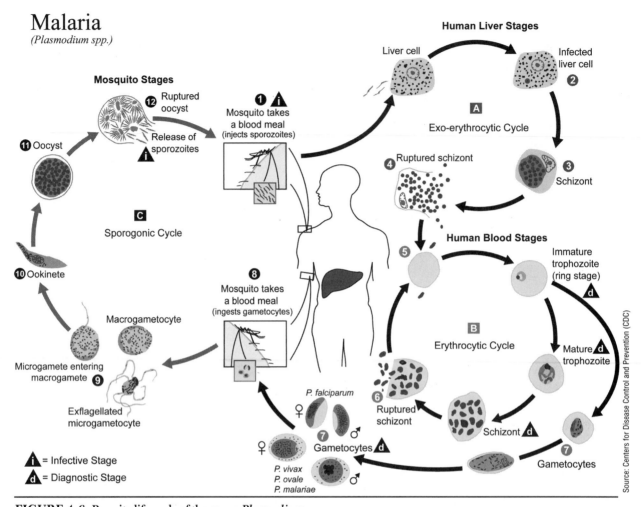

FIGURE 4-6 Parasite life cycle of the genus *Plasmodium*

there is another phase of multiplication that results in the production of sporozoites that reach the salivary glands to be injected into a new host. The parasites in the blood were first seen in 1880 by French army surgeon Alphonse Laveran, who was looking for a bacterial cause of malaria. He immediately realized that parasites rather than bacteria were responsible for the disease (Cox, 2002).

Disease Transmission

The female *Anopheles* mosquito is the chief vector and the most common means for transmitting malaria to humans. Some 60 species of this mosquito have been identified as vectors for malaria and the vector for a given geographic region will vary. The infection is transmitted by the bite of an infected female *Anopheles* mosquito. The mosquito most frequently bites at dawn and at dusk,

as this is the most active feeding times for mosquitoes. The mosquito is infected by biting a patient infected with malaria, where it aspirates the sexual forms of the parasite, the gametocytes, along with the victim's blood. These gametocytes continue the sexual phase of the cycle and the sporozoites fill the salivary glands of the infested mosquito. Once the mosquito becomes infected, it is destined to remain so for life.

Laboratory Diagnosis

Thick and thin peripheral blood smears stained with Giemsa or Wright-Giemsa stain are the methods of choice for diagnosing infections with a *Plasmodium* species. The diagnosis can only be definitely confirmed by the presence of the organism as an intracellular inclusion of the RBCs. Careful timing of the collection of blood samples is necessary to successfully demonstrate the presence of the organisms. Blood drawn just following the onset of a paroxysm (sudden recurrence of symptoms) such as a rapidly rising temperature should contain free merozoites, which if visible do not provide a means for identification of the species. The greatest number of parasites is present toward the end of a febrile episode. All asexual stages will be found for *P. vivax, P. ovale,* and *P. malariae* infections. For *P. falciparum,* the infections will yield only ring forms and gametocytes as an aid for identification of the species.

Multiple blood films, both thick and thin, must be thoroughly examined for the identification of the species. The thick smear is a screening procedure for the presence of parasites, and the thin smears are used for species identification. A diagnosis cannot be ruled out on the basis of one or two sets of negative smears. Multiple samples over a 48-hour period may be necessary before the patient can be considered negative for malaria infection. Although not used routinely, serological tests and DNA probes are also available for the diagnosis of malaria.

Treatment and Prevention

Upon the discovery that the mosquito acted as the sole vector of malaria, efforts to prevent and destroy the breeding grounds for the carrier became the focus, because no effective medication was available to destroy the organism, only to prevent it. The research that led to the realization of the role of the mosquito is credited to Patrick Manson, whose observations were instrumental in controlling the disease. Manson had already earlier and correctly shown that filarial worms, some of which are also blood parasites, were transmitted by mosquitoes. His postulation that the vector of the malaria parasite might also be a mosquito was derived partly from his knowledge of the life cycle of filarial worms. His assumptions that both diseases commonly developed in marshy areas were also partly due to the known association he had developed between the disease and marshy places in which mosquitoes breed (Cox, 2002).

Manson was unable to undertake the entire responsibility for this investigation himself, so he persuaded Ronald Ross, an army surgeon, to carry out the work in India. In 1897, Ross had observed what is now known to be the oocysts of *P. falciparum* in an *Anopheles* mosquito that had fed on a patient with these crescent-shaped malarial parasites in the gametocyte stage in his blood, but he too was unable to follow this up at the time

(Cox, 2002). Manson then turned his attention to bird malaria, where the fowl had contracted a species that does not infect man, that of *P. relictum. Culex* is a genus of mosquito where several species of this genus are vectors of important diseases that greatly affect man, such as **West Nile virus, filariasis,** Japanese **encephalitis,** St. Louis encephalitis, as well as avian malaria, a strain not known to infect man (Figure 4-7).

In this mosquito, Manson found all the stages of the parasite in culicine (term refers to those of the genus *Culex*) mosquitoes that had fed on the mucous membranes of sparrows infected by *P. relictum* (Figure 4-8). For almost half a century, the life cycle of the malarial parasite in humans was not wholly understood. During the stage following infection, the parasites could not be viewed microscopically in the blood for approximately the first 10 days after infection. It has been shown that a phase of division of the parasites in the liver precede the development of parasites in the blood (Cox, 2002). An American clinician, Wojciech Krotoski, working with other teams, also showed that in some strains of *P. vivax* the stages in the liver could remain dormant or nonactive for up to several months. This discovery led to an understanding of the life cycle of the malaria parasite (Cox, 2002).

An important component of the treatment for malaria lies in the prevention of infection by the use of quinine as an antimalarial therapy. A synthetic and somewhat nontoxic, drug, chloroquine, was developed around the beginning of World War II and has been quite effective in prevention. In an optimum situation, all stages of the malarial organisms, from sprorozoite to gametocyte, should be destroyed without harming the patient. Resistant strains of the *Anopheles* mosquito as well as resistant strains of *P. falciparum* and *P. vivax* have developed,

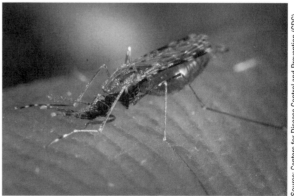

Source: Centers for Disease Control and Prevention (CDC)

FIGURE 4-7 Female *Anopheles* mosquito feeding on a human host

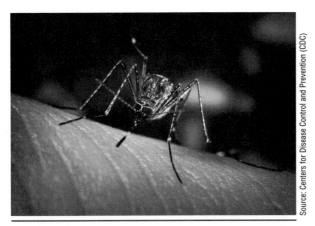

Source: Centers for Disease Control and Prevention (CDC)

FIGURE 4-8 *Culex tarsalis* mosquito, known to spread encephalitis, begins feeding on human host

partly from poor compliance or incomplete treatment regimens. More than a dozen vaccines are currently under development to possibly immunize large segments of individuals in endemic areas against this serious disease.

TOXOPLASMA SPP., TOXOPLASMOSIS, AND INFECTIONS CAUSED BY RELATED ORGANISMS

Toxoplasmosis is one of the most common and widespread parasitic infections but is relatively little known because in the majority of cases, infections are asymptomatic. The disease is usually a self-limiting infection due to a parasite called *Toxoplasma gondii*, and is often a recurrence of a mild infection that may be subclinical in that no signs or symptoms are apparent. However, for a fetus and for an immunodeficient person, it can be a serious cause of mortality and morbidity. The parasite that causes the infection, *T. gondii,* was discovered independently by the French parasitologists Charles Nicolle and Louis Herbert Manceaux while looking for a reservoir host for the organism that causes *Leishmania* in a North African rodent, the gundi, a natural host. Gundis are found in rocky outcroppings in desert-like environments of the northern parts of Africa. They first came to the notice of Western naturalists in Tripoli in 1774 and were given the name *gundi mice* (Cox, 2002).

The toxoplasmosis parasitic disease is capable of infecting almost all species of warm-blooded animals, including humans, but the primary host is the various members of the cat family. Animals are infected by eating infected meat, by ingestion of fecal matter of a cat that has itself recently been infected, or in some cases by transplacental transmission from the mother to her fetus (Figure 4-9). It should be understood, however, that cats have been shown as a major reservoir of this infection.

The prevalence of toxoplasmosis is considerable around the world. According to various statistics based on testing of blood donors, perhaps as many as one-third of the world's population may carry evidence of a *Toxoplasma* infection. The CDCP established rates in the United States based on random specimens collected by the National Health and Nutritional Examination Survey (NHANES) during a five-year period of 1999 to 2004. The infective rate for the general population was 10.8 percent, and for women of childbearing age (15 to 44 years), the rate was 11 percent (Jones, *et al.*, 2007). During the first few weeks, the infection typically causes

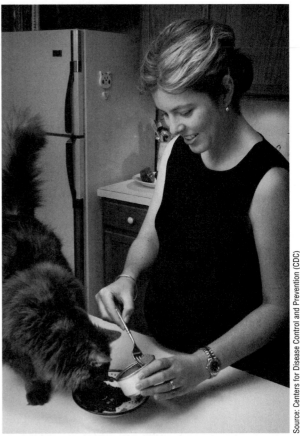

Source: Centers for Disease Control and Prevention (CDC)

FIGURE 4-9 Pregnant woman feeding her cat "canned" cat food, in order to prevent infection with the parasite, *Toxoplasma gondii*

a mild flulike illness or in many cases causes no outward manifestations of illness occur at all. After the first few weeks of infection have passed, the parasite rarely causes any harm or symptoms in healthy adults. However, those with a weakened immune system, and those infected with HIV or that are pregnant may become seriously ill, with sometimes fatal results. This parasite may also cause encephalitis (inflammation of the lining of the brain), which includes a number of sensory organs, including the eyes and ears along with the heart and liver.

Morphology

Toxoplasma gondii varies in its morphology during the developmental cycle. Forms of the parasites that may be ingested with food contaminated by the organism often appears as a curved banana shape or a crescent shape. The parasite enters the body through the mucus membranes of the intestinal and pharyngeal structures. In humans and intermediate hosts these parasites multiply during the acute phase of infection by cell division and during this rapidly dividing stage of development the protozoa are known variously as *tachyzoites*, *trophozoites*, or *endozoites*. Early in the infection, the tachyzoites are actively multiplying and may be seen as intracellular inclusions within many tissues of the body. These forms, 4 to 7 μm long and 2 to 3 μm wide, of the pathogen contain a nucleus toward the bottom half of the cells that are distributed by the lymph system and the circulatory system to the entire body. There the infected cells may lyse (be destroyed) and move to nearby cells that become infected. This process eventually results in damage to the tissue as necrosis with surrounding inflammation. It is possible that permanent damage may occur in vital organs that contain skeletal muscle. If intracellular cysts are formed in skeletal muscle, they may occur in the diaphragm, heart muscle, and the brain, affecting the tissue functions of these organs.

In human infections, most frequently if not solely, nonintestinal forms will be found. If the infected organism forms antibodies to the pathogen, the free and intracellular forms of the parasite disappear and, as a means of protection, are replaced by tissue cysts with a diameter of 100 to 300 μm. These cysts are walled off and each can contain several thousand bradyzoites that are also known as *cystozoites*. This condition causes clinically inconspicuous infection and can persist in the host for years because the cyst formation protects the parasites from attack by the immune system. It is highly probable

that infection is always followed by lifelong persistence of cysts and by a positive serology test for antibodies against the toxoplasmosis organism.

Symptoms

For healthy individuals an infection may only be evidenced by lymphadenopathy. Many immunocompromised patients such as victims of AIDS may show neurological involvement with confusion, neurological deficits, weakness, seizures, and decreased levels of consciousness. In addition, elevated temperatures may be experienced.

Life Cycle

While these developments were taking place, there were increasing numbers of records of toxoplasma infections in virtually all species of mammals and includes many species of birds. But the nature of the parasite remained obscure until the life cycle had been fully defined. The life cycle of *T. gondii* is a very complex one and it was not until 1970 when scientists from the United States and several European countries managed to independently show that this parasite was a stage in the life cycle that occurred as a common intestinal coccidian of cats (Figure 4-10). In the simplest form of the life cycle, cats become infected when they swallowed oocysts, a resistant infective stage containing sporozoites. These forms invade and multiply in intestinal cells, where sexual stages are produced, fertilization occurs, and more infective oocysts are produced.

However, there is an alternate life cycle. If the oocysts are swallowed by a nonfeline host, such as a mouse, multiplication occurs in the intestinal cells. But instead of sexual stages being produced, a disseminated infection follows during which resistant stages form in the brain and the muscle. The life cycle in the mouse halts at the asexual stage, but if a mouse is eaten by a cat or another mammal that preys on mice, the life cycle reverts to its basic sexual pattern. Humans are infected in the same way as are mice if they consume oocysts. But they can also become infected by eating any kind of meat containing the resistant forms of the organism. It is therefore not surprising that the life cycle remained a secret until William McPhee Hutchison, working in Glasgow in 1965, showed that the infectious agent was passed in the feces of cats (Cox, 2002).

At the time Hutchison thought that it was transmitted along with a nematode worm, as are some other flagellates and nematodes in fowl. Hutchison then identified

Toxoplasmosis
(Toxoplasma gondii)

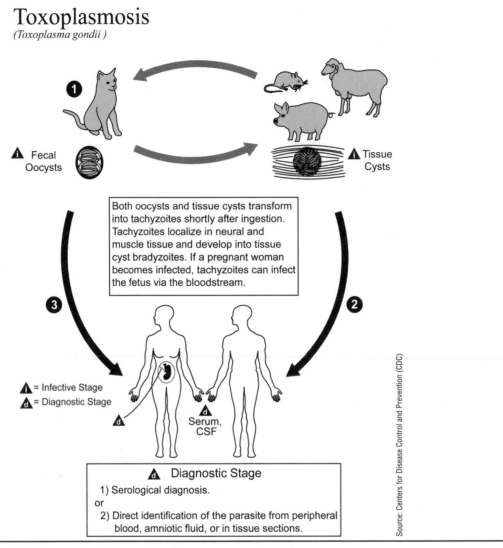

Both oocysts and tissue cysts transform into tachyzoites shortly after ingestion. Tachyzoites localize in neural and muscle tissue and develop into tissue cyst bradyzoites. If a pregnant woman becomes infected, tachyzoites can infect the fetus via the bloodstream.

Fecal Oocysts

Tissue Cysts

= Infective Stage
= Diagnostic Stage

Serum, CSF

▲ Diagnostic Stage
1) Serological diagnosis.
or
2) Direct identification of the parasite from peripheral blood, amniotic fluid, or in tissue sections.

Source: Centers for Disease Control and Prevention (CDC)

FIGURE 4-10 Life cycle of *T. gondii*, the organism that causes toxoplasmosis

protozoan cysts in a coccidian's feces as those related to *Isospora,* a common parasite of cats (Cox, 2002). During this same time period, other groups were following up Hutchison's 1965 observation of the presence of infectious agents in the feces of cats, with the result that there was independent confirmation by others that concurred with Hutchison's findings. With the discovery of the *T. gondii* life cycle, a concerted and massive search for similar phases in the life cycles of other coccidian parasites resulted. A number of protozoa that had previously not been properly identified were classified as mere stages in the life cycle of other poorly understood coccidians. It was determined that in many cases transmission depended on a predator–prey relationship, where the predator ingested infected meat from the prey (Cox, 2002).

Disease Transmission

Because *T. gondii* is carried by many mammalian and bird hosts, the disease is commonly transmitted to humans by inadequate handwashing following the handling of cats and their feces wastes from litter boxes and by eating uncooked or poorly cooked meat, particularly pork and lamb. From the intestines, once infected, the organisms travel through the blood and lymph system to other organs of the body, where damage may occur to tissues and organs.

Laboratory Diagnosis

Most *T. gondii* infections are not diagnosed, because individuals who are exposed never feel ill or become symptomatic or through a mistaken belief that a febrile disease such as a cold or flu as an innocuous viral infection. Serological testing for IgM antibodies against *T. gondii* is currently the most commonly employed diagnostic test for acute infections. Convalescent IgG antibodies will occur late in the infection after the acute phase has passed. Stained histological slides may reveal trophozoites and cysts containing bradyzoites from surgically obtained tissue biopsy samples. In the immunocompromised patient the presence of parasites in bronchoalveolar lavage or cerebrospinal fluid (CSF) from a spinal tap may be used effectively. Indirect testing for antibodies by an indirect fluorescent antibody test (IFA), a Sabin-Feldman dye test, indirect hemagglutination test, complement fixation, and antigen detection tests (direct tests) are available. These tests are not routinely performed in a clinical laboratory, and are most often referred to a reference laboratory which specializes in these techniques.

Treatment and Prevention

Prevention is accomplished through proper personal hygiene and avoiding the feces of cats and certain other animals such as pigs and sheep. Meat should be properly cooked before eating to ensure that the organisms are destroyed. It might be added that a great deal of exposure occurs in daily life, as up to one-third of the world's population shows antibodies against the organism.

TRYPANOSOMES AND SLEEPING SICKNESS

Trypanosoma cruzi, Trypanosoma brucei gambiense, and *Trypanosoma brucei rhodensiense* are three organisms that are responsible for several similar diseases by these blood-and-tissue parasites. *Trypanosoma cruzi* is the causative agent in the United States and parts of South and Central America for Chagas's disease, whereas *Trypanosoma brucei gambiense* and *Trypanosoma brucei rhodensiense* are responsible for the disease in Africa. A different group of vectors is responsible for transmitting this disease in each of the two hemispheres of the world, which will be discussed later in this section. These related diseases are indeed serious, and the WHO estimates that up to 16 to 18 million people may be infected with this parasite and many others are at risk for contracting the disease.

Trypanosoma cruzi

Trypanosoma cruzi is the causative organism for the American or New World variety of trypanosomiasis called Chagas's disease, named for Carlos Chagas who discovered the disease in 1909. Also called South American trypanosomiasis, the disease is found from the United States to as far south as Argentina, which extends south to the tip of the South American continent. The causative organism, *T. cruzi*, infects both wild and domestic animals which may gain contact with each other, and makes it difficult to control the spread of the disease. Poor personal hygiene and unsanitary conditions combine to place many poor farmers who handle animals

MICROSCOPIC DIAGNOSTIC FEATURE

General Classification—Sporozoan

Organism	*Toxoplasma gondii*
Specimen Required	Generally by tissue biopsy specimens, cerebrospinal fluid
Stage	Trophozoites or cysts are diagnostic
Size	Cysts measure from 12–100 µm
	Oocysts in feces and soil range from 9–14 µm
Shape	Oocysts are somewhat oval
Motility	None
Nucleus(i)	Long, spherical nucleus at one end of trophozoite
Cytoplasm	Smooth
Other Features	Tissue cysts contain large numbers of slow-growing trophozoites

at risk for becoming infected by this parasite. Infection may also occur through blood transfusions of infected blood donors, because the parasite is found in the blood. *T. cruzi* has also been implicated as the causative agent for encephalitis and as an opportunistic infection in immunocompromised patients such as those with HIV infections and other chronic illnesses. Victims may suffer from chronic infection by *T. cruzi* with serious medical consequences because no effective medication is available for an effective cure for the disease.

Morphology

Trypanosoma cruzi is a flagellate of the family Trypanosomatidae. The organism possesses one flagellum and a single mitochondrion in which the kinetoplast is situated, consisting of a specialized DNA-containing organelle. The identification of this parasite by morphological and biological features does not offer difficulties. Differentiation between *Trypanosoma rangeli*, a nonpathogenic flagellate that infects humans in some areas of Central and South America, and pathogenic strains is necessary. The organisms are transmitted by some of the same vectors that transmit *T. cruzi*.

Symptoms

Most frequently the disease ranges from mild to no symptoms, and usually the symptoms are confined to fever, facial edema, and hepato- and splenomegaly. But the infection is sometimes accompanied by myocarditis, cardiomyopathy, megaesophagus, megacolon (massive dilation of the colon), and eventually death may ensue.

Life Cycle

The trypanosomes of *T. cruzi*, found in the Western Hemisphere, are now known to be spread mainly by one of the "true" bugs (not all insects are correctly labeled as "bugs"). Various **triatomid** species belong to the order **Hemiptera** and include the reduviid bug, the insect responsible for transmitting the parasite in the Americas (Figure 4-11). These insects have efficient biting and piercing mouthparts and are often called "kissing bugs," commonly known by this name because of their tendency to bite the lips and face. During the time period between 1907 and 1912 the Brazilian scientist Carlos Chagas, gave the common name of the disease to the world. His research shows that the disease is from a

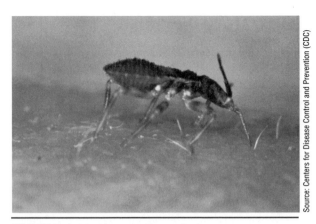

FIGURE 4-11 Chagas's disease is due to a protozoan, *T. cruzi,* transmitted by the true bug

T. cruzi infection and also proved that the trypanosome *T. cruzi* is transmitted by the previously mentioned "kissing bugs." These transient infective forms of the trypanosome organism circulate in the bloodstream and are taken up by the bloodsucking bugs as they feed on a mammalian host. After the parasites multiply in the gut of the bug, the infective forms are passed in the feces of the insect.

Disease Transmission

Chagas's first observation that the bloodsucking bugs infesting the poorly constructed houses harbored these flagellates appeared to be a well-reasoned possibility as a host for the *T. cruzi* protozoan. He also determined that the disease organism is not mechanically spread merely through a bite but is accomplished through the liquid feces that is excreted around a bite mark by the insect. A stage called the *epimastigote state* migrates to the anus of the bug and is deposited with its feces as the reduviid bug feeds on the victim (Figure 4-12) often in the mouth region. Organisms are able to enter the host by passing through the bite wounds and the victim rubs or scratches the bitten area, allowing the organism to enter the body of the potential victim. Although Chagas thought that without a doubt the link between the bites of the bugs and contraction of the parasitic infection was indisputable, his thesis was later supported by the French parasitologist, Emile Brumpt. Brumpt, in 1909, definitively demonstrated the transmission of the disease through contamination of the area with the feces of the bug. He proved that transmission of the protozoan did not occur during the biting process itself, but instead the organism entered the wound the bite left behind.

Trypanosomiasis, American (Chagas disease)
(Trypanosoma cruzi)

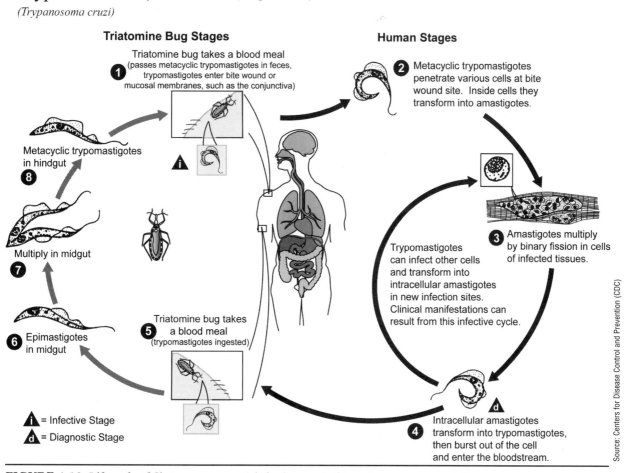

FIGURE 4-12 Life cycle of *Trypanosoma cruzi*, infective agent of American trypanosomiasis

The severity and progression of the disease depends on the tissues and organs involved and the most noticeable signs are massive distension of the intestinal tract, especially the esophagus and colon, and destruction of cardiac muscle. Consequences of the disease can result in death many years after the initial infection. American trypanosomiasis is often characterized by fever, lymphadenopathy, hepatosplenomegaly, and quite noticeable edema of the face (Figure 4-13). *T. cruzi* infections are common in many mammals on the North American continent but cases of human disease now occur for the most part in both South and Central America. This is due to increasing sanitation efforts in North America with improved housing, control and treatment of herd animals, and the use of insect control to prevent the vectors of this disease from spreading.

Laboratory Diagnosis

Invading trypanomastigotes may be found in histiocytes (a monocyte that has migrated from the blood to the tissue), which are phagocytes of the reticuloendothelial system as well as in other types of cells. The parasites transform as amastigotes and begin to multiply by the simple process of binary fission. Giemsa-stained smears will yield very small round or ovoid forms that are 1.5 to 4 µm and will contain a red nucleus with a dark rod-shaped kinetoplast. Peripheral blood films stained with Giemsa stain may show "U"- or "C"-shaped trypomastigotes that average up to 20 µm in length. The trypomastigote ingested by the reduviid bug during its blood meal is a delicate and slender organism with an undulating membrane similar to other protozoans and that runs

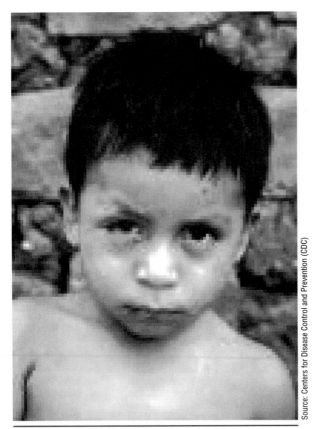

FIGURE 4-13 Chagas's disease manifested as an acute infection with swelling of the right eye

the length of the organism, extending as a free flagellum to the anterior portion of the organism.

Treatment and Prevention

Drugs currently available for the treatment of trypanosomiasis may be to some extent toxic. Melarsoprol is usually administered to those with more advanced stages of the disease. Pentamidine is sometimes prophylactically used during epidemics but the key to prevention is the control of the vectors involved in transmitting the organism and reconstruction and repair of homes to prevent the entry of triatomid insects.

AFRICAN TRYPANOSOMIASIS

African trypanosomiasis is spread by the tsetse fly (there are at least twenty-two species of the insect) in two separate geographic locations of Africa and demonstrate

MICROSCOPIC DIAGNOSTIC FEATURE

General Classification—Sporozoan

Organism	*Trypanosoma cruzi*
Specimen Required	Blood, tissue, or serological evidence of infection
Stage	Trypomastigote forms in circulatory system are diagnostic
Size	Amastigotes are 1.5–4.0 μm; trypomastigotes average 20 μm in length
Shape	Oocysts somewhat oval; "U"- or "C"-shaped trypomastigotes in blood smear
Motility	Flagellar motility of invading trypanomastigotes
Nucleus(i)	Large red nucleus with dark-stained rodlike kinetoplast in Giemsa-stained specimen
Cytoplasm	Smooth
Other Features	Tissue cysts contain large numbers of slow-growing trophozoites

Source: Centers for Disease Control and Prevention (CDC)

two distinctly different clinical pictures. The diseases are caused by infection with either of two subspecies of trypanosomes, *Trypanosoma brucei gambiense,* which causes Gambian (West Africa Sleeping Sickness) or chronic sleeping sickness, and *T. brucei rhodesiense,* which causes Rhodesian (Eastern African Sleeping Sickness) or acute sleeping sickness. The trypanosomes multiply in the blood and are taken up by tsetse flies when they feed on an infected human or other domesticated or wild mammal. The life cycle within the tsetse fly includes a period in which multiplication and development results during the formation of infective trypanosomes in the salivary glands of the fly after it feeds on an infected host. The infective trypanosomes are injected into a new host when the fly again feeds on an uninfected host. The infection itself causes a number of symptoms including anemia, wasting, and lethargy, and in some cases the parasites pass into the brain and cerebrospinal fluid, resulting in coma and death.

The disease is widespread because similar parasites are found in a large variety of both wild and domesticated animals. The first definitive accounts of sleeping sickness were by an English naval surgeon, John Atkins, in 1721 and Thomas Winterbottom in 1803 (Cox, 2002) showing humans as a reservoir for the organism (Figure 4-14). An appreciation of the real cause of the disease was not possible until Pasteur had established the germ theory toward the end of the nineteenth century as microorganisms were not yet discovered. Besides herd animals, trypanosomes have been discovered in the blood of fishes, frogs, and smaller mammals. Knowledge of the disease was well established by 1843, and in 1881 Griffith Evans found trypanosomes in the blood of both horses and camels where the tsetse fly abounded. This infection resulted in a wasting disease called surra in some areas of Africa and Evans suggested that the parasites might be the cause of this disease (Cox, 2002). Upon the completion of these observations by Evans, the most important discoveries about human and animal trypanosomiasis followed a short time afterwards.

Two years after Evans's discovery, David Bruce, a British army surgeon, was investigating an outbreak of nagana, a disease similar to surra, in cattle in Zululand. He was looking for a bacterial cause but instead found trypanosomes in the blood of diseased cattle, but proceeded to show that the organisms caused nagana in cattle and horses and that the same organisms also were capable of infecting dogs. He determined that all the infected cattle had stayed for a period of time in the fly-infested "tsetse belt" and that the disease was similar to that in humans. Common names for the disease included "negro lethargy" and "fly disease of hunters."

Morphology

The causative organisms for the two species of human infections in Africa, *T. gambiense* and *T. rodesiense,* are part of the *T. brucei-gambiense-rhodesiense* complex. *T. brucei* is believed to be responsible for a wild type of the organism found chiefly in wild game that over time has evolved to a form that gave rise to the two variants. The "tsetse fly belt" widely confines and limits the extent of infections by the two strains of the organism. The *Glossina* genus, the tsetse fly, serves as both the intermediate host and vector for the two forms of the disease. For the Gambian version of the disease, two species of *Glossina*, those of *G. palpais* and *G. tachinoides*, are vectors and intermediate hosts. A large portion of the African continent is known as the "fly belt" and for this reason is almost uninhabited by both humans and domesticated animals because of the danger of trypanosomiasis. The wet lowlands and rainforests found in West and Central Africa provide breeding grounds for the tsetse flies, contributing to widespread infection. The infection often leads to central nervous system derangement and eventually death ensues after several years.

Symptoms

Three stages ensue upon infection through the bite of an infected tsetse fly. Symptoms differ slightly between the East African and West African strains. In the East African variety, the tsetse bite is often painful and therefore readily noticed. The site of the bite develops into a red sore called a *chancre*. After 1 to 4 weeks other symptoms arise including fever, irritability, headache, extreme fatigue, muscle and joint pain, and swollen lymph glands. These signs and symptoms are often accompanied by weight loss and body rash. Infection of the central nervous system (CNS) may be manifested by confusion, changes in moods and affect (emotional reaction), slurred speech and even seizures, and difficulty walking and talking.

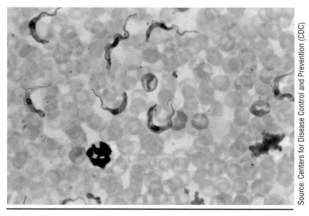

Source: Centers for Disease Control and Prevention (CDC)

FIGURE 4-14 Humans are the main reservoir for *Trypanosoma brucei gambiense*, but animals are also susceptible

If left untreated, the condition worsens and leads to death within weeks to months.

Symptoms of those with West African trypanosomiasis include the development of a chancre, usually in a slightly shorter time than in East African trypanosomiasis (1 to 2 weeks rather than 1 to 4 weeks) after the tsetse fly bite. Other symptoms occur several weeks later than the East African strain, and include a fever, rash, swelling around the eyes and hands, severe headaches, fatigue, and painful muscles and joints. Some people develop swollen lymph glands at the back of the neck. Weight loss occurs as the illness worsens. Infection of the CNS also causes personality changes as does the East African variety, characterized by irritability, loss of concentration, confusion, slurred speech, seizures, and difficulty with communicating and walking. As the common name implies, a number of patients sleep during the day but conversely have trouble sleeping at night. Without treatment, the illness gets worse and results in death several months to years following the infection. West African trypanosomiasis usually runs a longer disease course than that found in the East African trypanosomiasis.

Life Cycle

The life cycle of both *T. b. rhodesiense* and *T. b. gambiense* in man is similar, with the *Glossina* vector transmitting the organisms for both strains. Transfer of the organisms from host to host occurs when an infected tsetse fly who has taken a blood meal from an infected mammal injects metacyclic trypomastigotes from its salivary gland into the skin tissue of its intended host. The parasites enter the lymphatic system and pass into the bloodstream and into the CSF if the disease runs its course. Inside the host, they transform into bloodstream trypomastigotes and are carried to other sites throughout the body. They reach other blood fluids (e.g., lymph, spinal fluid) as they are circulated and continue reproduction by means of binary fission. These trypomastigotes then leave the midgut of the fly and are transformed into epimastigotes. The epimastigotes reach the fly's salivary glands and continue multiplication by binary fission in preparation for infecting another host.

Disease Transmission

Transmission of the disease is through the bite of an infected tsetse fly, of the two species of the genus *Glossina*. Blood transfusions and organ and tissue transplants, as well as transmission from a pregnant mother to the fetus, occurs in rare instances. The reservoir hosts are most likely wild game animals, particularly antelope, other ungulates (joint-footed), and domestic cattle.

Laboratory Diagnosis

Diagnostic measures are similar for West African and East African trypanosomiasis. Trypomastigotes in blood, lymph fluid, lymph node aspirates, and direct wet mounts are effective forms for identification. Centrifugation often leaves the organisms in the buffy layer (WBCs and platelets) of a blood sample, where they are effectively concentrated and can be stained with Giemsa stain for the presence of parasites. In patients with CNS involvement, CSF may be used to find the organisms. Some serologic techniques are designed for screening for the two strains of the organism but antibody detection by serological methodology has extreme sensitivity and specificity that may be too unpredictable for clinical decisions, providing false positive results in some instances.

Treatment and Prevention

Early patient management is vital for West African trypanosomiasis. Avoiding CNS involvement greatly increases the prognosis for one infected by the organism. Some medications that are effective in the hemolymphatic stage, in particular pentamidine isothionate usually cures the Gambian variety. In later stages with CNS involvement, the "blood-brain barrier" effectively prevents the medication from reaching the brain. Control, management, and avoidance of the tsetse fly is the most effective measure for preventing transmission of the disease. Clearing of moist breeding grounds and drainage of swampy areas helps to control the numbers of flies and therefore minimizes the potential for transmission. Travelers to endemic areas should wear deep but bright colors, avoiding pastels, and use bed nets and insect repellent.

LYMPHATIC FILARIASIS

Primarily three species of microfilarial parasites infect the lymphatic system of the human host. But other systems such as the circulatory system and related tissues may also become involved. The three species that are considered as lymphatic filariforms are: *Wuchereria bancrofti, Brugia malayi,* and *B. timori.* Other species of filarial that infect the subcutaneous tissues of the body and those that invade the serous cavities will also be presented.

FILARIAL WORMS AND LYMPHATIC FILARIASIS (ELEPHANTIASIS)

A discussion of the basics of filariform larvae and the diseases they produce and the impact of these organisms on humans is provided first in this section. It is followed by specific organisms and details of those particular organisms and identification of them. A number of significant pathogens include small "worms" called *microfilaria.* The superfamily (a group that falls between an order and a family) Filarioidea contains a number of nematodal organisms that reside in tissues of the human body. Some species of microfilaria are are found only in animals, but three members of superfamily Filarioidea are commonly found in humans and will be presented in this section.

Filariasis is the general name for a group of tropical diseases caused by various threadlike parasitic round worms (nematodes) and their larvae. The larvae transmit the disease to humans most often through mosquito bites, but the disease may also be less frequently transmitted by sand gnats, tabanid flies, blackflies, and a few other miscellaneous insects. An outbreak of filariasis may be characterized by chills and fever, headache, and skin lesions in the early stages. If left untreated or if treatment is delayed, the disease can progress to a state of gross limb enlargement and often with enlargement of the genitalia. This marked condition is commonly called elephantiasis and when the tissue injury has occurred, it cannot be corrected with treatment with medications. But surgery can be performed to remove some of the misshapen and massive amounts of skin and other tissues generated by the disease in the affected areas.

Life Cycle

The major species of causative organisms of filariasis in humans occupy certain niches of the body, which lead to their discovery and initial attempts at identification. The life cycles for each of the species that cause filariasis have slight variations from each other. Table 4-1 shows the general division of the organisms based on the tissue types each of the species typically invades. Organisms infect humans and other vertebrates through the bites of mosquitoes, gnats, and flies, depending upon the geographic location where each is found. Human filarial nematode worms have a complicated life cycle, which primarily consists of five stages. After the male and female worm mate, the female gives birth to live microfilariae by the thousands. The microfilariae are taken up by the vector insect (intermediate host) during a blood meal. In the intermediate host, the microfilariae molt and develop into third-stage (infective) larvae. Upon taking another blood meal, the vector insect injects the infectious larvae into the dermis layer of our skin. After approximately one year the larvae molt through two more stages, maturing into the adult worm. Adult worms can survive in the lymphatic system for 5 to 15 years.

Infected individuals do not always exhibit microfilaria in their blood. When microfilaria are demonstrated in stained blood smears, the victim of the infection is said to be *microfilaremic,* a term indicating a condition of the blood where the parasite can be visualized. A term, occult filariasis, may be used when an individual demonstrates the signs and symptoms of being infected by a microfilarial organism but no organisms are found during an examination of a blood sample. In some cases, as serological test for antigens (proteins) of the organism are found in the blood, although no visible organisms are observed.

The organisms migrate throughout the body, and infect a variety of tissue types. *Wuchereria bancrofti, Brugia timori,* and *Brugia malayi* are the most common organisms causing filariasis in humans. Filariasis is classified into three distinct types according to the parts of the body that become infected. Lymphatic filariasis affects the circulatory system that moves tissue fluid and immune cells (lymphatic system) and may cause gross enlargement of areas of the body due to the inability to reabsorb tissue fluids into the occlude blood vessels. Subcutaneous filariasis infects the areas beneath the skin and in some cases the whites of the eye. The third type of filariasis is that of infections of the serous cavities, where the filaria infect body cavities but does not cause serious disease. Several different types of worms, or filarial, can be responsible for each of these types of filariasis. But the most common species that infect humans include those found in the following table (Table 4-5).

TABLE 4-5 Parasitic Species Producing Filariasis

LYMPHATIC FILARIASIS	SUBCUTANEOUS FILARIASIS	SEROUS CAVITY FILARIASIS
Wucheria bancrofti	*Onchocerca volvulus*	*Mansonella perstans*
Brugia malayi	*Loa loa*	*Mansonella ozzardi*
Brugia timori	*Mansonella streptocerca*	
	Dracunculus medinensis	

Species of Causative Organisms for Filariasis

These species are divided into three groups according to the tissues and cavities of the body they impact upon and occupy, as shown at the top of the page.

The life cycles, the transmitting vectors, and in particular the tissues affected by these organisms, dictate the category into which they are placed. The worms that cause lymphatic filariasis are found chiefly in the lymphatic system, including the lymph nodes, and in chronic cases these worms lead to the disease called *elephantiasis*. Subcutaneous filariasis caused by *Loa loa* (the African eye worm), *Mansonella streptocerca,* Onchocerca volvulus, and Dracunculus medinensis (the guinea worm) result in invasions by the small worms or filaria of areas just beneath the skin, including the layers of tissue in the eye in the case of Loa loa and the fatty layers slightly deeper in the organ. Onchocerciasis is the term for "river blindness" and the chief vector of the organism responsible for this condition is the *Simulium* sp. of flies, or "blackfly" (Figure 4-15). Serous cavity filariasis caused by the worms *Mansonella perstans* and *Mansonella ozzardi* occupy the serous cavity of the abdomen that results in pronounced distension of the stomach. In all categories the transmitting vectors are either bloodsucking insects (fly or mosquito) or **copecod** crustaceans in the case of *Dracunculus medinensis.*

Epidemiology of Filariasis

It is probable that up to 170 million people in mostly tropical and subtropical areas suffer from some sort of filariasis, as there are several species which cause this disease. The continent of Africa, islands of the Pacific, areas

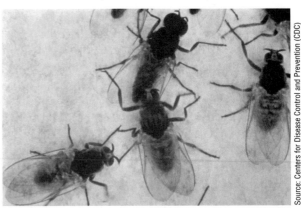

FIGURE 4-15 *Simulium* sp. of flies, or "blackflies," a vector of the disease, **onchocerciasis,** or "river blindness"

Source: Centers for Disease Control and Prevention (CDC)

of South America, Southeast Asia, and a few other areas of the world harbor most of the filarial diseases. Filariasis is often disabling and certainly figuratively damaging for many, but the disease is rarely fatal. However, it is one of the leading causes of both permanent and long-standing disability throughout the world. In 2002, an ambitious program to rid the world of six diseases within 20 years was undertaken by a number of organizations. The WHO, the Bill and Melinda Gates Foundation, the Carter Center, and the International Task Force for Disease Eradication (ITFDE) united their efforts to accomplish this worthy goal, toward which some modest gains have been achieved.

Along with lymphatic filariasis, five other diseases are earmarked as having the probability of becoming extinct within two decades. The remaining five potentially eradicable diseases, with the exception of the viral disease of polio, are all parasite infections and are identified as targets of these efforts. They include the guinea worm, polio, **trachoma**, **schistosomiasis**, and river blindness (onchocerciasis), all of which are found predominantly in parts of Africa and Latin America. In all of these diseases, a mosquito first bites an infected individual before biting another uninfected individual, and in the process transferring some of the worm larvae to the new host. Once within the body, the larvae migrate to a specific area or organ of the body where they mature to adult worms.

The two most common types of the disease are bancroftian and Malayan filariasis, which are both differing forms of lymphatic filariasis, a parasitic worm that lives in human lymph nodes and ducts (Figure 4-16). The bancroftian variety is found throughout the Africa continent, the Pacific Islands, southern and southeastern Asia, and the tropical and subtropical regions of South America and the Caribbean Malayan filariasis occurs only in southern and southeastern Asia as well as the southern area of the Thai peninsula, Borneo, and the major islands of the islands of the South China and Java seas. Filariasis is occasionally found in the United States and most particularly may be present among immigrants from the Caribbean and Pacific Islands. *W. bancrofti* was actually prevalent in Charleston, South Carolina, at one point in history and was contracted through slave trade and transmitted by mosquitoes capable of carrying the disease in the region. The disease had largely disappeared from the region by the early 1920s.

Lymphatic filariasis is a term that refers to a condition caused by infection with the nematode worms

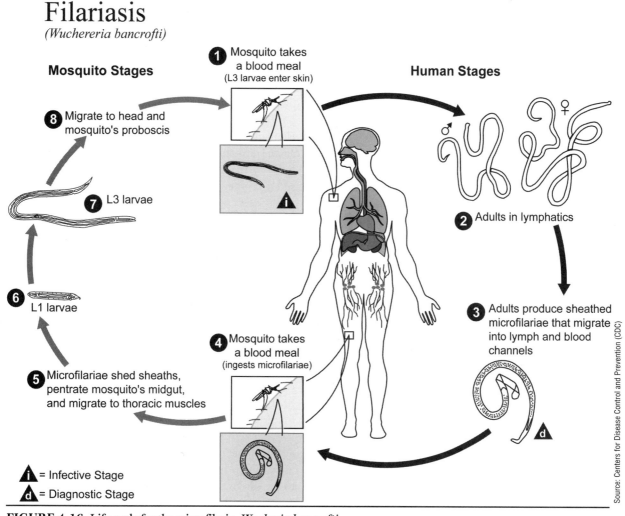

Filariasis
(*Wuchereria bancrofti*)

Mosquito Stages

Human Stages

1 Mosquito takes a blood meal (L3 larvae enter skin)

8 Migrate to head and mosquito's proboscis

7 L3 larvae

6 L1 larvae

5 Microfilariae shed sheaths, pentrate mosquito's midgut, and migrate to thoracic muscles

4 Mosquito takes a blood meal (ingests microfilariae)

2 Adults in lymphatics

3 Adults produce sheathed microfilariae that migrate into lymph and blood channels

i = Infective Stage
d = Diagnostic Stage

Source: Centers for Disease Control and Prevention (CDC)

FIGURE 4-16 Life cycle for the microfilaria, *Wucheria bancrofti*

Wuchereria bancrofti, Brugia malayi, and *B. timori,* which are transmitted by mosquitoes. The discovery of the life cycle by a Scotsman, Patrick Manson, in 1877 is regarded as one of the most significant discoveries in tropical medicine, but in the context of the history of parasitology it is better perceived as a logical extension of much that had gone before. Like *Dracunculus,* the adult filarial worms live in subcutaneous tissues, but unlike *Dracunculus,* the larvae, called *microfilariae*, produced by the female worm pass into the blood and are taken up by a bloodsucking mosquito when it feeds. After development in the mosquito, the microfilariae are injected into a new host upon which the mosquito feeds again. The microfilaria, when present in the circulatory system, are readily visible in a stained blood smear (Figure 4-17).

Clinical Signs of Filariasis

Elephantiasis, in which the lower limbs are misshapen and appear similar to that of elephants with little definition and with loose skin, was a particular form of the disease that has been met with a great deal of attention throughout the history of mankind. This grotesque swelling of the limbs may also include that of breasts and the genitals, particularly for the scrotum of men (Figure 4-18). The disease was obviously present since before recorded history, as artwork from early man shows drawings and statues of persons who may have been suffering from lymphatic filariasis. However, some of the drawings were highly stylistic and included exaggerations of certain physical characteristics, therefore, depictions of swollen

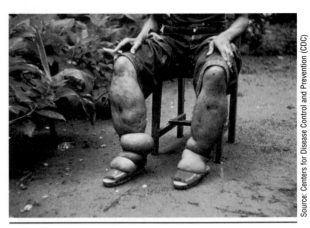

FIGURE 4-18 Elephantiasis of leg due to filariasis

limbs and genitalia may have been the artists' expressions of creativity in at least some of the ancient artistic renderings. Lymphatic filariasis has been found along the Nile River from past evidence as well as current victims of the infection. Some prominent figures from ancient civilizations show the swollen limbs of a victim of microfilariasis. The statue of the Egyptian Pharaoh Mentuhotep II from about 2000 BC shows evidence of possible elephantiasis in grotesquely enlarged limbs. In addition, small statuettes and gold weights from the Nok culture in West Africa from about AD 500 depict the enlarged scrota characteristic of elephantiasis (Cox, 2002).

Greek and Roman writers as well as Arabic physicians were careful to point out the differences between the physical effects of leprosy and those of elephantiasis from infection with the microfilaria (small worms). The first definitive reports of lymphatic filariasis only began to appear in the sixteenth century. The condition of filariasis was so well known that the common name "the curse of St. Thomas," was named after those who killed St. Thomas. His death occurred during a visit to Goa between 1588 and 1592, and the incident was documented when a Dutch explorer named Jan Huygen Linschoten recorded that the descendants of those that killed St. Thomas were "all born with one of their legs and one foot from the knee downwards as thick as an elephant's leg" (Cox, 2002). References to the disease of filariasis are available in other areas of Africa and Asia, including China, where Patrick Manson's studies in 1877 led to the discovery of the life cycle of the filarial parasites. Another pathological condition associated with lymphatic filariasis is chyluria, in which the urine appears

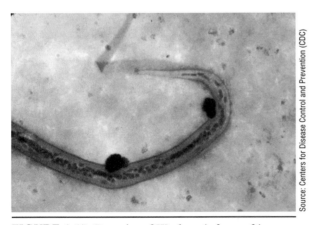

FIGURE 4-17 Posterior of *Wuchereria bancrofti* microfilaria in blood smear

milky. This condition was recorded by William Prout in his 1849 book *On the Nature and Treatment of Stomach and Renal Diseases* (Cox, 2002).

The larval microfilariae were first seen in the fluid from a hydrocele by the French surgeon Jean-Nicolas Demarquay in 1863 and in urine by Otto Henry Wucherer in Brazil in 1866 (Cox, 2002). However, the role of the microfilariae in urine and blood remained a mystery until Timothy Lewis, a Scottish physician working in India confirmed the presence of microfilariae in both urine and blood and showed their significance in the development of elephantiasis. The adult worm was described by Joseph Bancroft in 1876 and named *Filaria bancrofti* in Bancroft's honor by the British helminthologist Thomas Spencer Cobbold (Cox, 2002).

Disease Transmission

In an interesting development, while working on the life cycle of the organisms causing filariasis, Manson was led astray regarding the finding of an intermediate host. This assumption was based on the belief that the infection leading to filariasis was caused by drinking contaminated water. Later, when working in China, Manson found microfilariae in the blood of dogs and humans and hypothesized that these parasites in the blood might be transmitted by a bloodsucking insect such as the mosquito. Following this lead, he fed mosquitoes with the blood of his gardener, who was harboring the parasites, and found larval stages in the mosquitoes (Cox, 2002). But Manson erroneously thought that the parasites escaped from the mosquito and into the water and that humans acquired infection from this contaminated water by drinking the parasitic-laden water or by penetration of the skin. But the true mode of transmission was not certain until assumptions made by the Australian parasitologist, Thomas Bancroft, were followed up by Manson's assistant, George Carmichael Low, who demonstrated the presence of microfilariae in the mouthparts of mosquitoes in 1900, completing the history of the development of lymphatic filariasis (Cox, 2002).

How the Disease of Filariasis Is Contracted

The larval form matures into an adult worm within six months to one year and can live between four and six years. Each female worm can produce millions of larvae,

and these larvae only appear in the bloodstream at night, when they may be transmitted, via an insect bite, to another host. But a single bite is usually not sufficient to transmit an infection by one of the species of the causative organisms; therefore, for the most part, short-term travelers to an endemic region are usually safe. A series of multiple bites over a period of time is required to establish an infection. As a result, those individuals who are regularly active outdoors at night and those who spend more time in remote jungle areas are at an increased risk of contracting the filariasis infection.

Causes and Symptoms of Filariasis

In cases of lymphatic filariasis, the most common form of the disease, the disease is caused by the adult worms actually living in the lymphatic vessels near the lymph nodes. There they distort the vessels and cause local inflammation. In advanced stages, the worms can completely obstruct the blood and lymph vessels, causing the surrounding tissue to become enlarged. In bancroftian filariasis, the legs and genitals are most often involved, whereas the Malayan variety affects the legs below the knees. Repeated episodes of inflammation lead to blockages of the lymphatic system, especially in the genitals and legs. This causes the affected area to become grossly enlarged, with thickened, coarse skin, leading to elephantiasis.

In conjunctival filariasis, the larval forms of the worms migrate to the eye and can sometimes be seen moving beneath the skin or beneath the white part of the eye (conjunctiva). If untreated, this disease can cause river blindness, or onchocerciasis (Figure 4-19). Symptoms vary, depending on what type of parasitic worm has caused the infection, but all infections usually begin with chills, headache, and fever between three months and one year after the insect bite. There may also be swelling, redness, and pain in the arms, legs, or scrotum. Areas of pus (abscesses) may appear as a result of dying worms or a secondary bacterial infection.

Laboratory Diagnosis

The disease is diagnosed by taking a patient history, performing a physical examination, and by screening blood specimens for specific proteins produced by the immune system in response to this infection (antibodies). Early

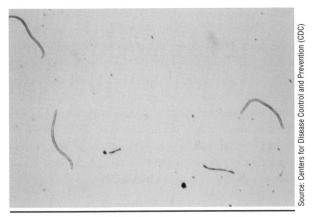

Source: Centers for Disease Control and Prevention (CDC)

FIGURE 4-19 Microfilarial pathogen *Onchocerca volvulus* in its larval form, causative agent for river blindness

diagnosis may be difficult because, in the first stages, the disease mimics other bacterial skin infections. To make an accurate diagnosis, the physician looks for a pattern of inflammation and signs of lymphatic obstruction, together with the patient's possible exposure in an area where filariasis is common. The larvae (microfilariae) can also be found in the blood, but mosquitoes which spread the disease are active at night, facilitating the spread of the disease because the larvae are usually only found in the blood between about 10 PM and 2 AM.

Treatment and Prevention

Several different medications and methods are used to treat a filariasis infection: eliminating the larvae by impairing the adult worms' ability to reproduce, and by actually killing adult worms. Unfortunately, much of the tissue damage that occurs in the condition of elephantiasis may not be reversible. The medication is started at low doses to prevent immune reactions caused by large numbers of dying parasites. Although effective, medications used in treatment can cause severe side effects in as many as 70 percent of patients as a result of either the drug itself or the massive death of parasites in the blood. Diethylcarbamazine is implicated in causing severe allergic reactions and the formation of pus-filled sores (abscesses). These side effects can be controlled by using **antihistamines** and anti-inflammatory drugs such as steroidal preparations called **corticosteroids**. In rare cases, treatment with diethylcarbamazine in someone with very high levels of parasitic infection may lead to a

fatal inflammation of the brain called *encephalitis*. In this case, fever is followed by headache and confusion, then stupor, and ensuing coma caused when massive numbers of larvae and parasites die. Other common drug reactions are merely nuisances, and may include dizziness, weakness, and nausea.

For medications that cause the wholesale death of the parasites, symptoms may include fever, headache, muscle pain, abdominal pain, nausea and vomiting, weakness, dizziness, lethargy, and even asthma. Reactions usually begin within two days of starting treatment and may last between two and four days. No treatment can reverse elephantiasis and surgery may be required to remove surplus tissue and to provide a way to drain the fluid from the damaged lymphatic system. Surgery may also be used to ease massive enlargement of the scrotum. Elephantiasis of the legs may also be aided by elevating the legs to lower the circulation of blood to the lower limbs and by providing support with elastic bandages. The prognosis for patients in the early stages or in mild cases is quite good, especially if the victim can avoid re-infection. The disease is rarely fatal, and with continued WHO medical intervention, with a goal of eliminating the disease by 2020, even gross elephantiasis is seldom seen even in the developing countries of the world.

IDENTIFICATION OF MAJOR MICROFILARIAL ORGANISMS

The three major species of causative organisms of filariasis listed earlier in humans occupy certain niches, which lead to their discovery and initial attempts at identification. Table 4-1 shows the general division of the organisms based on the issue types each of the species typically invade. Organisms infect humans and other vertebrates through the bites of mosquitoes, gnats, and flies, depending upon the location. Human filarial nematode worms have a complicated life cycle, which primarily consists of five stages. After the male and female worm mate, the female gives birth to live microfilariae by the thousands. The microfilariae are taken up by the vector insect (intermediate host) during a blood meal. In the intermediate host, the microfilariae molt and develop into third-stage (infective) larvae. Upon taking another blood meal the vector insect injects the infectious larvae into the dermis layer of our skin. After approximately one year the larvae molt through two more stages, maturing into the adult worm.

A clinical diagnosis may be complicated by the inability to isolate microfilaria from a patient's blood specimen. Even individuals who exhibit all of the signs and symptoms of having been infected by microfilaria may not contain the organisms in their blood when stained blood smears are microscopically examined. These individuals are considered *amicrofilaremic* in the absence of directly demonstrated infection. In this case, in addition to clinical observations, serological tests designed to detect circulating antigen in the blood may be effective in obtaining a definitive laboratory result.

WUCHERERIA BANCROFTI AND W. TIMORI

The *Wuchereria bancrofti* organism is named for a German physician, Otto Wucherer (1820–1873), for a genus of filarial worms of the class Nematoda (roundworms) and is commonly found in the tropical regions. *W. bancrofti* is one of the most important causative organisms for the condition of elephantiasis. Adults of this species inhabit the lymphatic ducts and the larger nodes, plugging up this important component of the body for draining tissue fluids and preventing swelling. Females give birth to "sheathed" microfilaria, and which remain in various internal organs of the host during the day. But at night they circulate in the blood, when mosquitoes most often feed on the blood of the infected humans. The development of the *W. bancrofti* organisms continue for about two weeks, when the larvae become infective, and are then passed to other uninfected humans through the bites of infected mosquitoes.

Morphology

The adult worms of these nematodes are long and slender, and smooth with rounded ends. It has a shortened head (cephalic) region and its nuclei are arranged throughout the length of the body except for the caudal or tail region. *W. bancrofti* is characterized by considerable sexual dimorphism. Sexual dimorphism means that there are systematic differences in the morphology between members of the two genders of the same species. Examples of sexual dimorphism include such factors as color, size, and the presence or absence of parts of the body. Some males of other species are even more dimorphic, with displays of ornamental horns or feathers used

in courtship displays, but the differences are more subtle in the filaria of *W. bancrofti*. The male worm is 40 mm long and 100 µm wide with a curved tail, whereas the female is much larger than the male. The female worm is 6 to 10 cm long and 300 µm wide or nearly three times longer and larger in both diameter and length than the male. Females are ovoviviparous, meaning reproduction by the hatching of eggs inside the mother organism, a process that can produce thousands of juveniles known as *microfilariae*. The microfilariae of *W. bancrofti* are approximately 245 to 300 µm and retain the egg membrane as a sheath and are sometimes considered embryonic stages.

Symptoms

Early in the course of the infection for Bancroftian filariasis, fever and chills may be accompanied by lymphadenitis and eosinophilia. Inflammation of lymphatic vessels (lymphangitis) or inflammation of the lymph nodes (lymphadenitis) may impact the lower extremities and sometimes the genitals and breasts. Lymph engorgement by the worms may become fibrotic and distended, producing considerable pain. The hardening and thickening of the skin follows with skin abscesses that drain to the outside of the body.

Life Cycle

W. bancrofti was the first organism discovered to be transmitted through an arthropod vector. The organism carries out its life cycle in two different hosts. The definitive host is a human and mosquitoes are the intermediate host. Adult parasites live in the lymphatic system of the human host, but the microfilariae found in the circulatory system are transported throughout the host. *W. bancrofti* is a periodic strain that exhibits nocturnal periodicity by residing in the deep veins during the day and during the night they migrate to the peripheral circulation between 10 PM and 2 AM. Next, the microfilariae are transferred into one of three common vectors which are of the mosquito genera: *Culex, Anopheles,* and *Aedes,* depending on the geographic location. Inside the mosquito vector, also known as the *intermediate host*, the microfilariae mature into motile larvae called *juveniles*.

The microfilariae obtained by the feeding mosquito penetrate the stomach wall and then migrate to the thoracic region of the mosquito. In the thoracic musculature of the mosquito the larvae grow and develop into an infective stage over a period of perhaps 10 days. The infective larvae, which range from 1 to 2 mm long, then move to the proboscis of the mosquito and during the next blood meal the insect infects the next host the mosquito bites. The larvae injected into a new host then move through the lymphatic system to regional lymph nodes, predominantly in the legs and genital area. There the larvae develop into adult worms where they undergo two molting stages over the course of 6 to 9 months before they reach sexual maturity in the regional lymph nodes and afferent lymphatic vessels. These adult worms may have a life span of up to 7 years and when they mate, the female deposits sheathed microfilariae into the blood. The sheaths are remnants of the egg that developed into a larval stage inside the female. After mating, the adult female worm can produce thousands of microfilariae that migrate into the bloodstream. A mosquito vector can bite the infected human host, ingest the microfilariae, and thus repeat the life cycle of *W. bancrofti.*

Disease Transmission

Depending on the geographic location, the *Culex, Anopheles,* or *Aedes* mosquito infected with *W. bancrofti* larvae infect the human host during a blood meal. The larvae separate from the proboscis (mouthpart) of the mosquito and invade the puncture wound. Following the cycles in which the larvae mature and reach an infective stage, the human host again is the source of infection for the next host upon which the mosquito feeds.

Laboratory Diagnosis

Samples should be taken between 10 PM and 2 AM to provide the optimum blood sample for the detection of microfilariae. The presence of microfilariae in peripheral blood or from lymphatic fluid is the most definitive diagnosis. Thick and thin smears of blood stained with Giemsa stain will show the presence of microfilariae. Concentration methods through centrifugation of samples fixed with 2 percent formalin will provide a buffy coat containing the organisms in light infections. Filtration of a fluid sample through a microfilter will yield microfilariae that appear as sheathed organisms that are 245 to 300 μm in length and with numerous nuclei that do not extend to the tip of the pointed tail are considered definitive for *W. bancrofti.*

MICROSCOPIC DIAGNOSTIC FEATURE

General Classification—Microfilaria

Organism	*Wuchereria bancrofti*
Specimen Required	Peripheral blood, lymphatic fluid
Stage	Microfilariae
Size	245 to 300 μm
Shape	Round and elongated with pointed tail
Body Nuclei	Extends to tip of tail
Other Features	Stained microfilariae appear "sheathed"
	Specimen should be collected between 10 PM, 2 PM

Serological testing results where elevated levels of serum IgE (antibodies) as elevated antifilarial antibodies and the presence of eosinophilia would support a diagnosis of lymphatic filariasis. Some individuals may not exhibit microfilariae in their blood samples, and in these cases, diagnosis may be based on the presence of circulating antigens of *W. bancrofti* and on the presence of clinical findings.

Treatment and Prevention

Antihistamines and analgesics are used to treat related inflammation, discomfort, and allergic responses. Several medications are available for various types of microfilarial infections depending upon the species. The treatment of choice for lymphatic filariasis is diethylcarbamazine over a period of three weeks. Surgical procedures may be necessary to relieve the lymphatic obstruction leading to extreme swelling and enlargement of parts of the body.

Prevention of infections by *W. bancrofti* is in the form of protection against the vectors of the disease. Insect repellent and protective clothing when travelling to endemic areas of the world are effective, but for year-round residents of the area, these measures are not practical. Bed netting when used conscientiously will prevent bites from the vectors, but the most effective measures for disease control lies in control of the vector populations. This includes removal of breeding sites and killing of the large populations of mosquitoes by insecticides. Because humans are the only host for this species of parasite, removing infected persons to other nonendemic regions will also stifle the source of infected victims for the insect vectors.

BRUGIA MALAYI

Brugia malayi is found in rural areas of Asia, in addition to isolated pockets in countries extending from the west coast of India to New Guinea, the Philippines, and Japan. (Amaya, 2003). The habitat in which *B. malayi* flourishes is in the rural freshwater swamp forests in Southeast Asia, and its intermediate host is that of one of several genera of mosquitoes. In open swamp and irrigated fields and hill forests of South and East Asia, *B. malayi* uses the mosquitoes of the genera *Mansonia*, *Aedes*, *Anopleles*, and *Culex*. In the intermediate host, *B. malayi* occupies the stomach, thorax muscles, and the proboscis or piercing part of the mosquito. The only definitive hosts the organism utilizes that may be bitten by the mosquito include human, monkeys, forest carnivores (meat-eating creatures), and domestic cats. The organism enters the wound before migrating to the lymphatic system through the bloodstream where it remains throughout its adult life (Amaya, 2003).

The impact of *B. malayi* on human health can be considerable. Infections by *B. malayi* frequently contribute to both physical and mental disabilities. The physical disabilities come in the form of the inflammation and marked swelling of the lymph nodes, normally from the waist down, due to the blockage of the lymphatic circulation. Mental disabilities often ensue and chiefly stem from psychological stress based on a lack of mobility and the attitudes they experience from social contacts when their physical appearance is drastically altered. Two genera of mosquito, *Mansonia* and *Aedes*, are vectors for *B. malayi*, which are also implicated in transmitting other diseases (Figure 4-20). For instance, *Aedes aegypti* is also known to transmit both yellow fever and dengue, among other diseases.

Morphology

The adult *Brugia malayi* is a long and slender organism with a smooth cuticle, kinked, and has a long cephalic space having a length-to-width ratio of about 2:1. The head is slightly swollen and has two circles of well-defined papillae. The tail of *B. malayi* is ventrally curved. Sexual differences exist, with the adult female *B. malayi* being approximately 8 cm long by 0.3 mm wide and the male about 2 cm long and 0.1 mm wide (Amaya, 2003).

Symptoms

B. malayi produces a condition marked by infection and swelling of the lymphatic system. The disease is primarily caused by the presence of worms in the lymphatic vessels and the resulting host response. Signs of infection are essentially the same as those seen in bancroftian (*W. bancrofti*) filariasis, including fever, lymphadenitis, lymphangitis, lymphedema, and potentially a secondary bacterial infection. Lymphadenitis, or swelling of the lymph nodes, is commonly a sign of many diseases and occurs as an early manifestation of filariasis, occurring frequently in the inguinal area before the worms mature.

Lymphangitis, inflammation of the lymphatic vessels, is in response to the infection and occurs early in the course of infection in response to worm development, molting, death, or accompanying bacterial and fungal infection. Abscess formation and ulceration of the lymph nodes occasionally occur during *B. malayi* infection. Repeated inflammatory reactions cause dilation of blood vessels and thickening of the affected lymphatic vessels, interrupting the fluid balance between tissues and the circulatory system. Elephantiasis resulting from *B. malayi* infection most often affects the lower extremities of the legs and arms. *B. malayi* infections rarely affect the genitalia as frequently as with bancroftian infection. Most infections appear asymptomatic but will vary among individuals. Those living in endemic areas with microfilaremia may never present with overt symptoms but in some individuals, the infective load is inconsequential as a severe inflammatory response may be elicited by only a few worms.

Life Cycle

The reproductive cycle of *B. malayi* begins when a mosquito, the intermediate host of a species in the genera *Mansonia*, *Anopleles*, and *Aedes*, acquires the sheathed microfilaria parasite in its blood meal. The microfilariae penetrate the gut wall of the mosquito where they lose their sheath and migrate to the muscles of the thorax. After 10 to 20 days, in which they undergo three

Filariasis
(Brugia malayi)

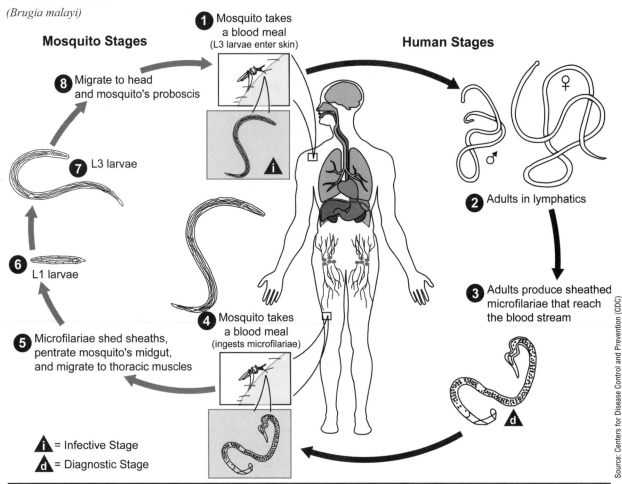

Mosquito Stages

1. Mosquito takes a blood meal (L3 larvae enter skin)

8. Migrate to head and mosquito's proboscis

7. L3 larvae

6. L1 larvae

5. Microfilariae shed sheaths, pentrate mosquito's midgut, and migrate to thoracic muscles

4. Mosquito takes a blood meal (ingests microfilariae)

Human Stages

2. Adults in lymphatics

3. Adults produce sheathed microfilariae that reach the blood stream

i = Infective Stage

d = Diagnostic Stage

Source: Centers for Disease Control and Prevention (CDC)

FIGURE 4-20 *Aedes aegypti,* which prefers to feed on humans, is the most common *Aedes* species

sequences of molts, they develop into the infective third larval stage. Once the third larval stage is complete the *B. malayi* migrate to the proboscis of the mosquito. During the mosquito's blood meal the larvae enter the wound of the definitive host, which consist of humans, monkeys, domestic cats, and forest **carnivores**. The larvae then migrate through the subcutaneous tissue to the lymphatic vessels of the definitive host. Within about a year they develop into mature adults (Figure 4-21). The sheathed microfilariae produced after copulation then enter the bloodstream, allowing the intermediate host to acquire the microfilaria and thus repeating the cycle again.

Nematode females appear to produce a phero- mone, a reproductive hormone, to attract the male and live chiefly in the lymphatic and subcutaneous tissues of the body (Figure 4-22). The male coils around a female as they complete the mating process, and there is no fur- ther contact by the parent organisms beyond mating and the laying of the eggs. *B. malayi*, as with other nematodes, only have longitudinal muscles that run the length of the body of the organism, so they use an S-shaped or serpen- tine (snakelike) motion during movement. Presence in the blood of the infective stages during the day or night vary due to geographic location, as some mosquitoes bite only at night, whereas others are able to feed around the clock.

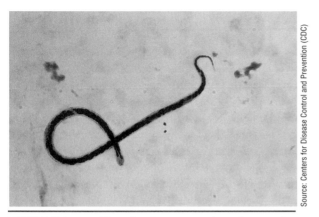

FIGURE 4-21 Life cycle of *Brugia malayi,* the causal agent of filariasis

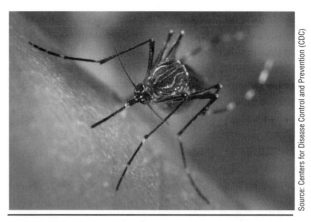

FIGURE 4-22 *B. malayi,* a nematode that can inhabit the lymphatics and subcutaneous tissues in humans, is one of the causative agents for lymphatic filariasis

Disease Transmission

A number of mosquito genera are able to transmit the predominantly night-feeding mosquitoes. The genera *Mansonia, Anopleles,* and *Aedes* are most capable of transmitting the organisms to human hosts, and the disease is confined to areas where these mosquitoes are prevalent. Usually a number of bites are required before transmission of the organism from the vector to the host.

Laboratory Diagnosis

The detection of microfilariae in the blood or from lymphatic fluid provides a definitive diagnosis. Microscopic examination of differential morphological features of microfilariae in stained blood films can aid diagnosis where Giemsa staining will uniquely stain the *B. malayi* sheath pink. The visualization of the tail portion where nuclei extend the length of the body with the presence of a sheath is sufficient to diagnose an infection by *B. malayi.* A distinctly obvious pair of nuclei should be seen near the tail and is separated from the other nuclei that run the length of the microfilaria. However, blood films can prove difficult given the nocturnal periodicity of some forms of *B. malayi*; same as for *W. bancrofti.*

Polymerase chain reaction (PCR)–based assays are highly sensitive and can be used to monitor infections both in the human and the mosquito vector. Lymphatic filariasis mainly afflicts the poor who live in areas without such resources. The two species of the genus *Brugia, B. malayi,* and *B. timori* can reasonably be differentiated between by the size of the microfilariae. *B. timori* averages 310 μm in length, whereas *B. malayi* averages 250 μm. A properly calibrated ocular and the measurement of several organisms to obtain an average length are critical to this differentiation. Some serological tests are available for elevated IgE titers of the victim's serum and a complete blood count to determine the presence of increased eosinophil percentages of the white blood cells would support the diagnosis. Tests using PCR technology are also available.

Treatment and Prevention

Treatment for *B. malayi* is similar to that of *W. bancrofti.* Antihistamines and anti-inflammatory drugs are used to treat related inflammation, discomfort, and allergic responses. The allergic response may also be mediated by the administration of corticosteroids. Several medications are available to eradicate the parasites, including Ivermectin, which must be administered as a single dose daily for a period of up to 6 months. Again, for serious changes in lymphatic and blood flow, surgical procedures may be necessary to relieve obstruction leading to swelling and enlargement of the limbs of the body.

Visitors to endemic areas for *B. malayi* to prevent infections are in the form of protection against the vectors of the disease. Insect repellent and protective clothing when travelling to endemic areas of the world, as well as netting that is permeated by insect repellents should be used in endemic regions of the world. Diethylcarbamazine (DEC) as a prophylactic may be combined with vector control for mass protection.

MICROSCOPIC DIAGNOSTIC FEATURE

General Classification—Microfilaria

Organism	*Brugia malayi, B. timori*
Specimen Required	Blood or lymphatic aspirate
Stage	Microfilariae
Size	Average for *B. malayi* is 310 μm, 250 μm for *B. timori*
Shape	Round and elongated with pointed tail
Nucleus(i)	Distinct pair of nuclei in the tail
Other Features	Stained microfilariae for both species appear "sheathed" but stain poorly in *B. timori*
	Time for collection for some species is at night, whereas others are subperiodic (modified circadian rhythm where the periods of appearance are not clear-cut)

SUBCUTANEOUS FILARIASIS

Four species of filarial parasites primarily infect the tissues beneath the epidermis of the human host. But other organs may be infected by specific species of those parasites producing subcutaneous signs and symptoms. The four species that are considered as subcutaneous parasites are: *Oncocerca volvulus, Loa loa, Mansonella streptocerca,* and *Drancunculus medinensis.*

DRACUNCULIASIS

The organism *Dracunculus medinensis*, better known as the guinea worm disease, dates back to at least the 1400s as documented in Egyptian writings. Two species of the organism of the genus *Drancunculus* exist: *D. medinensis* and *D. insignis. D. insignis* is a species of this genus, which primarily infects dogs and wild carnivores. But *D. medinensis* is the organism that has the greatest impact on the health of humans, and this section primarily relates to *D. medinensis.* These parasites received their respective names when it was seen by a European traveler in natives along the coast of West Africa, but the disease is prevalent today in India, Iran, Pakistan, and a large portion of Africa. It is also alleged to be the fiery serpent alluded to in the Bible. This parasite is also on the list of those slated for eradication by 2020, by efforts of the Carter Center, the Bill and Melinda Gates Foundation, and other national and international organizations.

DRANCUNCULUS MEDINENSIS

The *Drancunculus medinensis*, worms, members of the taxonomic order Spirurida, are long and thin worms that are often confused with other microfilarial worms, previously presented. *D. medinensis* worms belong to the order Camallanida and the suborder Camallanina.

Morphology

Dracunculiasis is widely known as the guinea worm disease. The condition is caused by the larvae that penetrate the stomach and duodenum where they are circulated through the body and the large female of the nematode invades the tissues of the body. The organism emerges slowly and painfully from the skin, from sites usually on the lower limbs. The disease can infect animals but the animal cycles that occur in North America and Central Asia but do not act as reservoirs of human infection. Adult female worms may measure from 70 to 120 centimeters but are only about 2 millimeters in diameter. The male worm is but 2 centimeters in length and 0.4 millimeters in diameter.

Symptoms

Redness and inflammation may occur at the site where the adult worm emerges from the skin. No symptoms associated with the copecod vector occur until the blister forms where emergence will occur. At this time, fever and allergic reactions appear with intense itching and sometimes asthmatic symptoms may occur. Periorbital swelling may become obvious along with nausea and vomiting. The symptoms are moderate at the time the adult worm penetrates the skin and the blister bursts.

Life Cycle

The life cycle for *D. medinensis* is quite simple in comparison with some other parasitic organisms. Ingestion of unfiltered water containing the infected copecod of the genus *Cyclops*, a tiny water flea which harbors the infective larvae of *D. medinensis*, begins the reproductive cycle. These crustaceans are the intermediate host for the causative organism for the disease of dracunculiasis. After ingestion of the copecods, these hosts die and release the larvae which penetrate the digestive organs and enter the abdominal and retroperitoneal (kidney cavities). After copulation, the male dies and the gravid (pregnant) female approaches the surface of the skin of an infected individual where a blister forms, then ulcerates and exposes the worm. This process takes approximately a year to complete. Upon contact with fresh water, the female worm emerges upon which her uterus prolapses (dropping down of an internal organ) and extremely large numbers of first-stage larvae are released into the surrounding water. These larvae are fed upon by a particular species of *Cyclops*, the intermediate host, and in about a week or slightly longer, the larvae are infective for humans who may ingest dirty water containing the infected *Cyclops* crustaceans (Figure 4-23).

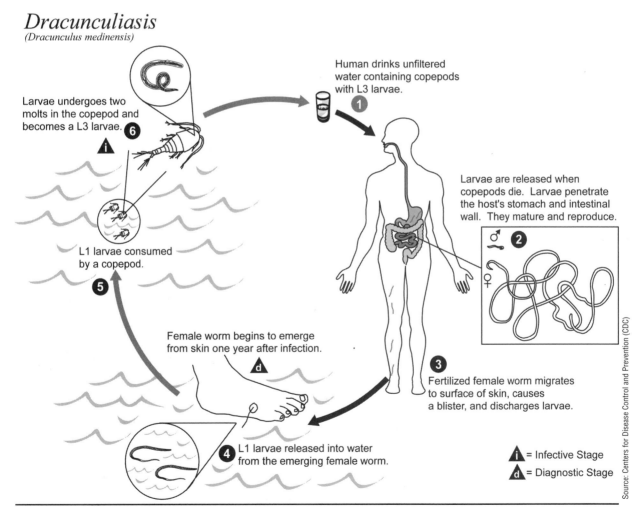

FIGURE 4-23 Life cycle of *D. medinensis*

Disease Transmission

The presence of dirty water from which humans obtain drinking water, such as step-down wells, cisterns to collect rain water, or open bodies of water, is required for transmission of the organism, producing dracunculiasis. The correct species of the genus *Cyclops* is essential for propagation of the population of infective larvae.

Laboratory Diagnosis

The best known organism of the genus *Dracunculus* is that of *D. medinensis*. This parasite is most commonly found in the subcutaneous tissues and muscles of humans and dogs, but may also be prevalent in herd animals. The condition dracunculiasis is characterized by open ulcers of the skin, particularly of the lower extremities. Identification of the disorder is accomplished chiefly by medical observation rather than a particular laboratory exam. At this point in the disease process, the caudal, or tail end, of the adult female worm begins to protrude from the host animal's body, frequently on the feet or other sites on a lower limb. The female is able to reproduce in the ulcerated area, after which she then releases an infective stage of her offspring into water, where the parasites can find new hosts.

D. insignis (also known as guinea worm, as well as *Dragon* or *Fiery Dragon*) is a species of this genus that infects dogs and wild carnivores, and like *D. medinensis*, also causes cutaneous lesions, ulcers, and sometimes heart and vertebral column lesions. The appearance of both species is much the same, and DNA testing is required to definitively differentiate between *D. medinensis* and *D. insignis*, a method necessary in order to effectively eradicate dracunculiasis.

D. medinensis may also infect the breast tissue, scrotum, or abdominal cavity. The adult female worm is quite large, and reaches lengths of up to 120 centimeters, or about 48 inches at the extreme (Figure 4-24). The male is somewhat smaller and lives in the subcutaneous tissues and are rarely seen, surviving only long enough, it is believed, to inseminate the female. No known animal reservoirs for this parasite exist, except for the *Cyclops,* which harbors the organism until the contaminated water is drunk. As a rule, all victims of this parasite have ingested water from a potentially infected source such as pools or ponds of standing water.

Treatment and Prevention

The traditional treatment for removing an adult *D. medinensis* worm consists of winding the worm slowly onto a small stick such as a match stick at a rate of only a few

MICROSCOPIC DIAGNOSTIC FEATURE

General Classification—Nematode (tissue)

Organism	*Drancunculus medinensis*
Specimen Required	Papule of loose connective body tissues from which organism is drawn
Stage	Adult
Size	70–120 cm by 2 mm in diameter
Shape	Round, slender, and extremely elongated
Motility	Relatively inactive as adult; movement toward emergence from the tissues of the body
Other Features	Off-white to pale yellow "worm" with pointed tail

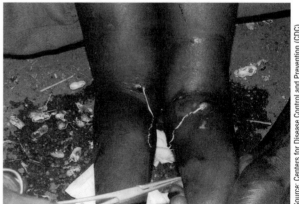

Source: Centers for Disease Control and Prevention (CDC)

FIGURE 4-24 Subcutaneous emergence of two female guinea worms, *D. medinensis*

inches per day to prevent breaking apart of the worm. This treatment is quite effective and is suitable for the geographic regions where the disease is endemic and living conditions are quite primitive. Medications such as metronidazole are effective in relieving symptoms but are not known to destroy the worm.

Prevention of the condition is possible by constructing facilities where safe drinking water and water for personal use can be obtained. This water may then be treated by chemicals and filtration to accomplish the goal of clean water. Water that may be contaminated with infected copecods should be boiled, filtered, or chemically treated. Global efforts by governmental agencies and private organizations have the potential of eventually eradicating the organism.

ONCHOCERCA VOLVULUS

Onchocerciasis is caused by the filarial nematode called *Onchocerca volvulus* which infects millions worldwide. The common name for onchocerciasis is "river blindness" based on the likelihood for blindness in those who are infected with *O. volvulus*. The condition is second only to trachoma, which is a disease resulting from an infection by *Chlamydia trachomatis*, in causing blindness on a worldwide basis. Those at risk for contracting onchocerciasis number into the tens of millions in 37 different countries spanning the continents and regions of Africa, Latin America, and the Saudi peninsula.

Morphology

The female worm may reach a length of 50 centimeters and measure one-half centimeter in diameter. The adult male is only about 5 centimeters in length and also is roughly one-half centimeter in diameter.

Symptoms

Clinical signs of the disease are pruritis (itching) and a rash. The skin may become swollen and painful, even increasing in temperature in the infected areas. Victims of the disease appear to be much older chronologically as the skin undergoes changes similar to aging. Loss of elasticity of the skin leaves a condition of thickened and wrinkled appearance. Sometimes pigmentation of the skin changes in response to the infection, particularly in the extremities.

But the most serious sign of the disease is visual damage, which is dependent upon the severity of the infections. Lesions occur in a part of the eye as migrating larvae invade the tissues there. When the dying microfilaria produce an acute inflammatory reaction, the sclera of the eye becomes opaque. Lymphadenopathy in both the inguinal and femoral areas may occur, leaving the victims at increased potential for hernias in the inguinal and femoral regions of the body.

Life Cycle

The infective larvae are transferred to a human host from a bite by one of the species of flies of the genus *Simulium*. During a period ranging from a half-year to 3 years following infection of a host, the female worms begin to produce microfilariae in nodules produced in the body, mostly in the dermis or subcutaneous tissues.

Disease Transmission

The disease is rampant and often devastating in the endemic areas populated mostly by agricultural settlements that are found on some of the most fertile farmland in the world, but the lands are sometimes abandoned due to the rate of infection of these residents. The organism is spread by the bite of the blackfly or the buffalo gnat of the genus *Simulium*, a vector that breeds in quickly flowing rivers and smaller streams.

Laboratory Diagnosis

Skin snips are used to determine the diagnosis of onchocerciasis from the skin biopsies. Tissue samples are placed in saline and the organisms are removed by use of microbiological needles in order to provide good visualization of the filarial. Microfilaria from this species are unsheathed and the nuclei do not extend to the tip of the tail as occurs in other species of microfilariae.

Treatment and Prevention

Ivermectin is a highly active antimicrofilarial drug and is furnished by the manufacturer at no cost in poor areas of the world. The medication does not actually kill the female worm but reduces the fertility of the female worms. Prednisone, a steroidal preparation, is used in the eyes to reduce the inflammatory reaction to the dying microfilariae.

Surgical extraction of the organisms from the eyes and head as they appear and treatment is available. Diethylcarbamazine is effective at killing the microfilariae, but side effects are considerable in heavy infections.

LOA LOA

Loa loa is the African eyeworm that is a species of filaria that resides in the subcutaneous tissues and conjunctiva (tissues around the eye). Approximately 3 million residents in Central Africa suffer from this condition, in which adult worms migrate through deeper tissues and into the conjunctiva of the eyes.

Morphology

Adult male worms average a range of 20 to 35 millimeters in length and 0.5 millimeters in diameter. The female adults are slightly longer in average size, and measure from 50 to 70 millimeters in length. Microfilariae are sheath-covered and are approximately 250 to 300 μm in length.

Symptoms

Localized inflammatory responses appear to be related to the host response to either the worm or its wastes from metabolic functions. Swollen areas as responses to the organism or its wastes are called *Calabar swellings*. These areas of edema may appear on any region of the body but are found mostly on the extremities. Localized lesions develop quickly and cause itching for several days. Lymphadenitis and moderate eosinophilia are also common. One important clinical sign is that of extreme eosinophilia, where 50 to 70 percent of the leukocytes of this type is common, with an average percentage for healthy individuals of only 5 to 7 percent.

Life Cycle

The vector for the disease organism is the *Chrysops* genus, known as mango or deer flies. The female bites the host and the infective larvae are injected into the wound site. After maturing, both the male and female adult worms migrate through subcutaneous and deep connective tissues. The microfilariae enter the vascular system and are found in the bloodstream predominantly at noon. The vector becomes infected when it feeds on the human host, the only host known for Loa loa, and ingests microfilariae. Development takes place in the thoracic muscles of the insect and in less than two weeks, the infective larvae appear in the mouth parts of the fly, which are then injected into another human host.

Disease Transmission

No environmental conditions give rise to the causative organism. The vectors (flies) must have access to infected hosts in order to transmit the organisms to others. Infective larvae are transferred to the human host by the *Chrysops* fly, and require 6 months or more for maturation. The worms move undetected through the subcutaneous layers of skin, and are seldom noticed in areas where the disease is endemic. Sometimes the first clue that a person is infected occurs when the larvae cause visual disturbances as they pass through the conjunctiva of the eye.

Laboratory Diagnosis

The microscopic study of blood samples is the simplest and most practical way of diagnosing Loa loa. Blood samples should be collected between 10 AM and 2 PM due to the diurnal cycle of the appearance of microfilaria in circulation. Thick and thin smears prepared and stained with Giemsa and sometimes concentration procedures are preferred. A sample of blood with 2 percent formalin as a fixative can be centrifuged and organisms will be concentrated into a small area. One basic feature of this species lies in the fact that nuclei will be visible to the tip of the tail, a characteristic valuable in differentiating between species of microfilariae.

Treatment and Prevention

Treatment includes surgical removal of the adult worm if seen in the conjunctiva of the eye or where it migrates near the skin's surface. Diethylcarbamazine is a therapeutic drug that kills both the adult worm and the filarial form. Drugs to combat inflammation are often used. Destroying or avoiding the vector is an effective way of preventing infections. Insecticides and protective clothing and clearing and draining of moist areas where the flies breed will accomplish a great deal in preventing infections.

MICROSCOPIC DIAGNOSTIC FEATURE

General Classification—Nematodes (tissue)

Organism	*Loa loa*
Specimen Required	Blood samples for microfilaria
Stage	Microfilaria are sheathed in stained specimens
Size	Adult males are 20–30 mm long; adult females are 50–70 mm in length
	Microfilariae are 250–300 μm in length
Shape	Ribbon-like and simple structure of head, body, tail regions
Nucleus(i)	Continuous to tip of tail
Other Features	Microfilaria are found most often in midday blood specimens as they are circulating to tissues

MANSONELLA STREPTOCERCA

Mansonella streptocerca also causes subcutaneous filariasis in humans, along with L. loa, O. volvulus, and D. medinensis, and is a common parasite of African rain forests. Because it may also be a parasite of chimpanzees, the pool of infected hosts may contribute to more widespread occurrences of infection.

Morphology

The adult worms of *M. streptocerca* produce microfilariae that measure 180 to 240 μm in length. The microfilariae are unsheathed and have body nuclei that extend to the tail's tip. The tip of the tail is called a "shepherd's crook" and appears as a partial coil.

Symptoms

Pruritis and poorly or hypopigmented macules are characteristic clinical signs and symptoms. Symptoms of arthralgia, fever, headaches, and hepatomegaly may occur but are attributed most frequently to infections by *Mansonella ozzardi*. Eosinophilia is often prominent in infections by all species of Mansonella. Inguinal adenopathy may also accompany an infection with *M. streptocerca*.

Life Cycle

The mature worms of *M. streptocerca* inhabit the layer of the dermis just beneath the exterior skin (around 1 mm). The microfilariae may be found in the skin and also in the circulating blood. Biting midges of the genus *Culicoides* are the vectors for this organism and there are two stages of the life cycle for *M. streptocerca*. The midge takes a blood meal from an infected host and ingests microfilariae into the midgut of the insect. The microfilariae then develop in the thoracic muscles of the midge into first-stage microfilariae larvae which travel to the midge's proboscis (biting apparatus). There it is capable of infecting a subsequent human host upon taking another blood meal ingestion, allowing a third-stage filarial larval form to enter the bite wound.

Disease Transmission

Streptocerciasis is acquired when bitten by an infected midge. An initial infection results in a pruritic dermatitis with hypopigmented (little associated color) macules. Streptocerciasis must be definitively identified, as other conditions including leprosy cause similar cutaneous symptoms and signs.

Laboratory Diagnosis

Infections with *M. streptocerca* should be suspected in patients from endemic areas or who have travelled there. Specific diagnosis may be made by finding microfilaria from skin snips or biopsies that are soaked in saline. Microfilariae are unsheathed and measure from 180 to 240 μm and possess body nuclei that reach the tip of a semicoiled tail.

Treatment and Prevention

Treatment is administration of the drug diethylcarbamazine and ivermectin has also shown promise as a treatment for the condition. But extreme itching of the skin

MICROSCOPIC DIAGNOSTIC FEATURE

General Classification—Nematode (tissue)	
Organism	*Mansonella streptocerca*
Specimen Required	Skin snips soaked in saline
Stage	Adult
Size	Adults are 180–240 μm in length
Shape	Unsheathed microfilariae
Body nuclei	Continuous in a single column to tip of tail
Other Features	Partial coil of tail is known as "shepherd's crook"

is a side effect of both of these drugs. In endemic areas, vector control would be advisable, but is rarely practiced. Insect repellent may prevent a great number of the bites but bed netting to prevent bites from the infected midges is not very effective as the midges are so small they can pass through the netting.

SEROUS CAVITY FILARIASIS

Two species of filarial parasites primarily infect the serous cavities of the human body. The two species that are considered to be parasites of serous cavities are: *Mansonella perstans* and *Mansonella ozzardi*. **Mansonella perstans** is another human filarial nematode transmitted by a fly called a midge, an extremely tiny bloodsucking fly. *Mansonella perstans* is one of the two parasites that lead to "serous cavity filariasis" in humans. *Mansonella ozardi* is the other parasite that produces serous cavity filariasis. Infections by *M. perstans* produce more benign conditions than those of *W. bancrofti, B. malayi,* and *Loa loa. Mansonella perstans* is prevalent in Sub-Saharan Africa, as well as areas of the New World (Central and South America, Caribbean) but both species occupy areas of the Congo River basin of West Africa.

MANSONELLA OZZARDI

Mansonella ozzardi is the only filarial infection by nematodes in the New World, and is found primarily in Central America and South America as well as in the Caribbean Islands. The organism invades the body cavities and the fatty tissue of the viscera and mesentery of and around the organs of the abdomen.

Morphology

The adult female worms of *M. ozzardi* measure 65 to 80 mm, whereas the male most often ranges from only 24 to 28 mm in length. The microfilariae are unsheathed but migrate through the tissues of the skin before entering the blood circulation. The larvae are nonperiodic and are roughly 88 μm in length.

Symptoms

Most victims of this infection are asymptomatic or experience rather mild symptoms. As with other filarial disorders, symptoms may be exaggerated in those who are not natives of the endemic area. Rarely, lymphadenopathy, fever, marked eosinophilia, pruritis, and skin lesions are experienced by the victims of *M. ozzardi* infections.

Life Cycle

The mature worms of *M. ozzardi* inhabit the mesentery and visceral fat surrounding the abdominal organs. The mature female worms produce unsheathed microfilariae, which migrate through tissues of the skin and enter the circulating blood, are ingested by the feeding midge (genus *Culicoides*) and are not periodic in their times of activity or appearance. In some regions, the blackflies (*Simulium*) are the primary vectors for the organism. Inside the insect the infective larvae ingested from the host undergo further development and are then passed on to the next host. Again, humans are the only known host for this organism.

Disease Transmission

M. perstans infection rates are high in endemic areas. The disease is acquired when bitten by an infected midge of the genus *Cullicoides,* except in the Amazon River basin where the vector is the blackfly.

Laboratory Diagnosis

The diagnosis of infections with *M. ozzardi* is primarily based on recovery of the unsheathed and nonperiodic microfilariae from blood specimens and skin snippings or biopsies for identification of the species. Thick and thin blood smears or centrifugal procedures for concentrating the parasites are also collected at any time of the day and prepared for examination.

Microfilariae of this species have nuclei that do not cover the entire length of the body to the tip of the tail, and they must be differentiated from the other blood-borne microfilariae.

Treatment and Prevention

Asymptomatic patients are not given therapy for the condition. Administration of the drug diethylcarbamazine is given three times per day for 10 days and has proven to be effective in eliminating larval microfilaria in patients who present with more serious clinical signs. In endemic area, insect repellent may prevent a great number of the bites. Again, bed netting to prevent bites from the infected midges is not very effective as the midges are so small they can pass through the netting. Eradication of breeding grounds in swampy areas and some other vector control processes have not proven effective in reducing the vector populations.

MANSONELLA PERSTANS

Mansonella perstans was previously known as *Dipetalonema streptocerca*, and is found in both humans and apes as a filarial infection. The infectious organism is found in most of central Africa and in the northeastern portion of South America. The organism resides primarily in the serous cavities of humans and apes.

Morphology

The adult worms of *M. perstans* are similar to those of *M. ozzardi*. The microfilariae are unsheathed but larger than *M. perstans,* measuring 190 to 200 μm and have body nuclei that extend to the tail's tip. The larvae are nonperiodic and appear at any time of the day. They have nuclei that extend to the tip of the tail.

Symptoms

Most victims of this infection are asymptomatic or experience rather mild symptoms. Calabar-like swellings have however been found in some cases. Where mature worms live in serous cavities, mild inflammatory changes may be noted in the host.

Life Cycle

The mature worms of *M. ozzardi* inhabit the serous cavities of the pleural, pericardial, and peritoneal regions of the body. The microfilariae (190 to 200 μm in length) are found in the circulating blood and are ingested by the feeding midge (genus *Culicoides*) and are not periodic in their times of activity or appearance.

Disease Transmission

M. perstans infection rates are high in endemic areas. The disease is acquired when bitten by an infected midge.

Laboratory Diagnosis

Infections with *M. perstans* may be accomplished through examination of blood or serosal effusions from body cavities. Blood samples are collected at any time of the day and prepared from skin snips or biopsies that are soaked in saline. Size is a chief criterion in differentiating the various species of bloodborne microfilaria along with other morphological characteristics. Because the disease may produce no symptoms or mild symptoms, the only clues for the infection by *M. perstans* may be an elevated serum antifilarial titer perhaps accompanied by considerable eosinophilia.

Treatment and Prevention

Administration of the drug diethylcarbamazine is standard treatment, but appears to be ineffective. Ivermectin also shows no activity against this infection. Metronidazole has been shown to be successful and is given for 30 days twice daily. In endemic areas, vector control would be advisable, but is rarely practiced. Insect repellent may prevent a great number of the bites but bed netting to prevent bites form the infected midges is not very effective as the midges are so small they can pass through the netting. Impregnation of protective clothing with permethrins appears to discourage bites from the midges.

SUMMARY

The varieties of parasites that infect cells of the blood are many. In addition, their life cycles are complex for many of them, and some stages may be lived outside the host and in the intermediate host. Examination of a stained smear with a combination of Wright-Giemsa or with Giemsa stain alone will yield the best information. Remember, the morphology of parasites is best seen with Giemsa stain, as the definition and clarity is not as good with Wright stain, which is best for blood cell morphology. These stains are useful for detecting various species of malaria *(Falciparum), Babesia, Trypanosoma, Leishmania*, and some species of microfilaria. Wet mounts are useful for certain characteristics observed in intracellular parasites, but permanent, fixed stains are also necessary for definitive identification. Thick smears, where the red blood cells are destroyed, are followed by stained, thin smears for most of these parasites.

Blood and other tissue flagellates include *Leishmania* and *Trypanosoma*, but these are quite different from the flagellated amoebae that may inhabit the intestines. A major difference is that a vector, an insect, is necessary for the transmission of these two organisms. *Trypanosoma cruzi* is the major organism of this genus and may include intracellular organisms in macrophages, liver cells, spleen cells, and bone marrow. Three major species of *Leishmania* exist, based on their geographic location. Dogs and various species of rodents are the reservoir hosts, whereas sandflies of two different genera are capable of transmitting the organism.

Malaria is the major category of parasitic infections that occur in the blood. These four species are prevalent based on their location, with *Plasmodium falciparum* as the major causative organism for the infection of humans. It should be remembered that there are many species of malaria, some of which are found in certain birds and animals, and are species from which humans possess natural immunity. The clinical symptoms of malaria are significant, with paroxysms of fever that include headaches, nausea, flulike sensations, and bone pain in more advanced cases. Fevers may cause shaking chills, followed by a fever of up to 40°C or 104°F. The fever cycle, along with blood smear examinations are useful in identifying species of malaria.

Babeosis is also a disease in which a number (more than 100) of various species exist. Only a few species, however, are responsible for the majority of disease from this organism, and vary by region. *Babesia microti* is primarily the species found in the northeast, the Midwest, and a couple of West Coast states. Another substantial contributor to this infection is blood transfusions and a few cases of intrauterine, transplacental transmission to fetuses. Babeosis is passed to humans through the bite of the deer tick, and symptoms are sometimes so mild as to be ignored, but fever, joint myalgia, arthralgia, nausea, and vomiting may be present.

Filarial worms and lymphatic filariasis sometimes cause a condition called elephantiasis. The superfamily *Filarioidea* contains a number of nematodal organisms that reside in tissues of the human body, of which the species *Wuchereria bancrofti* is the major infection causing the presence of microfilaria, or small roundworms. The larvae transmit the disease to humans most often through mosquito bites, but may also be transmitted by sand gnats, tabanid flies, blackflies, and other insects.

Another dreaded organism with widespread impact is that of the organism *Dracunculus medinensis*, which is known as the guinea worm. This parasite is common in the subcutaneous tissues and muscles of mostly humans and dogs. Dracunculiasis is a disease that causes cutaneous nodules which become open ulcers. At this time the caudal or tail end of the adult female worm begins to protrude from the host animal's body, most often involving the feet and lower limbs. The infective stage of the offspring of this organism is released into water, where the parasites can find new hosts.

CASE STUDIES

1. A middle-aged visitor recently arrived from the African continent for an extended visit in the United States with relatives. Her family became alarmed when she had extreme bouts of chills and fever that did not respond to aspirin or Tylenol. She was brought to the emergency department where blood samples were collected for both thin and tick smears. What would be the probable species of parasite involved in this medical condition?

2. Just before the fall semester began, two college sophomores from Connecticut decided to take a last break before beginning the rigors of study. After camping for a few days along the New England coast, they returned home to pack for a return to college. Two weeks after returning to college, both of the friends began suffering from a mild fever and headaches which were accompanied by fatigue. They had both heard of mononucleosis and made appointments at the student health center for potential treatment. Blood smears revealed intracellular inclusions that resembled malaria. What was the probable infective organism?

3. During the Desert Storm conflict, a number of National Guardsmen were deployed to northern Saudi Arabia and southern Iraq. They were issued an insect repellent but were eventually told not to use the material as it may be carcinogenic. Most of them reported numerous bites by sandflies, and a number of them had vague medical complaints upon returning to the United States, including sores on the skin, some of which extended into the subcutaneous tissues. With what condition would soldiers with these symptoms most likely be diagnosed?

4. After completing a veterinary assistant program, Julie obtained a position with a local veterinarian. The small animal practice involved a larger number of cats as patients. When Julie became pregnant, her obstetrician seemed concerned about her position where she had contact with cats, in particular. On what are his concerns founded?

5. A church group of college-age students from the southern United States organized a trip to Brazil. The purpose of the trip was to educate the natives of a remote village in the heavy forests of the country in matters of health and sanitation. Upon arrival, the group found no adequate housing, but a number of mud-walled thatched huts were empty and available for the two-week stay. Most of the meals were eaten outside as there were a number of insects with elongated bodies that could be easily seen near the tops of the mud walls. After a few nights, most of the students had reddened and itchy areas near the mouth, nose, and eyes. A topical ointment relieved most of the symptoms, but advanced medical care was not available in the village or even nearby. Shortly after returning to their homes, a number of those who had been on the trip to Brazil began to experience chills and fever. These symptoms were accompanied by glandular enlargement and a rash on the abdomen. Some complained of malaise and myalgia (muscle aches). One of the members of the church, a physician, suggested blood tests for all of those involved with the trip. What would be the most likely diagnosis obtained from these tests?

(continues)

CASE STUDIES (CONTINUED)

6. A recent undocumented immigrant from Guyana, on the northeastern coast of South America, visits the emergency room of a large hospital in the United States. He has vague symptoms and the only sign of disease is that of several localized areas that are inflamed and are manifested by pain and itching. Blood counts show a slight increase in the level of the percentage of a white blood cell called an eosinophil. Through an interpreter, the patient has experienced episodes of swelling in the extremities. What is the most likely cause of these signs and symptoms? Is the infection likely to occur in the United States?

7. A middle-aged Argentinian spent an extended vacation with relatives in the United States. While visiting, he developed a series of painful ulcers on his mucous membranes, particularly in the nose and mouth. He was taken to the family physician of his relatives and upon physical examination was found to have significant lymphadenopathy. Skin samples from the edges of some of the lesions revealed parasites when stained with Giemsa stain and examined microscopically. What is the probable name of this type of infection?

STUDY QUESTIONS

1. What do the terms *intercellular* and *intracellular* mean?

2. What are the symptoms of babeosis (sometimes are extremely mild)?

3. Why is the disease called leishmaniasis sometimes confused with malaria?

4. How is *Leishmania* transmitted?

5. What are the most common vectors of bacteria and other organisms in the world?

6. What are the four species of malaria that infect humans?

7. What kinds of organisms may be infected by the organism causing toxoplasmosis? What is the primary host for toxoplasmosis?

8. Oocysts are swallowed by a mouse, disseminated infection follows with resistant stages forming in the brain and the muscle; mouse is eaten by a cat and the life cycle reverts to basic sexual pattern; humans also eat meat infected with oocysts, contracting the disease.

9. In the Americas, *T. cruzi* is known to be spread mainly by the reduviid bug, Hemiptera, in Africa,

Gambian or chronic sleeping sickness, and *T. brucei rhodesiense* trypanosomes multiply in the blood and are taken up by tsetse flies when they feed.

10. Nematodes are threadlike, parasitic roundworms, usually small, that infect tissue and blood of humans and other animals.

11. Lymphatic, subcutaneous, and body cavity infections.

12. Lymphatic filariasis is caused by infection with the nematode worms *Wuchereria bancrofti*, *Brugia malayi*, and *B. timori*, all transmitted by mosquitoes. Microfilaria, particularly from *W. bancrofti*, affect the circulation of the extremities, called elephantiasis, where the lymph system is impacted, causing swelling of the legs, particularly, and also the scrotum.

13. Onchocerciasis is the name for the condition, and *Oncohocerca volvulus* is the cause.

14. Where was the parasite known as *D. medinensis* initially seen?

Epidemiology of Nematodes, Cestodes, and Trematodes

LEARNING OBJECTIVES

Upon completion of this chapter, the learner will be expected to:

- Describe in general terms the three classes of "worms" in the field of parasitology
- Relate the impact of hookworm infections on young children
- Describe the disease called bilharziasis and its origins
- Discuss the most common "worm" infection of children, with genus and species of organism
- Provide basic symptoms of a young child with an *E. vermicularis* infection

KEY TERMS

Anemia	Flukes	Mollusks
Arteriolitis	Fork-tailed cercariae	Perianal
Ascites	Granulomatous lesions	Periportal
Bilharziasis	Gravid proglottids	Platyhelminthes
Blood flukes	Ground itch	Progressive pernicious anemia
Cartilaginous	Helminthiases	Rhabditiform larva
Cercaria	Hematuria	Scolex
Cerebral cysticercosis	Hepatomegaly	Splenomegaly
Cestodes	Human hydatid disease	Swimmer's itch
Chlorosis	IgE	Teniasis
Cysticercosis	Lung fluke	Tetrachloroethylene
Dioecious	Lymphadenopathy	Thymol
Dysentery	Mesenteric veins	Tissue flukes
Embryonated eggs	Metacercariae	Urethral occlusion
Epsom salts	Miracidia	

INTRODUCTION

This chapter is intended to lay the groundwork for specific presentations of species of each of these three morphological types of "worms." The materials presented here basically discuss the history of major helminths and measures intended to eradicate them. Some of these parasites that inhabit various body organs have been well-known for centuries if not longer, and evidence of some of them exist in anthropological findings. When the student becomes acquainted in a general fashion regarding these types of parasites, it is easier to distinguish them as to general types during further studies in subsequent chapters. Some specific species are introduced in this chapter, but will be covered in depth later for information related to signs and symptoms, recovery of the organisms, and the identification of the various species.

The term *helminths* refers to worm-shaped organisms and are commonly referred to in lay terms as *worms* when one thinks of parasitic infections particularly of the gastrointestinal tract. There is a significant social impact placed on entire countries and regions of the world where these parasites are found. Ecological and environmental conditions that contribute to the increase of and prevalence of the "worms" are discussed in general in this chapter. Some of these organisms have complex life cycles that utilize a reservoir and a host in order to complete a life cycle and to infest other organisms. Some are even self-infective, where a human may serve in a manner as dual roles of both reservoir and host. Helminths consist of three basic groups: *round worm* (nematodes), *flat worm* (cestode), and *fluke* (trematode) (Table 5-1). These three groups are characterized by distinctive anatomic differences and will be discussed in general in this section.

TABLE 5-1 Classification of Helminths			
PHYLUM	**CLASS**	**ATTRIBUTES**	**EXAMPLES OF SPECIES**
Aschelminthes	Nematoda	Intestinal involvement of host	*Enterobius vermicularis* *Ascaris lumbricoides* *Trichuris trichiura (trichiura)* *Ancylostoma duodenale* *Necator americanus* *Strongyloides stercoralis*
		Blood and tissues	*Trichinella spiralis* *Wuchereria bancrofti* *Dracunculus medinensis* *Brugia* sp. *Loa loa* *Oncocerca volvulus* *Mansonella* sp.
Platyhelminthes	Trematoda		*Fasciolopsis buski* *Heterophyes heterophyes* *Metagonimus yokogawai* *Fasciola hepatica* *Clonorchis sinensis* *Paragonimus westermani* *Schistosoma* sp.
	Cestoda		*Diphyllobothrium latum* *Taenia* sp. *Hymenolepsis* sp. *Dipylidium caninum* *Echinococcus* sp.

NEMATODES

The phylum Nematoda is a class of the phylum Nemathelminthes and includes the true roundworms as well as those called *threadworms*. Six separate orders of Nematoda contain species that infect humans and other mammals, and it should be noted that a number of species also are capable of infecting plants and other forms of life, such as mollusks and insects. Of the parasitic roundworms that are able to infect humans, the hookworm is of the most medical importance and also is the most prevalent form of the roundworm found as a parasite of humans. The hookworm is a parasitic nematode worm that lives in the small intestine of its host, which may be a mammal, including dogs, cats, and humans. *Ancylostoma duodenale* is found primarily in northern Africa and India, whereas *Necator americanus* is chiefly confined to the so-called New World, which includes North and South America.

Until somewhat recently, *A. duodenale* was found routinely in southern Europe but efforts toward eradication there have greatly diminished the numbers of cases of infection by this parasite. By international organizational estimates, hookworms are thought to infect perhaps as many as 800 million people worldwide. Species other than *A. duodenale* and *N. americanus* exist but do not affect humans to any appreciable extent. The A. *braziliense* and A. *tubaeforme* species commonly infect cats, but are not known to infect humans. A. *caninum* infects mainly dogs but it is possible for this organism to infect humans, especially children who have close contact with dogs and their excrement (Figure 5-1).

Especially in a number of the developing countries of the tropics and subtropics, hookworm infections are considered to be a major cause for both maternal and child morbidity. Considerable attention has been paid to endemic regions where hookworm infections are prevalent. Children of these regions are particularly at risk because their future development and potential mental and physical advancement are often stymied. Physical and intellectual development characterized by cognitive retardation, stunting of growth, poor fetal development leading to long-term health problems in low birth weight and premature births are prevalent in mothers who suffer from hookworm infections.

One of the first symptoms to appear following infection by hookworms is dermatitis of the skin where

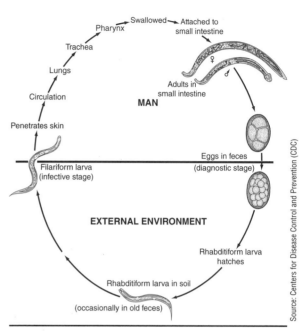

LIFE CYCLE of—

Hookworm

Source: Centers for Disease Control and Prevention (CDC)

FIGURE 5-1 Hookworm infection by direct contact with contaminated soil

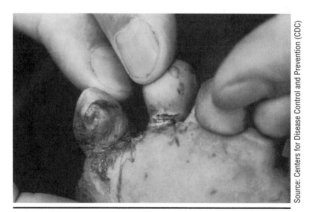

Source: Centers for Disease Control and Prevention (CDC)

FIGURE 5-2 Hookworm infection of toes the foot, also known as **"ground itch"**

the larvae penetrated the skin (Figure 5-2). Where sanitary facilities are not found in developing countries of the world, the organism enters the body through the feet, when the victim walks in contaminated soil. Seldom does death ensue even from heavy hookworm infections, but heavy economic and social costs are borne by the populations of the areas where hookworm infections abound. The inability of victims of this condition further exacerbate poor economic conditions and prevent further social development and improvement of the living conditions in the parts of the world where the diseases caused by hookworm infection are not controlled.

History of Hookworm Infections

As is the case for many other parasites, a number of symptoms are described in Egyptian literature from a century ago or more are similar to and could now be attributed to hookworm infestations. Some ancient physicians described conditions as a "derangement" accompanied by anemia. Over several hundred years, symptoms related to hookworm infection have been described in medical documents. In the case of Avicenna, a Persian physician from the eleventh century, the worm was discovered in several of his patients and the medical conditions of these patients were correctly attributed to an infection by a hookworm.

Several hundred years later, in 1880, after Avicenna's observations, a number of physicians correctly linked a hookworm infection to the conditions of diseased mine workers in the European countries of France; England; Germany; Belgium; and North Queensland, Australia. These workers, performing their tasks deep underground, were by nature forced to defecate inside the lengthy mining tunnels. Many of these miners were quite poor and wore worn-out shoes that exposed their feet to the contaminated ground and pooled water in areas where others had defecated.

Almost 20 years later, an epidemic of anemia and diarrhea among Italian workers constructing the Gotthard Rail Tunnel in Switzerland provided a breakthrough when it was confirmed that the skin was the major route of infection by hookworms. This knowledge, based on observations of those infected and the conditions under which they worked, led to the documentation that described the biological life cycle of the hookworm. Victims of hookworm infection suffered an initial skin rash that included signs of iron-deficiency anemia; nausea; abdominal pain; abdominal bloating; and pica, an abnormal craving for dirt to be ingested (Figure 5-3).

As is the case in much of medical research, a number of workers have contributed to the body of knowledge for many areas of health, including that of parasitology.

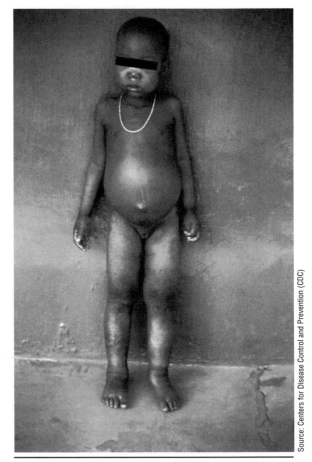

Source: Centers for Disease Control and Prevention (CDC)

FIGURE 5-3 Child with hookworm shows visible signs of edema, and was diagnosed with anemia

Prior to the definitive discoveries of hookworm infections and the signs and symptoms attributed to them in the latter decades of the 1880s, the Italian physician Angelo Dubini was credited with finding the worm during a postmortem exam of a peasant woman. The details of this discovery were published in 1843, and the name *A. duodenale* was no doubt due to the anatomic area of the body where the worm was found (duodenum). Upon finding numerous samples of these parasites when working in Egyptian medical facilities, a German physician named Theordor Bilharz in 1852 added to the body of knowledge of hookworm infection. Based on samples of these worms obtained during postmortem examinations (autopsies), he theorized that at least some of the occurrences of anemia found in the local region could be attributed to hookworm infections. The term used for anemia was *chlorosis,* which probably related to iron deficiency anemia, as it was attributed to low level of color of red blood cells, and is used today for a deficiency of chlorophyll in plants.

HOOKWORM INFECTIONS IN THE UNITED STATES

In 1899 an American zoologist named Charles Wardell Stiles, who was chief of the Division of Zoology of the U.S. Public Health Service, reported to the Pan-American Sanitary Congress that he had found the "germ of laziness" and that hookworm disease was common in the American South. Outdoor latrines and close proximity to contaminated soil by animals where rhabditiform larvae as a noninfective stage develop into filariform larvae are capable of infecting those coming in contact with the soil (Figure 5-4). Stiles, as a crusader for the health of the people of the South, identified the disease commonly called "progressive pernicious anemia" as being caused by *A. duodenale*.

But because *A. duodenale* is found primarily in northern Africa and India, the causative organism was most likely *N. americanus*, although African slaves could have brought the disease to the New World. Testing of school-age children in the 1900s revealed very heavy infestations in the group. Stiles noticed that the symptoms of the hookworm disease he saw in animals were similar to those of many poor Whites in the rural South. Stiles and Smith traded information by continually corresponding with each other as Stiles

made a trip through the Gulf-Atlantic states, hoping to confirm his theory that the poor medical conditions of many of the rural inhabitants were linked to hookworm infection.

Early Public Health Efforts Targeting Hookworm Infections

In 1902 Stiles made a strong case for an education campaign that he thought could be quite effective if implemented to completely solve the hookworm problem. So after several years of effort, Stiles was appointed in 1908 by President Theodore Roosevelt to the Country Life Commission, a group dedicated to improving farm life. At this time in U.S. history, farming was a way of life that occupied the majority of the population, and particularly so in the South. Through this appointment from the president, Stiles met Walter Hines Page, a southern crusader and journalist. Page had a working relationship with a number of members of the General Education Board, a philanthropic effort funded by industrialist John D. Rockefeller, and this coordination of a worthwhile project was successful.

With this impetus, John D. Rockefeller, Sr., bestowed a gift of one million dollars in the fall of 1909 to initiate an organization with a lofty title called the Rockefeller Sanitary Commission for the Eradication of Hookworm Disease. The result was a five-year program that proved to be a tremendous success for the public health of the United States. Efforts to eradicate hookworms were multipronged, and included public education, medication for those afflicted, field work to research effective projects, and the construction of modern government health departments in eleven southern states. But in the 1930s, an economically distressed period of time in the United States when the Great Depression reared its head, public officials again found that a great many children showed signs of hookworm due to a declining lifestyle.

Treatment of Hookworm Disease

Following efforts to rid the area where hookworms flourished in the warmer climates of the southern United States, the efforts were extended into the Caribbean nations and into Latin America in the 1920s. The move to

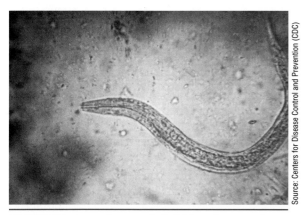

FIGURE 5-4 Hookworm rhabditiform larva, early, noninfectious immature stage

Source: Centers for Disease Control and Prevention (CDC)

remedy the widespread scourge of hookworm infections included the West Indies, where significant mortality rates were reported just before the end of the eighteenth century. The disease was also well established, as indicated by reports from Brazil and a number of other tropical and subtropical regions. Not only controlling the factors leading to contracting the disease and the spread of it, but treatment of existing infections was required to minimize the threat to new victims. Treatment from the turn of the century was with thymol, a mercury containing medication to kill the worms was used, followed by ingestion of Epsom salts to clear the body of the worms. Then, sometime later, a medication called tetrachloroethylene became available and replaced the thymol treatment as the preferred method for killing the organisms. In the mid-twentieth century new organic drug compounds that were even more effective and less toxic were developed and introduced for treatment of hookworm infections.

Many individuals with hookworm infection have no symptoms. Generally, very high loads of the parasite coupled with poor nutrition with inadequate intake of protein and iron will eventually lead to anemia. But many infected individuals are able to tolerate the condition for years while needlessly passing on the infection and showing no ill effects of the infection themselves. The symptoms can be linked to inflammation in the gut stimulated by feeding hookworms which is accompanied by nausea, abdominal pain, and intermittent diarrhea early in the disease, with progressive anemia occurring in prolonged disease. Old folk remedies were often followed, particularly in the southeastern United States. Impulsive eating of certain materials, perhaps accompanied by unreasonable desires for certain materials, such as pica (or dirt-eating) are present in some. Others exhibit prolonged constipation followed by diarrhea, heart palpitations from severe anemia, thready (weak) pulse, coldness of the skin, pallor of the mucous membranes, fatigue and weakness, and shortness of breath often occur in long-standing cases. Extremely grave medical conditions, including dysentery, hemorrhage, and edema, may culminate in eventual death.

In contrast to most intestinal **helminthiases**, where the heaviest parasitic loads tend to occur in children, hookworm prevalence and intensity can be even higher among adult males. The explanation for this is that hookworm infection tends to be occupational, so that plantation workers, coal miners, and other groups maintain a high prevalence of infection among themselves by contaminating their own personal work environment. However, in most endemic areas, adult women are the most severely affected by the accompanying anemia, mainly because they have much higher physiological needs for iron with regular menstrual cycles, repeated pregnancies, and also because they customarily have less access to adequate food than do men.

Life Cycle for Hookworms

This image for the biological life cycle of the hookworms is in areas where the organism thrives in warm earth with surrounding temperatures of over 18°C. Acid soil such as red clay or in muck found in much of the southern United States is not conducive to the survival of hookworm larvae. Hookworm larvae exist for the most part in sandy or loam soils. A rainfall average of more than 40 inches per year is almost mandatory for the reproduction of hookworms where a stage of the life cycle includes larvae that remain in the soil for a period of time. These environmental conditions are certainly met in many areas of the United States, especially the southeastern part of the North American continent and in other parts of the world. Eggs will not hatch if these conditions are not minimally met.

There is also a difference in survival of the two major species of the hookworm. Infective larvae of *N. americanus* can survive at higher temperatures than those of *A. duodenale*. This perhaps accounts for the fact that *N. americanus* is primarily found in the temperate zones of the southeastern United States and nearby regions, whereas *A. duodenale* is confined to Europe where the climate is cooler. As a general rule, these larvae live for only a few weeks in natural conditions suitable for their survival, and will die within a short time if exposed to direct sunlight, or if the conditions are too dry for the infective stage of the larvae. So as the United States and in particular the rural South moved from an agrarian society where almost everyone initially lived in close proximity to the soil and often raised animals, the incidence of these infestations have been greatly diminished. Diagnosis may be made by finding ova in the stool specimen of a victim, but *A. duodenale* and *N. americanus* are

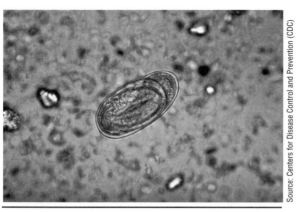

Source: Centers for Disease Control and Prevention (CDC)

FIGURE 5-5 Embryonated egg is indistinguishable between the *Ancylostoma duodenale* or *Necator americanus* hookworm

impossible to differentiate by examining the eggs of the two species (Figure 5-5).

CESTODES (TAPEWORMS)

The most important cestodes of clinical interest and that are pathogenic to man are *Taenia solium* (pork tapeworm), *T. saginata* (beef tapeworm), *Diphyllobothrium latum* (fish or broad tapeworm), *Hymenolepis nana* (dwarf tapeworm), and *Echinococcus granulosus* and *E. multilocularis* (hydatid). As is readily apparent from the names of some of them, these parasites are chiefly contracted through the diet and from contact with animals and their excrement. Infective larvae are able to infect the host by eating contaminated raw or undercooked meat, fish, or grains, depending upon the species of the parasite in question. *Taenia solium* cysticercosis or *Hymenolepsis nana* can be transmitted in a direct cycle via ingestion of eggs from human feces. *Echinococcus* eggs primarily from dog or fox hair cause **human hydatid disease** with humans as the intermediate host and with members of the canine family (dog and fox) as the definitive hosts. Reinfection with adult tapeworms is common but second infections with larvae are rare, which may be due to an immune response to the larvae stages of the parasite.

Epidemiology of Cestodal Infections

Epidemiologically, cestodes commonly found in humans have a worldwide distribution regardless of climate and environmental conditions. The general term in use where an infection by tapeworms has occurred is **taeniasis**. However, the incidence of a cestode infection is higher in developing countries, for obvious reasons such as the lack of sanitation and of food safety laws for protection of human health. The infection rate is lowest in North America, at approximately 1 infected person per 1,000 in most of North America. But the infection rate may be as high as 10 percent of the population in the poorest and least developed parts of the world. The pork tapeworm shows a higher rate of incidence than any of the others. But this is dependent on dietary habits because pigs are a main source of meat almost universally and may be raised in close proximity to dwellings in most of the population centers of the world.

Taenia solium, T. saginata (Taeniasis)

Unlike those of a number of other species of parasites, the eggs (ova) of the two species of the genus *Taenia* are virtually indistinguishable from each other. But fortunately for the medical laboratory professional or the parasitologist, identification of the two species is made possible by observing certain characteristic features of each of the adult forms and is accomplished as follows. **Gravid proglottids** (pregnant) are longer than they are wide in the two species. But *T. solium* and *T. saginata* differ in the number of primary lateral uterine branches as *T. solium* has only 7 to 13 lateral branches, whereas *T. saginata* possesses 12 to 30 lateral branches of the proglottid. Due to a slight overlap in the numbers of lateral branches, it is often necessary to examine several representative segments before arriving at a definitive identification. Adults of *Taenia* spp. can reach a length of 2 to 8 meters, but the hooked **scolex**, located at the head region, is only 1 to 2 millimeters in diameter. Humans are the only definitive hosts in the life cycle of these two tapeworm species (Figure 5-6).

Life Cycle of Tapeworms

Larval cysts of the tapeworm (cysticerci) are ingested with poorly cooked infected meat that contains these cysts and may lead to a disease generally called *cysticercosis*. Upon ingestion, the larvae escape the cysts and pass to the small intestine where they attach to the mucosa by the scolex

Cysticercosis

(Taenia spp.)

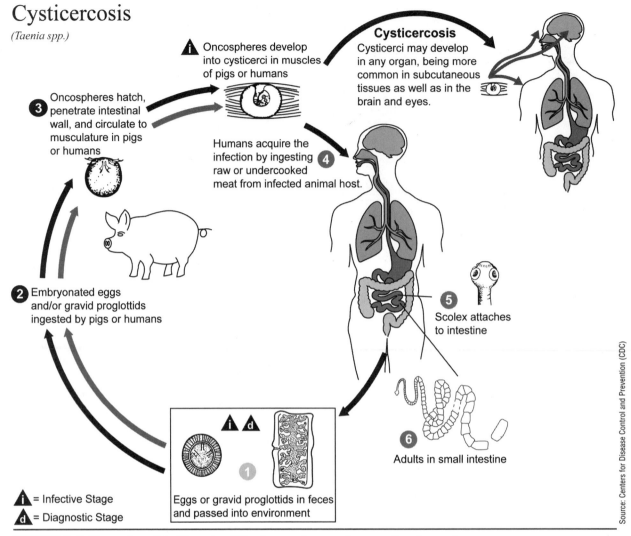

Cysticercosis
Cysticerci may develop in any organ, being more common in subcutaneous tissues as well as in the brain and eyes.

ⓘ Oncospheres develop into cysticerci in muscles of pigs or humans

3 Oncospheres hatch, penetrate intestinal wall, and circulate to musculature in pigs or humans

Humans acquire the infection by ingesting raw or undercooked meat from infected animal host. **4**

2 Embryonated eggs and/or gravid proglottids ingested by pigs or humans

5 Scolex attaches to intestine

6 Adults in small intestine

1 Eggs or gravid proglottids in feces and passed into environment

ⓘ = Infective Stage

ⓓ = Diagnostic Stage

Source: Centers for Disease Control and Prevention (CDC)

FIGURE 5-6 Illustration of the life cycle of *Taenia* spp., the causal agents of cysticercosis

suckers. The proglottids develop as the worm matures in the intestines over a period of 3 to 4 months. The adult tapeworm may live in the small intestine as long as 25 years and pass gravid (pregnant) proglottids with the feces (Figure 5-7). Eggs produced by the proglottids can persist on vegetation for several days and may be consumed by cattle or pigs, in which they hatch and form cysticerci, which may then be passed to other animals.

Cysticercosis

The symptoms for the disease vary with the intensity of the infection. Light infections may remain asymptomatic,

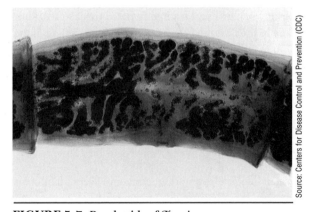

Source: Centers for Disease Control and Prevention (CDC)

FIGURE 5-7 Proglottids of *Taenia* spp.

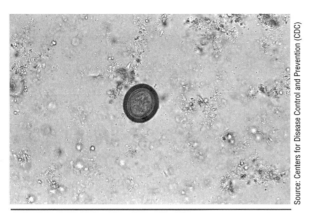

FIGURE 5-8 Eggs of two *Taenia* spp. species, *T. solium* and *T. saginata*, are indistinguishable from each other

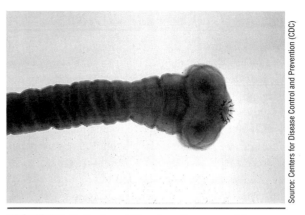

FIGURE 5-9 Scolex of *Taenia solium* cestodal tapeworm

whereas heavier infections may produce abdominal discomfort, epigastric pain, vomiting, and diarrhea. *T. solium* eggs can also infect humans and cause cysticercosis (larval cysts in lung, liver, eye, and brain), resulting in blindness and neurological disorders (Figure 5-8). The incidence of cerebral cysticercosis can be as high as 1 per 1,000 population and may account for up to 20 percent of neurological case in some countries (e.g., Mexico); cysticercosis ocular involvement occurs in about 2.5 percent of patients and muscular involvement is as high as 10 percent (India).

Prevention and control of cestodal infections requires proper harvesting, treatment, and storage of meat. A thorough inspection of beef and pork and adequate cooking or freezing of meat are effective precautions against transmitting the disease through the distribution of food, because cysticerci do not survive temperatures below –10°C and above 50°C. Treatment of breeding stock and exercising care in procuring food for these animals will aid greatly in controlling outbreaks. For an infected person, praziquantel is the drug of choice. Passage of the scolex or head of the tapeworm from the intestines must be accomplished in order to confirm a satisfactory treatment (Figure 5-9).

Pathology and Immunology of Tapeworm Infections

Gastrointestinal symptoms are due to the presence of the tapeworm. Cysticercosis symptoms are a result of inflammatory/immune responses. The chief method for diagnosing infestation with tapeworms is based on the recovery and identification of eggs by microscopy or visible proglottids in stool specimens or from the perianal area. Antibodies are also produced against the organisms found in cysticercosis and are useful epidemiological tools by immunological testing as an indirect method of identifying the causative organism. Cysticercosis may be confirmed by the presence of antibodies against the specific organism as a definitive diagnosis.

As members of the Platyhelminths, the cestodes, or tapeworms, possess many basic structural characteristics of flukes, but also show substantial differences. The single most striking difference, however, is that the cestodes consist of segments called *proglottids* and those of the flukes do not. And whereas flukes are flattened and generally leaf-shaped, adult tapeworms are flattened and elongated. In addition, tapeworms differ from flukes in that they may be quite long as they vary in length from 2 to 3 mm to 10 m, and may have as few as three segments up to several thousand segments. Edward Tyson, a British scientist and physician, was the first to recognize that the tapered end of the worm was the head. Although Tyson mainly concentrated on the roundworm called *Ascaris lumbricoides*, he contributed the first detailed work on the morphology of the tapeworms, or cestodes, of humans. His work can be considered as marking the beginning of a subdiscipline of parasitology called *helminthology*, which reached a peak in the nineteenth century. It was also during this period that the first real attempts were made to understand the infections caused by the various parasites and methods of diagnosis and treatment.

TREMATODES (FLATWORMS)

The class Trematoda is estimated to contain 18,000 or more species that are divided into two subclasses. These subclasses include Aspidogastrea and Digenea. Aspidogastrea, the smaller of the two, contains approximately 80 species. Digenea is the subclass that contains the majority of the diverse forms of trematodes. Nearly all trematodes are parasites of either **mollusks** or vertebrates (organisms with a backbone) but in some rare instances may infect cartilaginous fish which when poorly cooked or eaten raw may infect humans. All trematodes are parasitic but not all species are found in humans; mammals are the host for infections by these flatworms.

Life Cycle of Trematodes

Trematodes have characteristically complex life cycles and the larval form may inhabit different life forms than those where the adult trematode will parasitize as an adult. The most often recovered parasites from the class Trematoda are those of the liver fluke and the blood fluke, both of which commonly parasitize humans. The flukes, regardless of species, follow a similar path toward development into adults and the manner in which they reproduce.

When the adult fluke is living in the organs of a mammal for which it is adapted, eggs are produced as an immature stage. A female fluke may produce as many as three hundred eggs per day. These eggs pass from the digestive tract of their mammalian host into the water where they further develop. Following hatching of the eggs, a larval form called a **miracidium**, a free-swimming stage, will search for a snail as a suitable host. Almost all trematodes infect mollusks such as the aquatic snail in the first life cycle of infecting an intermediate host (Figure 5-10). The snail is the intermediate host and the larvae live in the blood vessels of the intermediate host until they are released from the intermediate host's body in either the urine or feces, dependent upon the species of the parasite.

While inhabiting the intermediate host, the fluke goes through a number of stages in their development into an adult. In the sporocyst stage, these cells divide quickly and the resulting sporocysts, called **rediae**, will become larvae. These parasitic larvae called **cercariae** develop in the mollusk host and will progress through stages called **mesocercaria** or **metacercaria** toward the adult form. These metacercariae may also become encysted in the skin or tissue of freshwater fish and is the route by which most humans become infected. Fish is a staple in the diet of those living in parts of Africa, Asia, South America, and the Middle East, where infections from fish carrying the parasite are contracted. In most species of flukes, the metacercariae will then become enclosed in a cyst and will survive on the surface of the water, except for the blood fluke (genus Schistosoma) which does not undergo this stage.

These cysts will become attached to vegetation and a mammal eats the vegetation that includes the cysts. In the digestive system of the mammal, the larvae will leave the ingested cyst and will pass through the intestinal walls and migrate to the specific organ which the particular species has an affinity for. While in the organ, the immature form of the fluke continues to develop into an adult capable of laying eggs. Blood flukes differ from the path where mammals eat infected water vegetation, as they become free-swimming cercariae and penetrate the skin of a host mammal, upon which they will reach the circulatory system of their hosts.

Flukes are often named by the environment in which they are found or by the primary host infected by the parasites. Some flukes are called "pond flukes," as they infect fish found in ponds. Tissue flukes infect the bile ducts, lungs, and many other specific organs. *Paragonimus westermani* is known as the lung fluke, and both *Fasciola hepatica* and *Clonorchis* sinensis are known as liver flukes. **Blood flukes** inhabit the circulatory system of mammals during some stages of their life respective cycles. The most significant trematodes from a clinical point of view may be the blood flukes *Schistosoma mansoni*, *S. japonicum*, and *S. hematobium*.

Schistosomiasis (Bilharziasis)

The three species of *Schistosoma* have different geographic distributions. *S. hematobium* is prevalent in Africa where the disease caused by the organism is called bilharziasis, and *S. mansoni* is primarily found in Africa and South America as well as some Caribbean islands. *S. japonicum* is more common in the Far East. It is estimated that up to 250 million people may be infected with the various species of schistosomes and 600 million more may be at risk due to contact with contaminated water in several areas of the world but primarily in Asia. The morphology of the adult worms is characteristic.

Opisthorchiasis
(Opisthorchis viverrini, O. felineus)

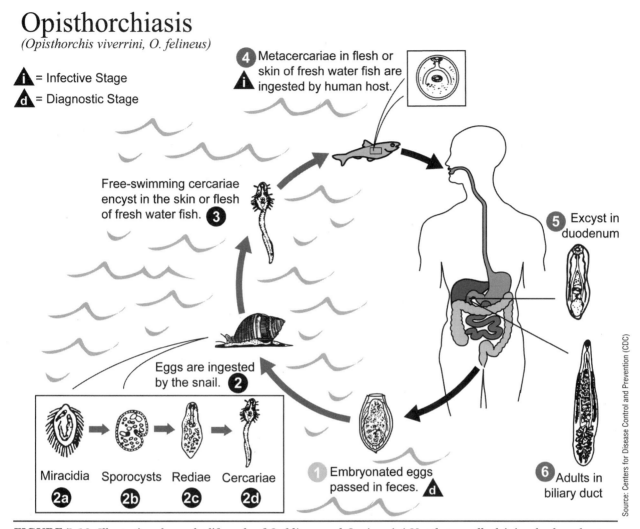

ⓘ = Infective Stage

ⓓ = Diagnostic Stage

4 Metacercariae in flesh or skin of fresh water fish are ingested by human host.

Free-swimming cercariae encyst in the skin or flesh of fresh water fish. **3**

5 Excyst in duodenum

Eggs are ingested by the snail. **2**

Miracidia **2a** Sporocysts **2b** Rediae **2c** Cercariae **2d**

1 Embryonated eggs passed in feces. **ⓓ**

6 Adults in biliary duct

Source: Centers for Disease Control and Prevention (CDC)

FIGURE 5-10 Illustration shows the life cycle of *O. felineus* and *O. viverrini*. Not that a mollusk is involved as a host

Adult worms are 10 to 20 mm long; the male has an unusual lamelliform (arranged in thin plates or scales) shape with marginal folds forming a canal in which the slender female worm resides. Unlike other trematodes, schistosomes may be divided by gender as they have separate sexes.

Life Cycle of Schistosomes

The life cycle of the schistosomes require fresh water in order to infect a host; interior lakes in the endemic areas of the world are often contaminated (Figure 5-11). Man is infected by cercaria in fresh water by skin penetration. After entering the body, the cercaria travel through the venous vessels of their human hosts to the heart, lungs, and portal routes of circulation. In about three weeks these forms mature and reach the mesenteric (*S. japonicum* and *S. mansoni*) or the bladder (*S. hematobium*) vessels where they live and ovulate for the duration of the host's life. Eggs germinate as they pass through the vessel wall into the intestine or bladder and are excreted in feces (*S. japonicum* and *S. mansoni*) or urine (*S. hematobium*). When in fresh water the larval miracidia hatch out of the egg and swim about until they find an appropriate snail. After two generations of multiplication in the snail, the fork-tailed cercariae emerge into the water and infect another human.

Symptoms may initially be merely a nuisance and scarcely noticed. Penetration by the cercariae may cause transient dermatitis (swimmer's itch). The symptoms

Schistosomiasis

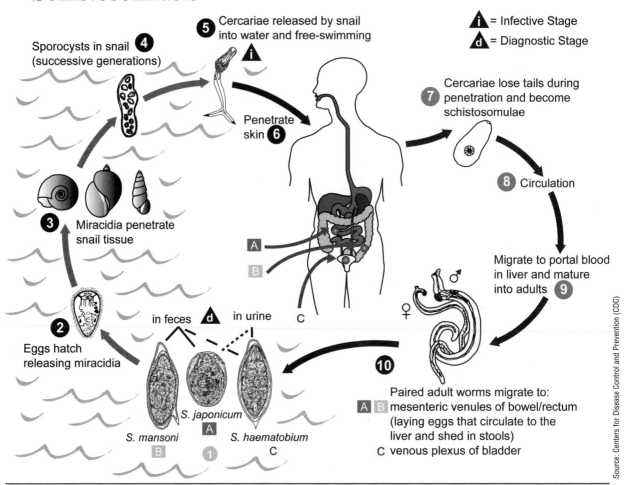

FIGURE 5-11 Illustration of the life cycle of the parasitic agents responsible for causing schistosomiasis

of schistosomiasis are primarily due to an allergic type reaction against the eggs and include splenomegaly (spleen enlargement), diarrhea, and lymphadenopathy. In the bladder they produce granulomatous lesions, hematuria, and sometimes urethral occlusion (Figure 5-12). Chronic infections with schistosomes may cause bladder cancers in endemic areas. In the intestine they cause polyp formation and in severe cases may result in life-threatening dysentery. In the liver the eggs cause periportal fibrosis and portal hypertension resulting in hepatomegaly, splenomegaly, and ascites. A gross enlargement of the esophageal and gastric veins may result in their rupture. *S. japonicum* eggs are sometimes carried to the central nervous system and can cause headache, disorientation, amnesia, and even coma.

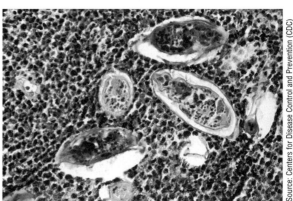

FIGURE 5-12 Histopathology of bladder shows eggs of *Schistosoma haematobium* with large numbers of eosinophils

Eggs carried to the heart produce arteriolitis (small vessel inflammation) and fibrosis resulting in enlargement and failure of the right ventricle. As in other parasitic infections, the infiltration of tissues of the body serve to stimulate production of large numbers of white blood cells called *eosinophils* which are produced during serious allergic responses.

Pathological reactions are stimulated by the cercaria upon contact with a potential host. The swimmer's itch is due to physical damage to the skin by proteases and other toxic substances secreted by the invading cercaria. A severe immunological reaction by the host may lead to severe hypersensitivity (allergic) reactions to schistosomal secretions and egg constituents. Embryonated eggs cause collagenase-mediated damage to the vascular endothelium. Host immune responses, both humoral (blood plasma antibodies) and cell mediated, have been shown to be of some protective value. IgE (immune globulin increased in allergic reactions) and eosinophil-mediated cytotoxicity have been hypothesized as a means of killing the adult worm.

Diagnosis of Schistosomiasis

The diagnosis is based on a history of residence in or travel to an endemic area, the development of swimmer's itch, or other symptoms. The eggs of each of the schistosomes are particularly characteristic and are used to confirm diagnosis. *S. hematobium* eggs in urine (55 to 65 by 110 to 170 µm) have an apical spine or knob. *S. mansoni* eggs in feces (45 to 70 by 115 to 175 µm) have a spine on the side. *S. japonicum* eggs (55 to 65 by 70 to 100 µm) are rounder than the other two of this genus, and possess a vague spine on the side (Figure 5-13). In order to prevent and control schistosomiasis, contaminated water should be avoided. All fresh water bodies in endemic areas should be avoided, as the possibility of contamination is high. Control measures include sanitary disposal of sewage that includes urine and the destruction of species of snails capable or being hosts. Medications are available to control the infection but there is no specific inoculation available to prevent becoming infected.

The egg of the *Schistosoma haematobium* trematode parasite has a unique posteriorly protruding, terminal spine unlike the vestigial remnant protruding from the lateral wall of the *Schistosoma japonicum* egg (Figure 5-14). These eggs are eliminated in an infected

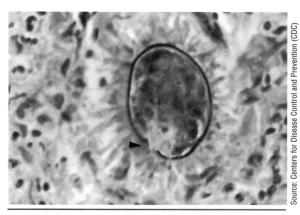

FIGURE 5-13 *Schistosoma japonicum egg*, and its vestigial spine (arrow) taken from a liver tissue biopsy. Eggs are smaller (55–65 µm by 70-100 µm) than those of the other species

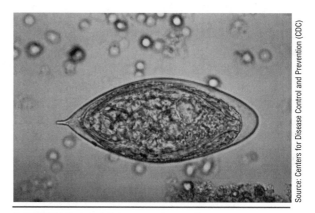

FIGURE 5-14 *Schistosoma hematobium* egg's posteriorly protruding, terminal spine

human's feces or urine, and under optimal conditions in a watery environment, the eggs hatch and release "miracidia," which then penetrate a specific snail intermediate host. Once inside the host, the *S. haematobium* parasite passes through two developmental generations of sporocysts and are released by the snail into its environment as "cercariae" (Figure 5-15).

Schistosoma mansoni parasites are found primarily in most areas of Africa and in tropical America, particularly the West Indies. Mesenteric veins of the connections of the small intestine to the posterior abdominal membranes lining the cavity provide an anatomic site for these organisms to colonize. Eggs may be emitted through either the bladder or through the intestine (Figure 5-16). *S. mansoni* eggs are larger than those of

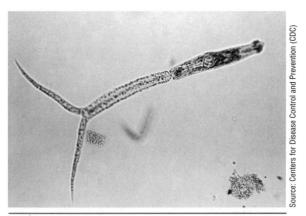

Source: Centers for Disease Control and Prevention (CDC)

FIGURE 5-15 Schistosomal cercaria, which is the larval stage of a parasite that causes swimmers' itch

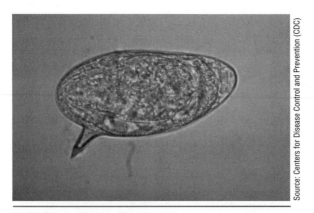

Source: Centers for Disease Control and Prevention (CDC)

FIGURE 5-16 Egg from *Schistosoma mansoni*

S. hematobium and *S. japonicum* and measure 115 μm to 175 μm as an average in length for these species. But other than the size, the greatest differentiating characteristic is that of its shape, with its very prominent lateral spine near their posterior end. The anterior end is tapered, as well as slightly curved.

Life Cycle of Pinworms

All parasites, including those termed as *worms*, require a host in order to survive. In the case of pinworms, the human serves as the host. The life cycle of a pinworm is quite simple in comparison with other parasitic organisms. Infections originate with the soiled fingers being placed in the mouth or when pinworm eggs are eaten, usually directly by contaminated hands or indirectly through contaminated food, bedding, clothing, or other personal items. The eggs are swallowed into the intestines where they hatch and mature. An adult pinworm is yellowish to white, somewhat slender, and is slightly less than one-half inch in length. The worms are readily visible in the feces of children with heavy infections.

Approximately one month following infestation of the gut, the adult female will move down the intestinal system and will exit the body through the anus. There she lays a batch of several hundred eggs on the skin surrounding the anus, usually during the night or early in the morning before light enters the bedroom. Upon depositing her eggs, the female pinworm has fulfilled her purpose in life so she then dies. Severe itching often accompanies the laying of the eggs, especially at night. In this way children are able to reinfect themselves by soiling their fingers and also accumulating eggs on the fingers and under the nails from the bed linens. The cycle of reproduction by transfer of the eggs to the mouth where they are again swallowed ensures a steady source of infection is present. Also, the eggs may remain viable for up to several days if the conditions are suitable.

SUMMARY

The organisms commonly called "worms" actually include three different morphological group, called nematodes, cestodes, and trematodes. Besides amoebal infections of the gastrointestinal tract, worms are a major contributor also. Nematodes are roundworms that include the much smaller threadworms with the major roundworm groups being the hookworms. The hookworm species of *Ancylostoma duodenale* are found almost exclusively in northern Africa and India, whereas the *Necator americanus* species is the main species seen in North and South America. The A. *braziliense* and A. *tubaeforme* species infect only cats but not humans, whereas A. *caninum* infects mainly dogs but sometimes humans, especially children.

Illnesses resulting from nematodal infections with a number of organisms called hookworms often include generalized anemia and the appearance of not being well. Hookworm infections are often merely referred to as "worms" or a symptom such as urticaria or itching of the skin.

Beginning just before and into the early part of the twentieth century, the U.S. Public Health Service concluded that the "germ of laziness" associated with hookworm disease had been found as a common malady in the American South. Progressive pernicious anemia seen in the southern United States was found to be caused by *A. duodenale*, and testing of schoolchildren in the 1900s showed heavy infections in the group. An investigator also noticed that symptoms of the hookworm disease in animals were similar to those of many poor Whites in the rural South. Philanthropist efforts by the industrialist John D. Rockefeller and President Theodore Roosevelt worked to diminish the rate of parasitic infections in the rural population through the Country Life Commission. Efforts to improve farm life through general sanitation and awareness of means for preventing the diseases began to bear fruit by a lessening of the cases of hookworm infections and resulting diseases.

But in the 1930s, during the Great Depression, public officials again found that many children again showed signs of hookworm. In the 1920s, a hookworm eradication program in the United States spread to the Caribbean and Latin American countries where well-established epidemics, particularly in Brazil, prevailed. Both control of new cases and treatment of existing cases were necessary.

Not only children but adult males who work in contaminated soil of farms and with a variety of farm animals were often heavily affected by hookworm infections. This life cycle for hookworms requires warm and sandy or loamy soil with substantial rainfall, conditions met in many areas of the United States. Infective larvae of *Necator americanus* survive at higher temperatures than *Ancylostoma duodenale* so the cooler climates of Europe are more favorable for propagation of *A. duodenale*.

The most important cestodes are the tapeworms *Taenia solium* (pork tapeworm), *T. saginata* (beef tapeworm), *Diphyllobothrium latum* (fish or broad tapeworm), *Hymenolepis nana* (dwarf tapeworm), and *Echinococcus granulosus* and *E. multilocularis* (hydatid). Diet and contact with animal excrement pose the greatest risks, where larvae infect a host by eating contaminated raw or undercooked meat, fish, or grains. *Taenia solium* cysticercosis or *Hymenolepis nana* are directly transmitted through ingestion of eggs from human feces and *Echinococcus* eggs come primarily from the definitive hosts, dog or fox, with humans as the intermediate host. Reinfection with adult tapeworms is common but second infections with larvae are rare, apparently due to developed immunity. There are literally thousands of trematodes, divided into two subclasses. The smaller subclass, Aspidogastrea, includes about 100 species as obligate parasites of mollusks that may also infect turtles and fish, including cartilaginous fish. The other subclass, Digenea, which shows the most trematode diversity, is obligate parasites of both mollusks and vertebrates and occasionally of cartilaginous fish.

Trematodes are known commonly as flukes and in the definitive host the eggs are shed along with feces from the host. Eggs shed in water release free-swimming larval forms infective to the intermediate host, where asexual reproduction occurs. Both tissue flukes that infect organs and systems of the body, and blood flukes are two major divisions of the trematodes. Blood flukes inhabit the blood in some stages of their life cycle and include the three main species of the genus *Schistosoma*: *Schistosoma mansoni*, *S. japonicum* and *S. hematobium*.

The life cycles of some of these flukes are complex, and may also be classified according to the environment in which they are found. The life cycle of schistosomes require fresh water in order to infect a host, so interior lakes in the endemic areas of the world are often contaminated. Humans become infected by cercaria from miracidia that infected the snails found in fresh water, where these cercaria penetrate the skin and travel through the blood vessels of their human hosts to the heart, lungs, and portal routes of circulation.

Severe symptoms and signs are routinely found that range from a mere nuisance splenomegaly (spleen enlargement), diarrhea, and lymphadenopathy. In the bladder, granulomatous lesions, hematuria, and sometimes urethral occlusion occur, perhaps leading to bladder cancer in chronic cases. In the intestine, polyps may form that result in life threatening dysentery. In the liver, the eggs cause periportal fibrosis and portal hypertension, resulting in hepatomegaly, splenomegaly, and ascites (swelling and distention of the belly).

CASE STUDIES

1. A young enlisted sailor has been living on the local economy in Thailand while attached to a U.S. embassy. Two months after his posting at the facility, he reported to the medical treatment facility complaining of diarrhea and somewhat severe abdominal pain. A stool specimen was cultured for pathogenic bacteria and yielded normal results. Upon his return to the treatment area an additional stool specimen was obtained and examined microscopically. Large operculated eggs that were broad and elliptical in shape were observed. What is the probable causative organism and what is another parasite that could be confused with the most probable diagnosed pathogen?

2. A female graduate student had worked and studied on Lake Victoria in Kenya for the past semester. Abdominal and flank pain spurred her to visit her physician. She denied any history of renal calculi in her family as well as abnormalities of the kidneys. A urine culture revealed no bacterial presence in the specimen but the urinalysis showed an abnormal level of protein as well as red blood cells and oval structures with terminal spines. What is the probable causative organism and how was the probable species determined?

3. A 58-year-old professor of sociology had returned from a vacation in Africa, where he began experiencing episodes of chills followed by fever. While considering a systemic viral infection, the physician ordered a complete blood count with thick and thin smears. The patient remembered that his urine had slowly darkened over the past few weeks and the blood count showed mild anemia. What disease was more than likely causing the symptoms and signs? What are some other parasites that may be diagnosed by study of blood smears?

STUDY QUESTIONS

1. What are the three classes of helminthes, the worms, of parasitology?

2. Name the three scientific names of worms that infect predominantly cats and dogs.

3. Name the two species of hookworm that infect humans in both the New and Old World.

4. List the clinical symptoms and signs for hookworm infections.

5. Nearly all trematodes are obligate parasites of _____ and _____.

6. Nearly all flat worms are also known as _____.

7. Flatworms or flukes can be classified into two groups. They are:

8. The organism of the genus that causes a disease called bilharziasis is:

9. Symptoms and signs of schistosomiasis are:

10. Complications of schistosomiasis that impact the liver may include:

11. A severe immunological reaction in the host who has contracted schistosomiasis and is life-threatening may include:

12. Where are the infective cercaria found in endemic areas of schistosomiasis?

13. What is the common name for a threadworm infection in children?

14. Besides an itchy anus at night, what are other signs and symptoms of pinworm infection?

Intestinal Nematodes

LEARNING OBJECTIVES

Upon completion of this chapter, the learner will be expected to:

- Trace the life cycle for *Ascaris lumbricoides*
- Describe the phenomenon where *A. lumbricoides* eggs may be found in the sputum
- Relate the health manifestations of a heavy infection by *A. lumbricoides*
- Discuss damage to the intestinal mucosa caused by *A. lumbricoides* and the two major hookworms

KEY TERMS

Ascariasis	Dysentery	Palpitations
Ascites	Edema	Protein deficiency
Bile	Emaciation	Pruritis
Biological life cycle	Eosinophilic enteritis	Sputum
Blastomeres	Eosinophils	Stratum corneum
Bronchi	Epigastric	Stratum germinativum
Bronchioles	Esophagus	Teres
Buccal	Folic acid	Thready pulse
Cardiac failure	Ground itch	Toe itch
Clay	Hemorrhage	Trachea
Coprolites	Hyaline shell	Translactational
Cryotherapy	Iron supplements	Vascular system
Cutaneous larva migrans	Loamy soil	Vitamin B_{12}
Defecate	Ovum	
Diarrhea	Pallor	

INTRODUCTION

The term *nematode* means "roundworm" because members of the phylum Nematoda can be viewed as a cross-section and may range from a few millimeters to more than 1 meter in length. A common characteristic found in nematodes is that both male and female representatives exist, unlike other parasites. As a general conclusion, the male roundworm is generally smaller than the female. Body development is rather complex with an exterior covering called a *cuticle* which covers several layers of underlying musculature, a complex nerve cord and a well-developed digestive system. Functional sexual organs are present in the male and in addition the body of the male ends in either a curved or coiled tail.

　　Humans are considered the definitive host for the species of roundworms that are considered medically important for the parasitic nematode infections. Where fertilized eggs or larvae are the means for reproducing adult roundworms, three routes are generally involved by which the host becomes infected. Depending on the species of nematode, the adult female nematode is able to produce an infection in the following ways:

- Ingestion of eggs by a susceptible host can result in immediate infection

- After a required period of external development, usually in the soil, either eggs or larvae reach an infective stage before developing the capability to infect a host, often by skin penetration

- Eggs or larvae are transmitted to a new host by insect vectors

PINWORMS

Pinworms are prevalent around the world, and although they are not a serious threat to the overall health of the individual, they do cause some discomfort through anal irritation and nervousness mostly in small children. The most prevalent type of human worm infection in the United States and perhaps around the world is by that of the pinworm. The term *worms* in children is a common lay term for pinworms. This frequently used reference to pinworms is almost universal as a descriptive name for this parasite, which is an organism of the genus and species *Enterobius vermicularis*. Because many children put their dirty fingers into their mouths, they are more susceptible to this type of infection. The condition is

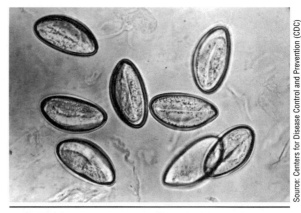

FIGURE 6-1　Eggs of the nematode, or roundworm *Enterobius vermicularis*

Source: Centers for Disease Control and Prevention (CDC)

most often confirmed by microscopic examination of the characteristic eggs where one side of the egg is flattened (Figure 6-1).

　　All parasites require a host and some may require up to three different hosts for development and infection, but for pinworms, only the human serves as a host, where the organism develops into an adult and serves as a vessel for transmission to others. The life cycle of *E. vermicularis* is quite simple when compared with many other parasitic organisms. Eggs are swallowed into the intestines, where they hatch and mature. Adult pinworms are a yellowish to white color and are slender, resembling a filament or a thick thread. It should be mentioned here that some commonly call the pinworm a "threadworm" but the term *threadworm* actually refers to a particular hookworm. A month after infecting the gut, the female worm moves down the intestinal system and exits the body from the anus. She then deposits up to several hundred eggs on the skin around the anus during the night or early morning.

　　After depositing her eggs, the female pinworm dies, as she has completed her life's mission of propagating the species. Itching often occurs after the eggs are laid. Children continue the cycle, reinfecting themselves by scratching their anus upon which eggs accumulate on the fingers and under the nails. The reproductive cycle starts again when the eggs are swallowed and begin to hatch. The eggs may remain viable for up to several days, if conditions are suitable. Treatment with medication is available to kill the parasites, and to be completely effective, all members of the family should be treated when a single family member is diagnosed with a pinworm infection. Personal hygiene and sanitary living conditions are necessary to avoid becoming infected and then reinfected. Although pinworm infections are relatively harmless, they are a nuisance but are easily treated, and ridding the entire family of the annoying symptoms of the disease is required to effectively control the infection.

ENTEROBIUS VERMICULARIS

Enterobius vermicularis is called a pinworm due to its long pointed tail that resembles a straight pin in the adult worm. These pinworms may be visible in the stools of those infected, and are readily visible in the feces of children with heavy infections, but the diagnosis is generally made by the presence of eggs.

Morphology

As a common trait in nematodes, the female worm is larger than the male and may reach a length of 7 to 13 mm, making the adult females easily visible in the stools from an infected individual. The adult males may be largely unnoticed because they are so small. The egg of the species is oval but flattened on one side. It has a thick and colorless shell and measures 50 to 60 μm in length by 20 to 30 μm in width. Larvae may be visible inside the egg due to the colorless shell of the embryonated eggs.

Symptoms

Symptoms often range from being ssymptomatic to any or several of the following signs and symptoms. An itchy anus due to an inflammatory response to the adult worm, especially at night, will be the most frequent symptom exhibited. In addition to this manifestation, any or all of the following may be present:

- Irritability may occur in children along with nervousness and disruptive behavior
- With severe scratching of the anus, the skin may break down and progress to a secondary bacterial infection
- Rare cases appear to cause anorexia, or loss of appetite
- Somewhat vague or ill-defined feelings of not being well may be present
- Female children may also have an itchy and inflamed vagina
- Adult worms may be seen in the stools

- Eggs may be seen with the naked eye, clinging to the skin around the anus
- Pinworms do not contribute to abdominal pain but have, perhaps erroneously, been attributed to cases of appendicitis as they have been observed in tissue specimens such as the appendix.

Life Cycle

Most infections originate from soiled fingers coming in contact with the mouth or when pinworm eggs are eaten, but they may occur through contaminated food, bedding, clothing, or other personal items. The pale-colored adult pinworm, of slightly less than one-half inch in size, is easy to visualize in the feces during heavy infections. Since the female dies upon laying her eggs, reinfection must occur cyclically in order to maintain an ongoing infection.

Approximately 1 month following infestation of the gut, the adult female will move down the intestinal system and will exit the body through the anus. There she lays a batch of several hundred eggs on the skin surrounding the anus, usually during the night or early in the morning before light enters the bedroom. Severe itching often accompanies the laying of the eggs, especially at night. In this way children are able to reinfect themselves by soiling their fingers and also accumulating eggs on the fingers and under the nails from the bed linens. The cycle of reproduction by transfer of the eggs to the mouth where they are again swallowed ensures a steady source of infection. Also, the eggs may remain viable for up to several days if the conditions are suitable.

Disease Transmission

The infection is spread via the fecal-oral route by ingestion or inhalation of embryonated ova. The disease may also be transmitted by fomites (inanimate objects that are contaminated by organisms) and from soiled fingers, dirty bed linens, toilet seats, and clothing. The disease is found throughout the world and spreads quickly through families and groups in close contact with each other, such as in day care centers for young children.

Laboratory Diagnosis

The "Scotch tape test" is the most economical, easiest, and effective means of diagnosing infection with *E. vermicularis*. Applying a piece of transparent cellophane tape over a tongue blade into the perianal folds late at night or before daylight affords the best opportunity of recovering evidence of infection. The slide is then examined microscopically for the typical ova and four to six slides collected at different times should be performed before ruling out the infection. Occasionally the adult worm will also be found on the slide along with the characteristic ova.

MICROSCOPIC DIAGNOSTIC FEATURE

General Classification—Pinworm, larval form

Organism	*Enterobius vermicularis*
Specimen Required	Feces
Stage	Diagnostic specimens include ova or adult female "worms"
Size	*Worms*—Male adult range from 2–5 mm with curved posterior and the adult female ranges from 8–13 mm with long pointed tail and three cuticle lips
Shape	Long, pointed, and pinlike morphology
Motility	Sluggish motility when viewed in fecal specimen
Other Features	May also be found in vaginal area of female children; occasionally female adults along with eggs may be found on Scotch tape prep

E. vermicularis

Adult Female worm

Delmar/Cengage Learning

MICROSCOPIC DIAGNOSTIC FEATURE

General Classification—Pinworm, (Nematode egg)

Organism	*Enterobius vermicularis*
Specimen Required	Scotch tape prep for eggs or worms
Stage	Egg
Size	Ova are 50–60 µm × 20–30 µm
Shape	Flattened on one side, with a C-shaped embryo in the egg
Shell	Thick, colorless
Other Features	Partially embryonated eggs may develop to an infectious stage within approximately six hours

E. vermicularis
Ovum, embryonated

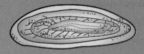

Delmar/Cengage Learning

Treatment and Prevention

The physician will most likely request a procedure to test a sample of the patient's feces to make a positive identification of pinworms as the cause for symptoms of infection. Medication is available to kill the worms and this is usually prescribed for the infected person and all members of the household. Usually one dose is followed up with a second dose 2 weeks later to take care of any surviving worms. Although safe for humans, a prescription from the physician is required before starting the medication. A repeat preparation should be examined following completion of treatment to ensure complete eradication. All family members should take the medication, regardless of whether they are experiencing symptoms, because the condition is quite contagious and some are asymptomatic, showing no evidence of the common symptoms and signs of infection. Treatment for relieving the itching of the anus can be effective with the use of various types of soothing anti-itch creams or similar preparations. Recurrence of the infection is likely if bed linens and bed clothes are not thoroughly washed to kill both eggs and worms, and if personal hygiene is not practiced, including thorough hand washing following trips to the bathroom and when playing with other children.

ASCARIS LUMBRICOIDES

Ascaris lumbricoides, sometimes considered the "large roundworm," is one of six worms classified by Linnaeus, who performed most of his observations and studies between the 1730s and 1750s. His work took him to countries throughout several areas of the world, which confirmed the widespread range of the parasite. Linnaeus is credited with giving the scientific name to *Ascaris lumbricoides,* along with other plants and animals. The names of some of the organisms he classified more than 270 years ago have remained unchanged. It has been stated in a number of publications by health departments and other health care agencies that up to one billion people or perhaps one-seventh of the world population are now infected with *A. lumbricoides,* because it is a parasite found around the globe.

The chief source of most of the infections by this parasite is the practice of using human feces to fertilize soil where food is grown. The adult worm lives in the intestine (Figure 6-2) and the female produces eggs that pass with fecal materials, where the larvae within the eggs develop and reach an infective stage in soil. Foods grown and gathered from agricultural areas where the soil is contaminated by feces containing eggs from this species may directly transmit the eggs to humans when

food contaminated with infective eggs is eaten and the larvae emerge from the ingested eggs in the intestine.

The history of ascariasis is long and has been determined to have been an infection plaguing humans since before recorded history. The eggs of *A. lumbricoides* have been found in human coprolites (stony casts of feces, also known as coproliths) from several regions in South America that, by various dating procedures, are believed to have been excreted several thousand years ago. In particular, the regions now known as Peru and Brazil have both yielded evidence of *A. lumbricoides* in ancient specimens (Cox, 2002). Throughout the countries of southwest Asia and China, there also is evidence of *A. lumbricoides* as well as in a Middle Kingdom Egyptian mummy dating from 1938 to 1600 BC and from China in the Ming Dynasty between AD 1368 and 1644 (Cox, 2002).

The evidence from Europe would most likely be scanty at best because human specimens are less well preserved than those in drier climates, accounting for little archaeological evidence of the organisms in human remains from the continent. In the late 1600s Edward Tyson, an English physician, wrote of and detailed a description of the worm itself, although ascariasis had been described and treatment documented from several centuries before Tyson's contribution. Tyson had learned from Veslius' book that described *Lumbricus teres* (teres means earth) as perhaps the cause of *A. lumbricoides* infections contracted from contaminated soil. Anatomical studies require good illustrations as well as verbal descriptions, and Tyson's work was spread broadly over a number of disciplines.

Tyson's work contained the first illustration of dissected internal parasites that depicted both males and females as well as the eggs of the female. But he greatly underestimated the number of eggs that may be produced, with the belief that only around 1000 eggs were laid by each parasite. But later investigations revealed that a single female worm is capable of producing up to 200,000 eggs per day during a 1- to 2-year life span (Figure 6-3). Therefore it is easy to see that an epidemic could easily start with only a few of the organisms. Tyson believed the worms reproduced sexually in the intestine, but he did not make the connection of how they arrived there.

Morphology

A. lumbricoides is a considerably large worm that may reach up to 35 cm (more than 12 inches) in length and that is often excreted in the feces, and is sometimes seen protruding from or emerging from the anus even when the victim is not

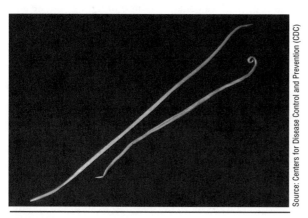

Source: Centers for Disease Control and Prevention (CDC)

FIGURE 6-2 *Ascaris lumbricoides* nematodes; larger female can reach over 12 inches

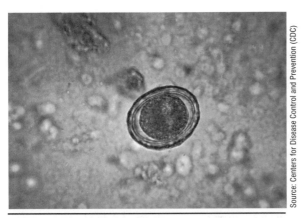

Source: Centers for Disease Control and Prevention (CDC)

FIGURE 6-3 Fertilized egg of the roundworm *Ascaris lumbricoides*

defecating. These organisms are readily visible and quite startling. Extensive written records of probable ascariasis have been found in sources including the Egyptian medical papyri, the works of Hippocrates in fifth century BC, Chinese writings from the second and third centuries BC, and texts of Roman and Arabic physicians (Cox, 2002).

The fertilized egg is broad and oval, and measures 45 to 75 μm in length and 35 to 45 μm in breadth. The thick but transparent shell is surrounded by a mammillated outer covering that is dark yellow to brown and is bile-stained with an appearance that is singularly characteristic for the species. If the mammillated covering is missing, the egg is said to be decorticated. Infertile eggs are longer than fertilized eggs, ranging from 80 to 90 μm long and the interior of the egg shows disorganization and no visible structures.

Symptoms

Adult ascarids normally cause few or no symptoms, but heavy infections may result in nutritional deficiencies, especially in children. In some patients, considerable flatulence (emission of intestinal gas) may be experienced with an infection by *A. lumbricoides*. Migration into the lungs may lead to hemorrhages and inflammatory infiltrations upon which hemoptysis (coughing up of blood) may be observed. Eosinophilia, an increase in a type of white blood cell occurring in allergic reactions and parasitic infections, is often concurrently observed with a set of signs that may include coughing, dyspnea (shortness of breath), and a mild fever. The intestinal phase includes abdominal discomfort and bloating along with nausea, vomiting, pains, and **diarrhea** may occur.

Intestinal obstructions are a serious consequence that may result from a heavy infection by this parasite.

Life Cycle

For the species of *Ascaris* that lives in the human intestine, the male is somewhat smaller than the 12-inch maximum length for the female. After eggs are passed with the feces, they require a period of 2 weeks' incubation in the soil before they are viable and are capable of causing an infection. After eating the eggs that have contaminated vegetables harvested from the soil, the eggs hatch in the intestine of the host and then enter the circulatory system (the veins) by means of the hepatic portal circulatory system. This circulatory route takes the blood containing the newly hatched larvae directly through the heart and into the lungs.

A. lumbricoides worms do not mature immediately upon hatching but are able to migrate around the body and eventually travel to the lungs. There they migrate up the respiratory passageways called the **bronchioles** and **bronchi**, where they are coughed up in **sputum** from the respiratory system and then swallowed. By this means the larvae enter the intestines (the portion called the **jejunum**) where they continue infecting the body as they develop into adult worms in the intestine (Figure 6-4). After approximately 2 months of infection, the eggs are deposited and are passed in the feces where they become infective in warm, moist soil within 2 weeks. Females lay infertile eggs when males are not available for mating.

Disease Transmission

Humans are infected when they ingest embryonated eggs from contaminated soil where feces have been deposited. The eggs in feces usually include first-stage larvae and maturation takes place in the soil, particularly hard clay soil. The second stage is reached in 2 weeks and is capable of causing ascariasis during which the person becoming infected by swallowing the embryonated eggs.

Laboratory Diagnosis

Diagnosis most often is made by the identification of either or both fertilized and unfertilized eggs of *A. lumbricoides*. Adult worms may also be identified, as they may pass from any body orifice including the anus, nose, or mouth. The larvae may also be found in sputum or gastric washings from infected individuals.

LIFE CYCLE of—

Ascaris lumbricoides

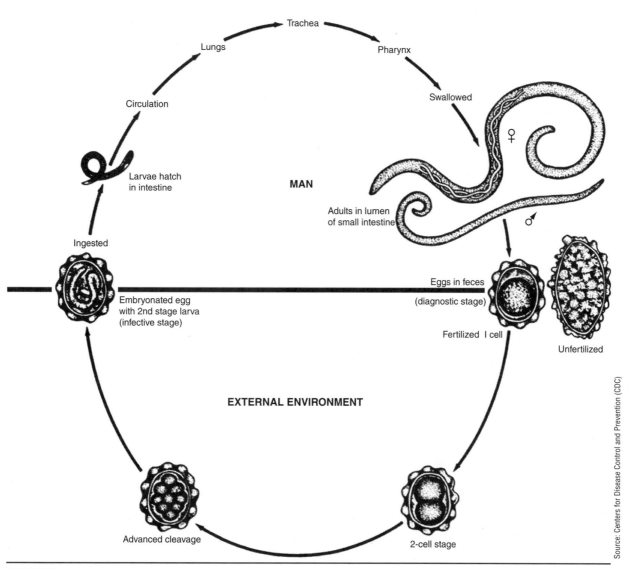

FIGURE 6-4 Various stages in the life cycle of the intestinal roundworm nematode _Ascaris lumbricoides_

Treatment and Prevention

Treatment is available using a variety of antihelminthic drugs such as mebendazole and piperazine. Larvae may not be affected by this treatment so repeat treatments may be required. Prevention of the infection by _A. lumbricoides_ includes the availability of sanitary facilities for defecating and the proper hand washing and cleaning of food materials such as those grown in the soil. The use of human feces as fertilizer, a common practice in some developing countries, should be avoided.

MICROSCOPIC DIAGNOSTIC FEATURE

General Classification—Ascarid (Nematode egg)

Organism	*Ascaris lumbricoides*
Specimen Required	Feces
Stage	Egg
Size	Fertilized egg: 45–75 μm
	Unfertilized egg: 80–90 μm
Shape	Broad and oval fertilized egg
	Infertile eggs are longer, 80–90 μm in length
Shell	Thick, yellow-brown, and mammillated
Other Features	Unfertilized eggs show disorganized internal contents

A. lumbricoides
Adult worm

Ova
Infertile egg

Fertile egg

Decorticated egg

MICROSCOPIC DIAGNOSTIC FEATURE

General Classification—Ascarid (Nematode worm)

Organism	*Ascaris lumbricoides* adult "worm"
Specimen Required	Feces
Stage	Adult
Size	15–35 cm and 2–4 mm in diameter
Shape	Round and elongated
Motility	Sluggish, curling movements
Other Features	Off-white to pale yellow "worm" with pointed tail
	Sometimes described by patients as "earthworms"

WHIPWORM INFECTIONS

Whipworms are a type of roundworm of which there are perhaps as many as 60 different species. Humans are infected chiefly by a species of whipworm originally called *Trichuris trichuris*, but currently identified as *T. trichiura*, where they inhabit the large intestine of humans and animals. The name of the organism refers to the characteristic shape of the adult organism.

TRICHURIS TRICHIURA

The human whipworm (*Trichuris trichiura or Trichocephalus trichiuris*) and previously known as *Trichuris trichiura*, is one of the most prevalent parasitic roundworms found worldwide. The existence of the organism has been documented for many years and in the older literature it was described as causing a condition called trichuriasis when it infects the large intestine of the human.

Morphology

The *Trichuris trichiura* parasite is commonly referred to as the "whipworm" because of its resemblance in the adult worm to a whip. The name refers to the shape of the worm with the appearance of an old-fashioned buggy whip with a long and slender thread-like anterior portion and with thicker, wider "handles" at the posterior end that is long and slender, described as a threadlike caudal portion. The male is characterized by a slightly coiled tail, whereas the female has a rounded and somewhat blunt posterior that is not coiled.

The adult worm ranges from 30 to 50 mm with a range of 35 to 50 mm for the female. The male is slightly smaller than the female, ranging from 30 to 45 mm in length. The eggs have a mucogelatinous plug at each terminal end of the elongated egg that is bile-stained and barrel-shaped. A smooth but thick shell covers the egg, which is from 45 to 55 μm in length and 20 to 23 μm in width.

Symptoms

Whipworm infections in humans can cause a range of symptoms, by presenting no symptoms at all to only mild symptoms that may progress to somewhat severe symptoms. As in the case with hookworm infections, severely heavy numbers of whipworms in humans can cause stomach pain with loss of appetite and iron deficiency, bloody diarrhea, weight loss, rectal prolapse (detached rectum), and fecal incontinence.

Life Cycle

A simple and direct life cycle for *T. trichiuria* involves the passage of feces containing eggs that mature in about 2 weeks and become infective. Embryonated eggs with first-stage larvae are ingested from contaminated and packed clay soil that clings to root vegetables and leaves of other vegetables in many areas of the world where environmental conditions suitable for the propagation of whipworms are present. Development of the larvae occurs in the duodenum and cecum, where the worm attaches to the mucosa of the intestine by its anterior mouthparts. In about 3 months, the adult is able to lay eggs. A female may produce 2,000 to 20,000 unembryonated eggs per day, which may be deposited in the human feces and into the soil.

These unembryonated eggs from the stool of the infected individual incubate in the soil and reach an infective capability when they achieve an embryonated stage after 2 to 3 weeks. The embryonated eggs contain the first stage of larval development and are contracted primarily from hard clay soil, where heavy rain fall may leach other organic nutrients from the soil. It is not uncommon to find a *T. trichiura* infection accompanied by a second parasite such as *A. lumbricoides*, and perhaps along with other common intestinal parasites.

Whipworm organisms are spread to humans through a fecal-oral transmission when contact with soil containing whipworm eggs occurs. Whipworm infections are more common in children through playing outside and introducing focally contaminated dirt containing whipworm eggs into the mouth. Although whipworms are distributed on a worldwide basis, they survive best in tropical or semitropical climates including the southeastern United States where the weather is warm and humid and plentiful rainfall is present. In addition, recent studies have shown a possible genetic predisposition to infection with the whipworm.

Disease Transmission

Ingestion of embryonated eggs from both contaminated water and food is the most common route leading to a whipworm infection. But direct infection from the soil contaminated with feces and close contact during activities such as gardening and farming also provides for a major portion of the cases of trichiuris. In addition to placing dirty fingers into the mouth, another common way of becoming infected is the ingestion of *T. trichiura* eggs due to poor preparation of foods (e.g., eating unwashed vegetables from soil that is contaminated).

Following ingestion, the eggs then hatch in the small intestine where the resultant larvae grow and molt (shed their skin periodically as they grow). These larvae then penetrate the villi of the small intestine and continue developing into young worms. The young worms then move to the cecum (first portion of the large intestine) and the duodenum where they penetrate the mucosa and complete their development to adult worms in the large intestine. The life cycle from time of ingestion of eggs to development of mature worms is approximately 3 months, at which time the female *T. trichiura* is capable of laying eggs. Adult worms can live up to 5 years and the female worm can lay up to 20,000 eggs per day for an entire lifetime. When these eggs from the feces are used as fertilizer or if an infected individual has defecated on the ground, the eggs incubate in the soil and become infective when they reach an embryonated stage after a period of 2 to 3 weeks. As with a number of parasitic infections, whipworms are frequently transmitted to a host either through eating vegetables grown in contaminated soil or by direct contact by an individual with the soil where infective eggs are introduced to the mouth. It is not uncommon to find a *T. trichiuris* infection accompanied by a second parasite such as *A. lumbricoides*.

Laboratory Diagnosis

Stool specimens and identification of the eggs, which are characteristic with their elongated shape and the polar plugs found in the terminal ends, are evidence of a *T. trichiura* infection. Identification and differentiation of eggs is the most common method for identifying an infection by the whipworm. Routine concentration methods may be necessary in order to recover both ova and adult parasites. Adult worms are rarely seen in fecal samples but are useful in identifying an infection of *T. trichiura*; if seen, females are larger than males, as previously described, although this overlapping range provides for little diagnostic value. The females have a rounded posterior end compared to the male counterparts which possess a coiled posterior end. Their characteristic eggs have a smooth shell and are barrel-shaped, brown, and have bipolar plugs.

During the early stage of infection there may be only limited signs of infection in fecal samples. This is due to the cycles of periodic skin shedding and growth, which must occur for a period of approximately 3 months before adults mature and begin egg production. It should be remembered that the mature *Trichuris trichiura* has a narrow anterior esophageal end and shorter and thicker posterior anus, a characteristic necessary to differentiate adult worms from other species of parasites. These pinkish-white worms extend through the intestinal mucosa and attach to the host through their slender anterior end where they feed on tissue secretions. Mechanical damage may occur in the intestinal mucosa when toxic or inflammatory damage to the intestines of the host occurs, resulting in blood loss and anemia in victims with heavy infections. Whipworm infections may also be accompanied by concurrent infections with *Giardia, Entamoeba histolytica, Ascaris lumbricoides,* and hookworms. This fact requires that the parasitologist be especially careful in ruling out other infections upon identification of one particular species.

Treatment and Prevention

A drug commonly used is that of mebendazole but prevention is the best course as for most other parasites. Good personal hygiene and the avoiding of contaminated

MICROSCOPIC DIAGNOSTIC FEATURE

General Classification—Nematodal whipworm egg

Organism	*Trichuris trichiura*
Specimen Required	Feces
Stage	Egg most often diagnostic with occasional adult stages seen
Size	Egg ranges from 50–55 × 22–23 μm
Shape	Eggs are smooth-shelled and brown with barrel shapes and are unembryonated when passed; characteristic mucogelatinous plugs on opposite ends of elongated eggs
Shell	Smooth shell surface; may be thick and yellow-brown with staining by bile
Other Features	Pink to white larval forms

T. trichiuria

Adult worm

Ovum

Delmar/Cengage Learning

water and food and providing for safe disposal of human wastes will eliminate many of the cases. It is necessary to teach children to both avoid infection and reinfection. Changes in the lifestyle should be taught to the children that include hygienic practices and habits that are reinforced by the parents and others in authority, such as teachers. This is a practice that will stand them in good stead for many years, and will help to avoid other parasitic and bacterial infections such as pinworm as well as many infections. During treatment and following treatment, all family members should adopt the practice of thoroughly washing hands and cleaning fingernails thoroughly and regularly with warm water and soap. After using the commode, the seat of the commode should be sprayed with a disinfectant to prevent eggs on the surface of the seat from coming in contact with the hands when a family member is infected. Food preparation should be started only after careful washing of the hands. Keep finger nails short and clean, and avoid scratching the anus and genitals and nail biting will prevent reinfection. Daily bathing and showering are important, as well as washing bed linens and nightwear with hot water and laundry detergent.

HOOKWORM INFECTION

It should be noted that a large number of nematodes are capable of infecting humans. Another category of a widespread nematode is the hookworm (refers to a number of species), which is also a roundworm and lives in the small intestine of its host. Its eggs and worms are frequently found in the fecal specimens of those infected with hookworms (Figure 6-5). The two major species, *Ancylostoma duodenale* and *Necator americanus*, range over broad areas of both the Old and the New World. These two species are much smaller than the large roundworm called *Ascaris lumbricoides* and include additional physical complications in the infected victim through migration into the body's tissues. Obstruction of the gastrointestinal tract that may be experienced with an *A. lumbricoides* roundworm infestation is less frequent in hookworm infestations.

The most significant risk from hookworm infection is the development of anemia, which is caused by depletion of dietary iron, proteins, and iron supplements, that are absorbed in the digestive tract. The worms extract blood large amounts of blood and in addition may damage the mucosa of the intestinal tract and cause blood to appear in the feces. The blood loss through the stools

may require testing for occult blood, which is a condition caused by broken down red blood cells that are not visible to the naked eye. It is possible to become infected with hookworms by direct contact with contaminated soil, generally through walking barefoot, or accidentally swallowing contaminated soil.

ANCYLOSTOMA DUODENALE AND *NECATOR AMERICANUS*

Many individuals with hookworm infection have no symptoms. The two major hookworm species, those of *Ancylostoma duodenale* and *Necator americanus,* are similar in many ways. Therefore, they are treated jointly and comparatively in this section. *Strongyloides stercoralis* is another pathogen that must be differentiated from the hookworms, *A. duodenale* and *N. americanus*.

Morphology

The adult stages of *A. duodenale* and *N. americanus* are seldom seen for identification, but they are similar in appearance. The eggs are indistinguishable as there is only a slight difference in size between the two species. The eggs of *N. americanus* are slightly larger than those of *A. duodenale* and measure from 55 to 75 μm in length, with a width of between 35 and 40 μm. *A. duodenale* and *N. americanus* also differ in their mouthparts or buccal cavities (Figure 6-6). The buccal capsule of *A. duodenale* has visible teeth, whereas *N. americanus* has specialized structures called cutting plates.

Symptoms

The symptoms can be linked to inflammation of the gastrointestinal system that is stimulated by feeding hookworms. Inflammation is accompanied by nausea, abdominal pain, and intermittent diarrhea early in the course of the disease, and a common consequence of hookworm infections is that of progressive anemia that often occurs in prolonged infections. Patients with more severe infections may encounter the above symptoms as well as vomiting related to the nausea along with general fatigue. Old home remedies were often followed in many areas of the world, particularly in the southeastern United States. Impulsive or unreasonable appetite desires such as pica (or dirt-eating), led to the practice in the southern states

LIFE CYCLE of—

Hookworm

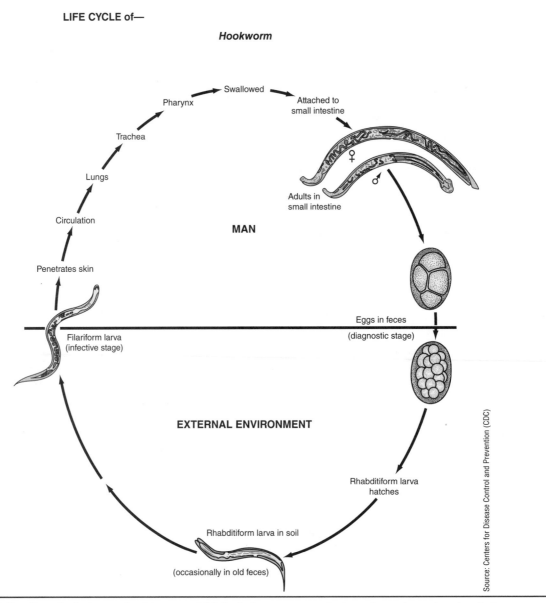

FIGURE 6-5 Life cycle for human hookworms, which includes two nematode (roundworm) species, *Ancylostoma duodenale* and *Necator americanus*

of selling small bags of white clay to satisfy these cravings. Prolonged constipation followed by diarrhea, **palpitations**, **thready pulse**, coldness of the skin, **pallor** of the mucous membranes, fatigue and weakness, and shortness of breath may occur in long-standing cases. The extremely grave medical conditions such as **dysentery**, **hemorrhage**, and **edema** may culminate in fatal consequences in cases of hookworm infections that are untreated.

Hookworm infections begin with larval invasion of the skin, particularly the lower extremities and feet. The lesions resemble bites of spiders and insects, and may produce blistering typically cause intense itching (**pruritis**) that is called "ground itch" or "toe itch." and may be accompanied by racking coughs, chest pain, wheezing, and fever for some people who have been exposed to extremely high levels of larvae. Epigastric pains,

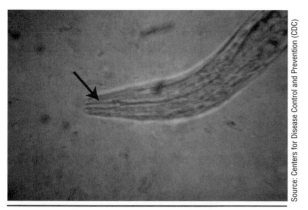

Source: Centers for Disease Control and Prevention (CDC)

FIGURE 6-6 Buccal (mouth) cavity morphology of a hookworm, during its rhabditiform, early noninfectious larval stage

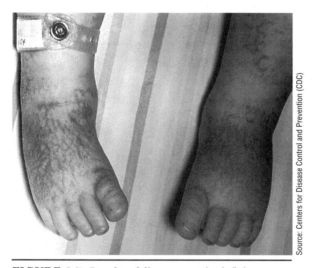

Source: Centers for Disease Control and Prevention (CDC)

FIGURE 6-7 Results of dietary protein deficiency including edema

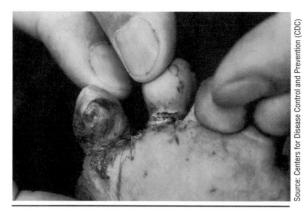

Source: Centers for Disease Control and Prevention (CDC)

FIGURE 6-8 A hookworm infection involving the toes of the right foot

nausea, vomiting, indigestion, constipation, and diarrhea can occur either in the earlier or in the later stages as well although gastrointestinal symptoms tend to grow less severe over a period of time. Advanced and severe infections that are not treated often progress to severe anemia and **protein deficiency** states. Characteristics of those suffering from chronic hookworm disease often include **emaciation** and wasting, **cardiac failure** or abdominal distension with *ascites*, a term indicating a fluid-filled cavity (Figure 6-7).

No specific symptoms or signs of hookworm infection and sometimes no symptoms at all are present until the health of the infected individual occurs. Clinical signs may occur from a combination of intestinal inflammation

and a progressive iron and protein-deficiency anemia. Often the first sign of having contracted a hookworm infection is that of the inflammation where the larvae penetrated the skin of the host (Figure 6-8), signs that may last for a week or more. However, as the health of the individual deteriorates, the more noticeable signs and symptoms will occur.

Upon penetrating the human skin, animal hookworm larvae may produce a slowly spreading skin eruption called **cutaneous larval migrans**. These nematodal larvae migrate through circuitous paths between the top two layers of the skin (**stratum germinativum and stratum corneum**), resulting in lesions called vesicles that contain serous fluids. With the advancing movement of the larvae over the body, the initial areas of the lesions appear dry and crusty. Often the first sign of infection is the associated itching followed by a rash at the site where skin was penetrated and became contaminated by soil or loamy sand. Penetration of the skin by these larvae may ultimately lead to anemia, abdominal pain, loss of appetite, diarrhea, and weight loss.

Life Cycle

The generalized biological life cycle of the hookworm requires environmental conditions conducive to its survival, and is able to proceed when the temperature of the earth reaches temperatures of over 65°F or 18°C. The larvae exist primarily in sandy or loamy soil and cannot survive in clay or boggy wet soil as this type of soil condition is not favorable for survival of the microfilaria

LIFE CYCLE of—

Strongyloides stercoralis

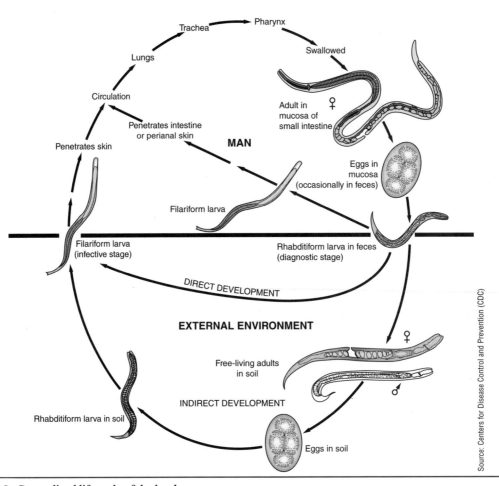

FIGURE 6-9 Generalized life cycle of the hookworm

in the ground (Figure 6-9). Rainfall averages must be more than 1000 mm or 40 inches per year. These environmental conditions are certainly met in many areas of the United States as well as in other parts of the world. Especially conditions in the southeastern part of the North American continent and other temperate zones in Latin and South America enable the organisms to thrive during the warm seasons. Only if these conditions exist can the eggs from fecally contaminated earth hatch to yield larvae. Infective larvae of _Necator americanus_ can survive at higher temperatures than those of _Ancylostoma duodenale_ which are better adapted for cooler temperatures. This fact accounts for the difference in the prevalence of the two species in certain areas of the world. Generally, the hookworm organisms live for only a few weeks at most under natural conditions and tend to die almost immediately on exposure to direct sunlight or drying out of the larvae, which is the infective stage. It is absolutely mandatory that these infective larvae be deposited in an environment of damp dirt, particularly sandy and loamy soil in order to both survive and develop.

Once in the gut of the infected host, the hookworm _Necator americanus_ is capable of causing a prolonged infection of several years. It has been observed that some adult worms have been known to live for up to 15 years or more, but it is known that a considerable number may die within a year or two after the initial infection of the host. But there is a difference in the life span of the two hookworms. *A. duodenale* adults live much shorter lives than *N. americanus,* as they usually survive for an average of only about 6 months. But the infection can be prolonged because there are always inactive or dormant larvae that can be drawn sequentially from areas of tissue storage over a substantial number of years in order to replace the dead adult worms. This will generate a rise in the population of the organisms on a seasonally fluctuating basis. A fluctuation in transmission during certain weather conditions such as warm and moist soil conditions may contribute to the prevalence and speed of transmission of the infection.

The mature hookworms mate inside the host and the females will often lay up to 30,000 eggs per day, which translates to several million eggs per female during a lifetime. Most of these eggs tend to pass out through the feces of the host. Because it takes 5 to 7 weeks for adult worms to reach maturity and then to mate and produce eggs, there may be few or no eggs detected in the early stages of very heavy infection. Therefore, several fecal specimens may be necessary to detect either eggs or worms following the appearance of acute symptoms. Diagnosis may be difficult unless care and diligence in collecting and processing specimens is practiced. Remember, the possibility of recovering eggs and larvae or mature worms of many parasites from known infections does not approach a 100 percent rate even under the best of circumstances and when an experienced and diligent laboratory practitioner is examining the specimens.

Disease Transmission

Infection by hookworm of the host is by the larvae and not the eggs from the adult organism. Although *A. duodenale* can be ingested and cause infection, the most common method of infection is through skin penetration of the larvae. Walking barefoot through contaminated water and soil containing fecal matter almost always results in contraction of the hookworm larvae. The scarcely visible larvae are able to penetrate the skin of those who walk barefoot in contaminated areas and once inside the body the microfilariae migrate through the vascular system to the lungs. From there they are coughed up into the trachea before being swallowed. As the organisms pass down the esophagus they are safely equipped to pass

through the hostile environment of the stomach and to enter the small intestine, a process that takes about a week to complete.

Upon entering the digestive system the parasites complete their life cycle in the intestine and during this time the larvae mature into adult worms. A third hookworm of dogs, *Ancylostoma caninum*, is currently becoming more familiar as a parasite of humans. It has been found in a number of countries in both tropical and temperate areas that include North America. It was always considered a host-specific canine parasite that very rarely invaded humans and, when it did, caused essentially asymptomatic infections. It is difficult to rid the body of *A. caninum* once the adults are attached to the intestinal mucosa (Figure 6-10).

In contrast to most intestinal parasites, where the heaviest parasitic loads tend to occur in children, hookworm prevalence and intensity can be even higher among adult males. The explanation for this is that hookworm infections tend to be occupational so that plantation workers, coalminers, and certain other groups maintain a high prevalence of infection among themselves by contaminating their work environment. However, in most endemic areas adult women are more severely affected by anemia than men, mainly because they may have much higher physiological needs for iron because of menstruation and repeated pregnancies. But an additional factor that contributes to poor health in women is that they customarily have access to much poorer food than the men who may hunt and work in the fields providing greater access to food. The larvae of hookworms and those of *S. stercoralis* are quite similar and may easily be confused

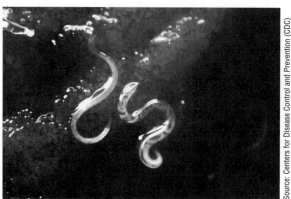

FIGURE 6-10 The hookworms, *Ancylostoma caninum*, attached to the intestinal mucosa

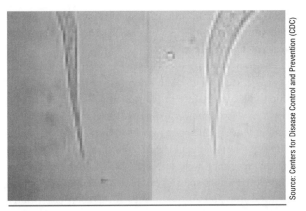

Source: Centers for Disease Control and Prevention (CDC)

FIGURE 6-11 Hookworm (L), and a *Strongyloides* (R) filariform infective stage larvae

with each other, especially because both are contracted in the same manner, from contaminated soil. It may be important to differentiate between the two filariform larvae (Figure 6-11).

An interesting consequence of *Ancylostoma duodenale* infection is that of translactational transmission of the infection in humans where a breast-feeding mother passes the infection to the infant. The larvae are able to pass into the mammary glands of the mother, so that the newborn baby can receive a large dose of infective larvae through its mother's milk. This possibly explains cases of heavy and sometimes fatal hookworm infections in children a month or so of age, in places such as China, India, and in other more isolated population groups that include the aborigines of northern Australia. *Ancylostoma caninum*, a related organism, also causes infections in dogs. The organisms may be passed through the milk of the mother dog and the newborn pups may even die of hemorrhaging from their intestines. This phenomenon may lend credence to those who associate parasitic infections of similar organisms in both domestic animals and humans as confirming a close evolutionary link between some species of human and canine parasites.

Laboratory Diagnosis

Recovery of ova (eggs) or larvae may not be possible in the early stages of the infection, until the disease has progressed to a more advanced stage. Diagnosis depends on finding characteristic worm eggs on microscopic examination of the stools. The eggs are oval or elliptical and measure roughly 60 μm by 40 μm, are colorless with a brownish-yellow tint, and have a thin transparent hyaline shell membrane that is not normally bile stained. When released by the worm in the intestine, the egg contains an unsegmented ovum. During its passage down the intestine, the ovum develops and thus the eggs passed in feces have a segmented ovum, usually with 4 to 8 blastomeres.

Because the similarity of the ova of both agents is so strong, a report of "hookworm ova" is sufficient without differentiating between the two species. *S. stercoralis* hookworm larvae require an entirely different treatment, so the differentiation between hookworm and *S. stercoralis* must be made. In a number of parasitic infections, blood tests in early infection often show a rise in numbers of eosinophils, a type of white blood cell that is preferentially stimulated by worm infections in tissues (large numbers of eosinophils are also present in the local inflammatory response). Falling blood hemoglobin levels will be seen in cases of prolonged infection with sometimes severe anemia as well as a general appearance of illness and perhaps a loss of weight. The victim is often listless from the anemic condition and presents a picture of generally poor health when infected by large populations of hookworm parasites.

Differentiation of species between *A. duodenale* and *N. americanus* requires the presence of the rhabditiform larvae as well as other factors (Table 6-1). Sometimes the ova hatch in the feces and both ova and larvae will be found in a fecal sample. Distinguishing features for differentiation of species is made by the morphology of the buccal capsule and presence of copulatory bursa in the male. The buccal capsule of *A. duodenale* is equipped with teeth, whereas that of the *N. americanus* reveals cutting plates. Three developmental stages of hookworm larvae are as follows:

1st stage—the rhabditiform larva is the free-living form

2nd stage—filariform larvae not capable of independently living in the environment and must find a host; possess shorter esophagus than that of the rhabditiform larvae

3rd stage—infective form capable of penetrating the skin through contact with soil

Treatment and Prevention

Topical solutions for treatment of dogs and cats are available, a critical component of preventing the disease from being contracted by humans. It utilizes moxidectin for control and prevention of roundworms, hookworms,

MICROSCOPIC DIAGNOSTIC FEATURE

General Classification—Ova of nematode (hookworm)

Organism	*Ancylostoma duodenale* and *Necator americanus*
Specimen Required	Fecal specimen
Stage	Most diagnostic stage is the ova, as adult larvae are seldom found in stool samples
Size	50–75 μm for ova
Shape	Eggs are slightly oval in shape
Shell	Colorless and thin-shelled
Other Features	Eggs identical except for slight differences in size for both *Ancylostoma duodenale* and *Necator americanus* and are colorless with an embryo in a 4–8 cleaved pattern

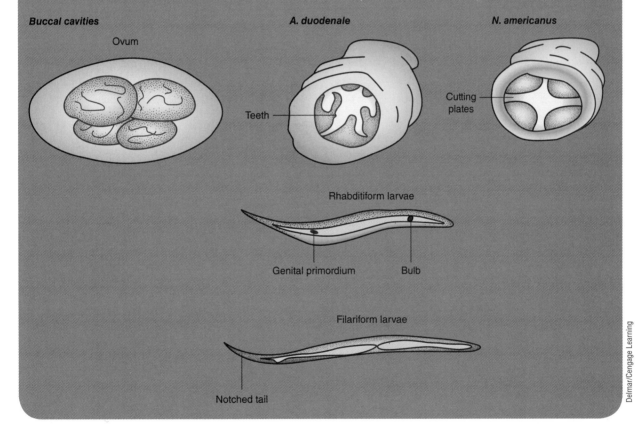

Buccal cavities · Ovum · A. duodenale · N. americanus · Teeth · Cutting plates · Rhabditiform larvae · Genital primordium · Bulb · Filariform larvae · Notched tail

Delmar/Cengage Learning

heartworms, and whipworms. In the late 1800s and early 1900s many southerners, particularly rural residents of Mississippi, were plagued by hookworms. Many homes in the state at that time did not have indoor plumbing or proper sanitation facilities for adequate personal hygiene and for disposal of urine and excrement and coupled with the sandy and loamy soil, the parasites were bountiful (Figure 6-12).

As a result, hookworms, spread by fecal contamination of the environment, had become quite prevalent during this period along with other associated diseases caused by lack of sanitation. Eggs hatch in the soil and

TABLE 6-1 Differentiation Between *N. americanus* and *A. duodenale*

GENUS AND SPECIES	*NECATOR AMERICANUS*	*ANCYLOSTOMA DUODENALE*
Common Name	New World hookworm, American murderer	Old World hookworm
Etiologic Agent of	Necatoriasis, Uncinariasis	Ancylostomiasis, Wakana disease
Infective Stage	Filariform larva	Filariform larva
Definitive Host	Humans	Humans
Portal of Entry	Usually via skin penetration rather than ingestion	Usually via ingestion rather than skin penetration
Mode of Transmission	Skin > Mouth	Mouth > Skin
Habitat	Small intestine (jejunum, ileum)	Small intestine (duodenum, jejunum)
Maturation in Host (days)	49–56	53
Mode of Attachment	Oral attachment to mucosa by sucking	Oral attachment to mucosa by sucking
Mode of Nutrition	Sucking and ingesting of blood	Sucking and ingesting of blood
Pathogenesis	Larva—ground/dew itch, creeping eruption; adult—IDA Microcytic, Hypochromic Anemia	Larva—ground/dew itch, creeping eruption; adult—IDA Microcytic, Hypochromic Anemia
Laboratory Diagnosis	Concentration methods and Direct Fecal Smear	Concentration methods and Direct Fecal Smear
Treatment	Albendazole, mebendazole, or pyrantel pamoate	Albendazole, mebendazole, or pyrantel pamoate
Length of Adult	5–9 for males; 9–11 for females	8–11 for males; 10–13 for females
Shape	Head curved opposite to curvature of body, giving a hooked appearance to anterior end	Head continuous in same direction as the body
Temperature at which 90% of eggs hatch (C)	20–35	15–35
Diagnostic Feature—Adult	Semilunar cutting plate; bipartite dorsal ray	Male–Tripartite dorsal ray
Diagnostic Feature—Egg	Morula	Same

the larval stages can penetrate the skin of those not practicing proper sanitation and care in avoiding exposure (Figure 6-13). Diagnostic characteristics of a hookworm egg are its thin shell with an oval or ellipsoidal shape ranges from 57 to 76 μm *x* 35 to 47 μm in size.

Hookworms cannot survive, except in ideal soil conditions and temperatures which place a geographic restriction on where they are found. To control and prevent infections by hookworms, it is necessary to practice preventive measures outlined by health departments and other authorities. Continued adherence to preventive measures is necessary to prevent reinfection. Common rules to practice to ensure protection from parasitic infections include the following instructions:

■ Do not defecate outside latrines or toilets that are provided for convenience and safety. Even burying the feces in soil may allow propagation of the parasites in the soil and cause infections to other hosts weeks later.

MICROSCOPIC DIAGNOSTIC FEATURE

General Classification—Hookworm adult

Organism	*A. duodenale* and *N. americanus*
Specimen Required	Feces
Stage	Adult
Size	Females 10–12 mm in length; male slightly shorter
Shape	Round and elongated with a long pointed tail
Motility	Not reported
Other Features	Well-developed mouthparts for attaching to intestinal mucosa

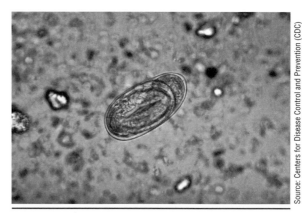

FIGURE 6-13 Egg *of Ancylostoma duodenale* or *Necator americanus hookworm*

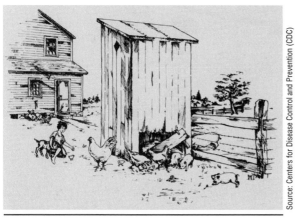

FIGURE 6-12 Hookworm infection by direct contact with contaminated soil

- Do not use human excrement or raw sewage as fertilizer in agricultural practices. This is practiced in some cultures and is called "night soil." Fruits and vegetables that are normally eaten raw and come from developing countries are a ready source of parasitic infections and mere rinsing of the food is not sufficient to remove or destroy the organisms.

- Deworming of the family pets, both dogs and cats, will aid the pets in remaining healthy and

may help to avoid infecting humans. Some canine and feline hookworms, such as *caninum,* known as the common dog hookworm, may in rare cases develop to adulthood in humans and when they do, they may result in eosinophilic enteritis in people. Their invasive larvae can also cause an itchy rash called *cutaneous larva migrans* on the skin of humans.

STRONGYLOIDES STERCORALIS, DIFFERENTIATING FROM HOOKWORM LARVAE

Since it is sometimes difficult to differentiate between the eggs of *Ancylostoma duodenale* and *Necator americanus* along with most other hookworm species in order to identify the genus, additional steps may be necessary. The eggs must be placed in an appropriate environment in the lab to allow the larvae to hatch out, at which time the larvae are easier to identify due to the morphology exhibited. If the fecal sample is left for a day or more under simulated tropical conditions, the larvae will have hatched out, allowing speciation, and eggs might no longer be evident. It is paramount to distinguish hookworm larvae from *S. stercoralis* larvae, because infection with *S. stercoralis* has a more serious impact on the victim and requires different treatment. This species also is known as *threadworms* and are capable of living in the small intestine or as a free-living worm (Figure 6-14). Although the larvae of the two hookworm species, *A. duodenale* and *N. americanus,* can be distinguished microscopically, this is not typically done except for research purposes. Adult worms would

Strongyloidiasis
(Strongyloides stercoralis)

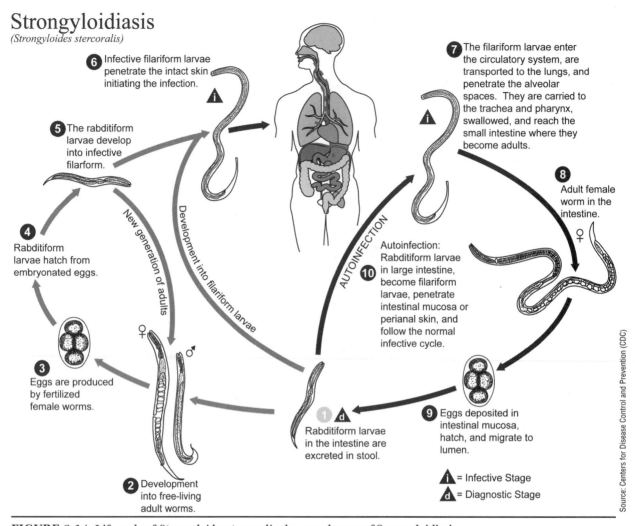

6 Infective filariform larvae penetrate the intact skin initiating the infection.

5 The rabditiform larvae develop into infective filarform.

4 Rabditiform larvae hatch from embryonated eggs.

3 Eggs are produced by fertilized female worms.

2 Development into free-living adult worms.

New generation of adults

Development into filariform larvae

7 The filariform larvae enter the circulatory system, are transported to the lungs, and penetrate the alveolar spaces. They are carried to the trachea and pharynx, swallowed, and reach the small intestine where they become adults.

8 Adult female worm in the intestine.

AUTOINFECTION

10 Autoinfection: Rabditiform larvae in large intestine, become filariform larvae, penetrate intestinal mucosa or perianal skin, and follow the normal infective cycle.

1 **d** Rabditiform larvae in the intestine are excreted in stool.

9 Eggs deposited in intestinal mucosa, hatch, and migrate to lumen.

i = Infective Stage
d = Diagnostic Stage

Source: Centers for Disease Control and Prevention (CDC)

FIGURE 6-14 Life cycle of *Strongyloides stercoralis*, the causal agent of Strongyloidiasis

normally only be obtained through a surgical procedure but if the surgical procedure is done, definitive identification of the species is possible.

STRONGYLOIDES STERCORALIS

Rhabditiform (L) larvae that hatch from eggs are 250 to 300 μm long, and approximately 15 to 20 μm wide. They have a long **buccal** canal, and the rhabditiform larvae are usually not found in the stool (Figure 6-15). But if examination of the stool is delayed, eggs may hatch and there may be abundant larvae present. If larvae are seen in stool, these larvae of *Stronyloides stercoralis* must be differentiated from that of the hookworms *N. americanus*

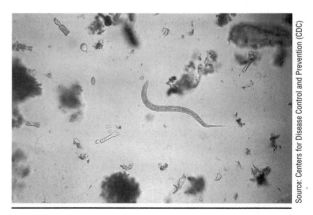

FIGURE 6-15 Morphologic structure of a hookworm rhabditiform larva of *Stronyloides stercoralis*

Source: Centers for Disease Control and Prevention (CDC)

TABLE 6-2 Differentiation of *S. stercoralis* and Hookworm Larvae

	BUCCAL CAVITY	BULB	TAIL	GENITAL PRIMORDIUM
Hookworm—rhabditiform	Long	Yes		Small
Hookworm—filariform	Long	No	Pointed	
Strongyloides—rhabditiform	Short	Yes		Large
Strongyloides—filariform	Short	No	Notched	

and *Ancylostoma duodenale* (Table 6-2). This is necessary because the clinical manifestations of an overwhelming systemic infection with *S. stercoralis* are severe fever and abdominal pain, respiratory problems, shock, and possibly death. These medical complications are in addition to the common problems associated with a general common hookworm infection. In addition, the treatment for the two groups is radically different.

Morphology

The adult forms of the worm called *Strongyloides stercoralis* are also called *threadworms*. The adult female is rarely seen in fecal specimens and is roughly 2 mm long, with a short buccal cavity and a long and slender esophagus. The worm produces thin-shelled eggs that are a bit smaller than those of hookworms, but in most respects are the same as and are indistinguishable from those produced by hookworms. The noninfective rhabditiform larvae are released from the eggs in the intestine following ingestion but are seldom found in stool specimens. The diagnostic stage of *S. stercoralis* larvae is that of the first stage, which is usually passed in the feces and ranges from 200 to 400 μm and 15 to 20 μm in width. The buccal cavity is short and the organism has a prominent genital primordium, which is a primary means of differentiating it from the hookworm larvae. The third stage is the infective stage, where the filariform larvae develop from the rhabditiform larvae in the soil in most instances. The third stage is somewhat larger than the rhabditiform stage and reaches a length of up to 680 μm. This form has a longer esophagus than does the hookworm and has a notched tail in direct contrast to that of the pointed tail of a hookworm larva.

Symptoms

Some itching may be experienced during skin penetration but there are few symptoms associated with this stage until the intestinal phase is reached. During the intestinal phase, diarrhea and abdominal pain occur with vomiting and weight loss in some individuals. Pulmonary symptoms may occur when the filariform larvae enter the lungs via the circulatory system, causing coughing and shortness of breath, particularly in heavy infective loads of organisms. This condition may progress to bronchopneumonia in severe cases. Sepsis and meningitis may develop where multiple forms of bacteria develop with a spread of the organisms into the blood stream and to the brain, a condition that is more common in immunocompromised individuals.

Life Cycle

Most commonly the direct route is the transmission route where infective filariform larvae from the soil penetrate the skin and then pass into the circulation. In the blood stream the larvae are transported to the right heart, the lungs, trachea, and pharynx where they are swallowed and mature into adult worms in only 2 weeks. The adult females then produce eggs that upon hatching release rhabditiform larvae into the intestine. These noninfective larvae develop into an infective stage and are capable of infecting a new host. An indirect cycle may be implemented where the rhabditiform larvae develop into free-living adult male and female worms. They mate and produce eggs and noninfective larvae that then develop into infective larvae upon incubation in the soil.

Disease Transmission

Strongyloidiasis is transmitted from one host to another host when the skin is penetrated by the infective filariform larvae living in contaminated soil. Because hookworms are contracted in a similar manner, the *S. stercoralis* larvae must be differentiated from the hookworm larvae. *S. stercoralis* is equipped to undergo a unique process called *autoinfection*. This phenomenon involves the development of the first larval form into infective larvae in the host's intestine. The infective larvae

MICROSCOPIC DIAGNOSTIC FEATURE

General Classification—Nematodal threadworm

Organism	*Strongyloides stercoralis*
Specimen Required	Feces
Stage	Most often the adult larval form is the primary infective form as the rhabditiform larva
Size	Two forms of larva; rhabditiform larva are 200–250 μm, which show short buccal capsule (mouth), prominent genital primordium; filariform larva are approximately 500 μm in length and possess notched tail with equal lengths of esophagus and intestinal tract
Shape	Larva are elongated and slender, hence the term *threadworms* as the filariform larvae are more slender than the rhabditiform stage
Motility	Rhabditiform larvae are motile in the soil and penetrate skin of those coming in contact
Other Features	Free-living cycle in the soil may revert to production of infective filariform larvae

S. stercoralis

Larvae

Bulb

Long buccal cavity

Genital primordium

Rhabdifiform

Delmar/Cengage Learning

are able to penetrate the walls of the colon, ileum, or perianal skin, giving access to the circulatory system. These larvae migrate in the blood to the lungs, are coughed up, and then swallowed where they repeat the cycle. This autoinfective ability leads to long-standing and lifelong infection unless effective treatment destroys all adult parasites as well as the migrating infective larvae.

Laboratory Diagnosis

The diagnosis for *S. stercoralis* is most frequently made by identification of the rhabditiform larvae appearing in human feces. Occasionally filariform larvae may also be seen in feces. Differentiation between hookworm larvae and *S. stercoralis* larvae are made by comparison of the forms based on anatomic differences in the larvae of the species (Table 6-2). In widely disseminated cases larvae have also been recovered from sputum for identification of the larvae. Threadworm ova are rarely seen in the feces. Eggs must be allowed to hatch before the larvae are available for identification. When found, the eggs (ova) are thin-shelled, measure 54 × 32 μm, and may be segmented.

It is necessary to distinguish subtle morphological characteristics of these larvae. Sometimes the course of treatment is predicated upon the species of parasite inhabiting the body. The few species of hookworms that commonly infect the human can be differentiated through the use of these tables.

Treatment and Prevention

Treatment for the hookworm may include treatment with local cryotherapy (cold treatment) when it is still in the skin and has not invaded the other organs and tissues. Medications are available that are effective both in the intestinal stage and during the migrating stage when the parasite is still under the skin. It is often necessary to treat the host for anemia when the disease is quite advanced by the administration of supplements to increase the red blood cell count. Other essential supplements that may also be required to restore nutritive health include vitamins such as folic acid or vitamin B_{12}. The treatment for the two hookworms is the same, but academic interest often requires the differentiation between the two species of hookworms (Table 6-1).

Prevention of hookworm infections and those of *S. stercoralis* are accomplished through proper sanitation, with effective sanitary facilities for disposal of human wastes. Good and effective personal hygiene are essential for preventing and managing infections. The medication of first choice is that of ivermectin, which has fewer side effects than some of the other preparations. The second line medication is albendazole, but none of these are effective for autoinfective larvae that are migrating through the body, so repeat administrations of medications is required to rid the body of the parasite.

SUMMARY

Besides the hookworms, *Ancylostoma duodenale* and *Necator americanus* were briefly described in the previous chapter. Another roundworm called *Ascaris lumbricoides* is of such epidemiological proportions that it requires its own section. *A. lumbricoides* is a large roundworm, one of six worms classified by Linnaeus who began a classification system for plants and animals.

Up to one billion people, or an estimated one-seventh of the world population, are thought to now be infected with a worm called *A. lumbricoides*. Soil contamination by feces where food is grown causes most of the infections by this parasite. The adult worm lives in the intestine, but eggs pass out with fecal materials and eggs develop in the soil where they mature and reach an infective stage. Foods contaminated by feces containing eggs may directly transmit the eggs to humans, where the larvae hatch from the infective eggs that have been eaten.

Ascaris species that inhabit the human intestine may grow to a length of more than 12 inches. A 2-week incubation period must occur before the eggs can cause an infection. After eating these eggs, the eggs hatch in the intestine and then enter the circulatory system (the veins), which takes the blood and the newly hatched larvae directly through the heart and into the lungs. In the lungs, they are coughed up in sputum and then swallowed. Here the larvae enter the intestines (the jejunum) where they continue infecting the body while developing into adult worms in the intestine.

Ascariasis has been determined to have infected humans prior to recorded history. If the disease occurred in Europe during this early period in human history, evidence has been destroyed by climactic and soil conditions, but eggs of *A. lumbricoides* have been found in casts of human feces from several regions in South America that date to several thousand years ago. *A. lumbricoides* is a large worm that may reach up to 35 cm (almost 14 inches) in length and may emerge from the anus even without defecation occurring.

Ancylostoma duodenale and *Necator americanus* range over broad areas of both the Old and the New World, are much smaller than *A. lumbricoides*, and are capable of passing into a human's body tissues. Those two species are much smaller than the large roundworm called *Ascaris lumbricoides*, and include additional physical complications through migration into the body's tissues. Obstruction of the gastrointestinal tract, as is common with *A. lumbricoides*, seldom happens in hookworm infections.

Eosinophilia occurs in response to a number of parasitic infections that include hookworm infections as an immune response to an invasion of the tissues themselves. Falling hemoglobin levels in the blood are often found in cases of prolonged infections, as well as a general appearance of illness along with sometimes a considerable loss of weight. Hookworm prevalence can be higher among adult males due to plantation work and coalmining. Adult women have much higher physiological needs for iron than men because of menstruation and repeated pregnancies, but in many endemic areas, adequate nutrition is not available. As an additional risk, *A. duodenale* infections are also known to occur rarely through translactational transmission to the infant of the infection through breast-feeding by an infected mother.

The roundworms of *Ancylostoma duodenale*, *Necator americanus* (hookworms), and *Ascaris lumbricoides* are the most prevalent roundworms that cause nematode infections in humans. In addition, organisms similar to these that infect humans also infect cats and dogs. The close attachment of animal to human has been present since early civilization. This leads to the belief that these organisms were shared by man and animal and reflects the close living arrangements. Over the years, slight evolutionary changes may have occurred where the organisms became better suited to inhabit either the human or a lower animal. These organisms are chiefly spread by fecal contamination of the environment, which would explain the passing from humans to animal of these parasites.

Diagnosis of nematode infection by hookworms and *Ascaris lumbricoides* is achieved almost exclusively by the recovery of eggs or larvae. Eosinophilia does not occur until tissue invasion has occurred, so this clinical sign is also limited. And, in addition, early in the parasitic infection by roundworms, there may be few or no symptoms. When *A. duodenale* is suspected and eggs have been found, it is necessary to differentiate between the larvae of *A. duodenale* and *Strongyloides stercoralis* larvae, because infection with the less frequently diagnosed *S. stercoralis* has a more serious impact on the health of the victim and requires a different treatment.

It is also difficult to differentiate between the eggs of *Ancylostoma duodenale* and *Necator americanus*. The larvae of the two hookworm species, *A. duodenale* and *N. americanus*, can be distinguished microscopically but this differentiation is not typically done. The adult worms of these two hookworm species, unlike those of *A. lumbricoides*, can only be obtained through a surgical procedure, and if this is done a definitive identification of the species is possible. The best course of action is to avoid contamination of the soil for any of these species just presented. Food sanitation and personal hygiene will go a long way toward diminishing these infections.

CASE STUDIES

1. A 12-year-old boy from a semi-rural area in the mountains of the southeastern United States is out of school for the summer vacation. He plays in a small creek during the summer. Upon using the restroom, the boy chanced to see a long and slender worm in his stool. He had suffered from mild abdominal discomfort along with periodic bouts of diarrhea. When he called his mother's attention to an "earthworm" in his stool, she took him to his pediatrician. What was the probable diagnosis, and how would the diagnosis have been made?

2. A 70-year-old male farmer had experienced chronic weight loss, weakness, and dizziness as well as loose stools. The patient was previously diagnosed with hypertension heart disease and chronic alcohol abuse. The anemia could be attributed to blood loss from a recent mitral valve repair, but the patient denied any loss of appetite. Laboratory results that included a complete blood count confirmed a low hemoglobin of 9.1 g/dL (normal range should be 13 to 16 g/dL for a male). In addition to the low hemoglobin, a moderately high eosinophil count of 9 percent, a possible indication of either an allergy to an environmental factor or to the immune reaction to a parasitic infection. A stool specimen was sent to the microbiology laboratory for a routine culture to rule out a bacterial infection of the intestinal tract along with an ova and parasite (O&P) examination. The stool specimen visually resembled rice water stool. An abundant number of thin larvae morphologically confirmed the diagnosis of a parasitic infection. Distinguishing morphological characteristics of the larvae revealed a rhabditiform larval stage of a parasite. What was the probable diagnosis, and how would the diagnosis have been made?

STUDY QUESTIONS

1. How is ascariasis transmitted in most instances?

2. The estimate of worldwide infection with *A. lumbricoides* is:

3. During which period of history did signs of human infection with *A. lumbricoides* occur?

4. *A. lumbricoides* is a large worm that may reach up to what length?

5. How was it determined that a tapeworm was a single worm?

6. How many eggs can a single *A. lumbricoides* female produce in a day, as an estimate?

7. How do *A. lumbricoides* and the two major species of hookworm differ in their effects on the stomach?

8. What symptoms and signs are found in serious diseases of heavy hookworm infection?

9. How is *Ancylostoma duodenale* passed from mother to baby?

10. Approximately how many eggs are laid by the female hookworm per day, and where are these eggs eventually expelled?

11. Why does it take a considerable period of time before acute symptoms of hookworm infection appear?

Intestinal Cestodes

LEARNING OBJECTIVES

Upon completion of this chapter, the learner will be expected to:

- Describe the process by which cestodes reproduce
- Understand the role of an intermediate host in the life cycle of the parasite
- Define the development of cysticerci and the process of infecting definitive or final host
- Explain why humans are considered "accidental" or "incidental" hosts
- Discuss reproduction of cestodes and location of male and female reproductive systems
- Provide an explanation of how prevention of infection by tapeworms could be achieved

KEY TERMS

Accidental host

Acetabula

Bladderworms

Bothria

Cephalic ganglion

Cestodiasis

Coenurus larva

Coracidium

Corpus Hippocratorum

Cyclophyllidean

Cysticercosis

Cysticerci

Diphyllobothriid

Ellipsoidal

Flame cell

Flukes

Hemaphroditic

Hydatid larva (cyst)

Incidental host

Mature proglottids

Micro-crustacean copepod

Neurocysticercosis

Oncosphere

Operculum

Plerocercoid larva

Procercoid

Proglottid

Pseudophyllidean

Rostellum

Scolex

Strobila

Taenia saginata

Taenia solium

Taenia tapeworms

Taeniid

Unembryonated eggs

Uterine pore

CESTODIASIS (TAPEWORM INFECTIONS)

The terms cestodiasis and cystercosis are used synonymously in the tapeworm infection process of animals and humans. Humans can be infected by as many as 40 species of adult tapeworms and approximately 15 larval forms, mainly as accidental or incidental hosts. This means that the food source may be the primary host that is infected, and then is ingested by the accidental host. Uncooked meat from definitive hosts, when ingested, may result in infections of a number of tissues of the human body, including the formation of cysts in the heart, eyes, muscles, and even the brain. Patients with a history of eating uncooked or undercooked pork, beef, and fish and who exhibit signs of new onsets of seizures may be found to have lesions of the brain from cysts formed there.

CYSTICERCOSIS

Cysticercosis is a term related to infection of the pork tapeworm larvae *Taenia solium.* Neurocysticercosis is the most frequently encountered parasitic infestation of the central nervous system. In underdeveloped countries the disease has been endemic in Latin and South America, Africa, and rural areas of Eastern Europe and Asia. A recent increase in the condition has been observed in the United States and Canada, predominantly in the immigrant populations from South America and Asia. Humans are considered incidental hosts or accidental hosts for the larval stages of several tapeworm species contracted almost exclusively by ingesting contaminated meat or its by-products and wastes. The eggs hatch in the stomach before the larvae penetrate the wall of the intestine and are circulated throughout the system, with frequent involvement in the brain (Figure 7-1). It is

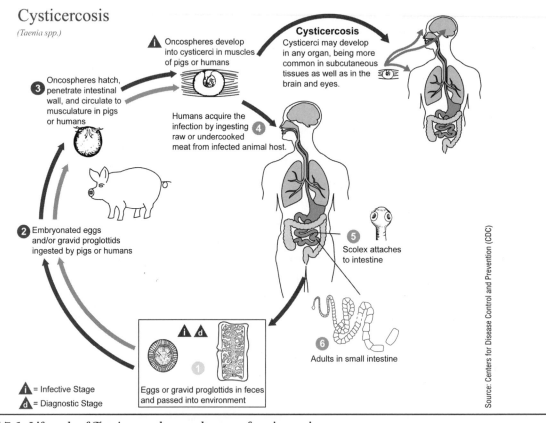

Source: Centers for Disease Control and Prevention (CDC)

FIGURE 7-1 Life cycle of *Taenia* spp., the causal agents of cysticercosis

common for asymptomatic infections to occur but a significant number of patients exhibit seizures, increased intracranial pressure, focal neurologic abnormalities, and various levels of altered mental status.

Four forms of neurocysticercosis are described as pathological conditions of humans: meningeal, parenchymal, ventricular, and mixed. In each of these anatomic areas, the death of the larval stages stimulates an extremely strong inflammatory response. Sizes of lesions vary from small ones of approximately 1.5 cm to larger cysts that range from 4 to 7 cm in diameter. Cysts may be visualized as calcified lesions most effectively and accurately by CT (computerized tomography) but the disadvantage of this method is due to significant exposure to X-rays. An imaging procedure called *magnetic resonance* (MR) is sometimes used for demonstrating these calcified lesions, a process that is beneficial when the lesions are surrounded by edema, which does not yield suitable images with CT.

The most important cestodes belong to two groups: the **taeniid** and **diphyllobothriid** tapeworms. The characteristic taeniid adults, which can reach a length of several meters, live in the intestine, attached by a **scolex** and shed **mature proglottids** ("segments") containing numerous eggs that pass out into the soil or water, at which time the enclosed eggs are released. When an intermediate host consumes the eggs, they hatch in the intestine and then release larval stages called **oncospheres**. These developmental forms burrow through the gut wall to reach various tissues of the host, where they develop into encysted cysticerci or **bladderworms**. The life cycle is complete when undercooked or raw meat is eaten and the **cysticerci** are released and attach to the gut wall of the final host, developing into adult tapeworms (Figure 7-2).

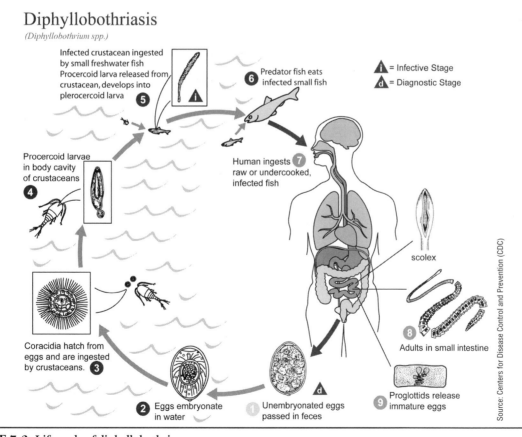

Diphyllobothriasis
(Diphyllobothrium spp.)

Infected crustacean ingested by small freshwater fish Procercoid larva released from crustacean, develops into plerocercoid larva **5**

i = Infective Stage
d = Diagnostic Stage

Predator fish eats infected small fish **6**

Procercoid larvae in body cavity of crustaceans **4**

Human ingests **7** raw or undercooked, infected fish

scolex

Coracidia hatch from eggs and are ingested by crustaceans. **3**

Adults in small intestine **8**

Eggs embryonate in water **2**

Unembryonated eggs passed in feces **1** **d**

Proglottids release immature eggs **9**

Source: Centers for Disease Control and Prevention (CDC)

FIGURE 7-2 Life cycle of diphyllobothrium spp.

Epidemiology of Cysticercosis

In the sixteenth and seventeenth centuries, structures resembling cysticerci were documented by several scientists, but none of the documentation of these observations initially suggested that parasites were responsible for the formation of these cysts. It was not until the late eighteenth century when Johann Goeze demonstrated that certain cysts were the larval stages of tapeworms. A major medical complication associated with infection of *T. solium* is cysticercosis, where the infected individual becomes the intermediate host and harbors the larvae in tissues throughout the body. Therefore, *T. solium* may be treated as an intestinal disorder as well as a contributor to infections of various tissues of the body.

In the late 1700s the German pastor, Johann August Ephraim Goeze, in his study of the pork tapeworm *T. solium*, hypothesized that an intermediate host was involved in the propagation of *T. solium*. Goeze observed that the scolices of the tapeworm in humans resembled cysts in the muscle of pigs, and attempted to make a relationship between the two. It was discovered that embryonated eggs were passed in human feces and then ingested by the intermediate host. In the intestinal tract of the host the oncosphere was freed before traveling through the walls of the intestines and then entering the circulatory system. The oncosphere finally gains access to the muscles of the host, and is transformed into a cysticercus.

Speciation of two commonly encountered tapeworms, *Hymenolepsis nana* and *Taenia solium* should occur due to the differing clinical presentations of each of these. This is accomplished by comparing anatomic features of the eggs of the two organisms. On the inner layer of the two membranes surrounding the *Hymenolepis nana* egg (40 to 60 μm x 30 to 50 μm) are two poles from which 4 to 8 polar filaments are spread out between the two membranes. The oncosphere of *T. solium* as a larval stage has 6 hooks in the egg (Figure 7-3).

The cysticercus resembles a bladder and was described by Aristotle (384 to 322 BC) as "bladders that are like hailstones" in a section on diseases of pigs in his book entitled *History of Animals* (Figure 7-4). These cysticerci are now known to form cysts in the heart, brain, or eye, in addition to the muscles. The most serious consequence of this condition is that of encysting in the brain where the cysticerci cause a number of serious neurological symptoms including seizures. Although the cysts in the muscle cause no apparent serious illness in humans, cysts that form in the brain may cause symptoms

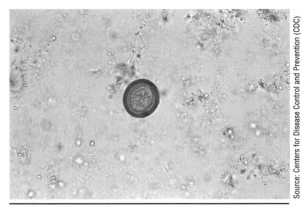

FIGURE 7-3 *Taenia solium* oncosphere, which is the larval stage with 6 hooks

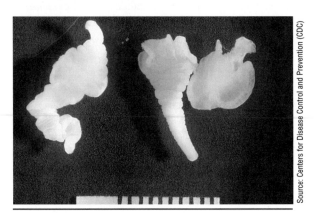

FIGURE 7-4 *Taenia solium* cysticerci, which represent the larval, or intermediate, immature developmental stages of this pork tapeworm

resembling epilepsy. More than likely this would have been a common occurrence in early civilizations when food was prepared under less than sanitary conditions. But no written evidence of this exists, even with the extensive works of Hippocrates, the father of medicine.

The adult stages of *T. solium* and *T. saginata* rarely cause any overt signs or symptoms and there are no early descriptions of diseases that might have been caused by these tapeworms. In addition to *T. solium*, humans are also not only susceptible to the larval tapeworm or cysticerci of the pork tapeworm *T. solium*, but to another organism that forms cysts in the tissues of the body. The hydatid or hydatiform cysts of the dog tapeworm *Echinococcus granulosus* also form similar structures in the tissues of the body. This includes cysts in the central nervous system that often cause seizures in the canine similar to the species of cestodes that may infect the brains of humans. The encysted larvae or cystercerci of *T. solium* in the flesh of pigs were known in ancient history as "measly pork" and appeared to be well known to the ancient Greek physicians, but the condition was never described as a disease of humans.

Evidence exists from early history in the Bible of the Jews regarding the dangers associated with eating certain foods. Certain dietary restrictions abound in the Jewish faith as well as for the Muslims as two religious groups that also observe similar proscriptions against eating pork and who practice the ritualistic preparation of foods. Indirect evidence from different cultures indicates that people were aware of the possible dangers inherent in eating the flesh of pigs because infections with cysticerci are rarely found in Jews and Muslims.

By the nineteenth century, animal experiments demonstrated without a doubt that cysticercosis was caused by the ingestion of *T. solium* eggs. These observations led to public health measures, which had a significant impact on the control of tapeworm infections in humans by restricting the amount infected meat on the market for human consumption. Because meat was required to be inspected before sale as long as 200 years ago, those who ate meat from the butcher shops may have been relatively safe. But many poor farmers raised their own meat and almost certainly fed their animals contaminated food, which their families ate and was a practice that propagated cysticercosis.

Identification of Cestodes

Anatomically, cestodes are divided into three parts. These parts include a scolex, or head, which bears the organs of attachment; a neck, which is the region of segment proliferation; and a chain of proglottids called the *strobila* (Figure 7-5). The strobila elongates as

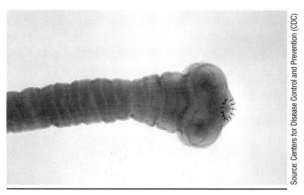

Source: Centers for Disease Control and Prevention (CDC)

FIGURE 7-5 Scolex of *Taenia solium*, a cestodal tapeworm

new proglottids form in the neck region. The segments nearest the neck are immature and in this region the sex organs not fully developed, whereas those closer to the posterior end are mature and are fully capable of reproduction. The terminal segments are gravid (pregnant) and the egg-filled uterus of each segment is the most prominent feature.

DIPHYLLOBOTHRIUM LATUM

Humans may also harbor the adults of *Diphyllobothrium latum,* the broad tapeworm that is also called the fish tapeworm, which lives in the intestine. Eggs are passed in the feces and the first larval stage, the *coracidium*, develops within the egg and when eaten by a copepod (a minute crustacean found in fresh water), it proceeds to develop into the second larval stage called the *procercoid*. When an infected copepod is eaten by a fish, the procercoid develops into the third larval stage, the *plerocercoid*, and when a human eats an infected fish, the plerocercoid develops into an adult tapeworm in the gut (Figure 7-6). This particular tapeworm was well known in ancient history and is mentioned, sometimes indirectly, in the major classical medical writings including the Ebers papyrus, the **Corpus Hippocratorum**, and the works of Celsus and Avicenna (Cox, 2002). However, there are no accurate early clinical records because there are few overt signs of the infection in most victims apart from abnormal hunger, malaise, and abdominal pain.

Morphology

Early descriptions of the worm tend to be unreliable because, as has already been mentioned, there was considerable confusion with the two common species of *Taenia*. Nevertheless, by the beginning of the seventeenth century, it became apparent that there were two very different kinds of tapeworms (broad and taeniid) in humans. Although no doubt others had studied the broad fish tapeworm *Diphyllobothrium*, it is suggested that the fish tapeworm was first recognized as being distinct from *Taenia* by the Swiss physician Felix Plater, who extensively described the disease (Cox, 2002). The first accurate description of the proglottids of cestodes was provided by another Swiss biologist, Charles Bonnet, in 1750, but unfortunately the worm he illustrated was

LIFE CYCLE of—

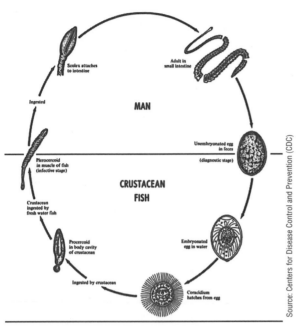

FIGURE 7-6 Various stages in the life cycle of the tapeworm *Diphyllobothrium latum*

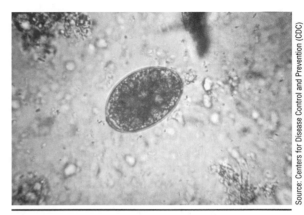

FIGURE 7-7 Egg from the cestode *Diphyllobothrium latum*

Symptoms

Most individuals infected with a fish tapeworm are asymptomatic. However, digestive disturbances including abdominal pain and cramps accompanied by weight loss may occur but few symptoms may be experienced by healthy individuals. Anemia ensues in these infections due to a vitamin B_{12} deficiency, due to the presence of the parasites infecting the intestine.

Life Cycle

By the middle of the eighteenth century, it was apparent that infections with *D. latum* occurred in humans whose diet was mainly fish. However, it was not until the life cycles of other tapeworms of biological interest had been described that further progress was possible. The complications posed by the inclusion of three different hosts (humans and various species of fish and copepods) in the life cycle served to confuse the life cycle of the parasites. An understanding of the life cycle of this parasite began in 1790, when the Dane Peter Christian Abildgaard observed that the intestines of a fish called the stickleback contained worms that resembled the tapeworms found in fish-eating birds; however, it was some time before there was any significant advance in our understanding of the life cycle of *D. latum*. The entire cycle begins with eggs in feces, upon which the eggs in the embryonic stage hatch in water and release coracidia, which are ingested by certain crustaceans.

The life cycle of *D. latum* is complex due to the requirement for two intermediate hosts. The adult

a *Taenia* scolex. He discovered his mistake in 1777 and later revised his works (Cox, 2002).

D. latum is the largest tapeworm found in humans with the strobila (entire length of the organism) reaching a length of up to 10 meters, with as many as 200 strobila involved. It is also the only tapeworm that produces operculated eggs and lays them in the feces. *Diphyllobothrium* sp. **unembryonated eggs** (58–76 μm **x** 40–51 μm) passed in the stool are oval or **ellipsoidal** (Figure 7-7). At opposite ends of the egg is a hardly discernible **operculum**, or lid, and at the other is a barely perceptible knob.

In place of the suckers or hooks found on most tapeworm scolices, the *D. latum* tapeworm has a structure called the **bothria**, which consists of two sucking grooves, and is the structure from which the name is derived (*di-* indicates two, and bothrium). The gravid proglottids are wide and contain a rosette-shaped uterus from which unembryonated eggs are released. The fish tapeworm, *D. latum*, is apparently unique as the only tapeworm that lays eggs and where these eggs may be recovered from the feces.

tapeworm lives in the small intestine and, because the organism is hermaphroditic, it can mate with itself. After self-fertilization occurs, eggs are produced and these un-embryonated eggs leave the human host while contained within the feces. Because no development has occurred until the eggs are released, the egg disintegrates in fresh water and a ciliated embryo called the **coracidium** is freed into the water where it infects the first intermediate host, a copepod crustacean of the genus *Cyclops*. A procercoid larval form develops in the copepod and the infected crustacean is eaten by a second intermediate host, which is a freshwater fish. If the undercooked or uncooked freshwater fish is eaten by a human or other mammal, infection occurs. A scolex emerges for attachment to the intestinal wall and the tapeworm matures in the small intestine.

Disease Transmission

Infections with the *D. latum* organism due to diet are endemic in some parts of the world including Alaska, the Great Lakes region, and countries of the Scandanavian peninsula, Latin America, Africa, and Asia where fish is a large part of the diet. If the first intermediate host, which is the copepod, is ingested by humans through contaminated water, the procercoid larvae may develop into a sparganum, a process called *sparganosis*, where the larvae migrate into the human's subcutaneous tissues.

Laboratory Diagnosis

Proglottids and the scolex of *D. latum* are seldom found in the examination of human feces. Definitive diagnosis is usually accomplished by detection of the characteristic eggs of *D. latum* from human feces.

Finding the characteristic eggs of *D. latum* is the most often used diagnostic feature and also enables differentiation from the eggs of the fluke *Paragonimus westermanni*. This tapeworm egg lacks the "shoulders" near the operculum that are found in fluke eggs.

Treatment and Prevention

Praziquantel and niclosamide are the drugs of choice for *D. latum* infections. If a sparganum (larval stage of certain tapeworms, especially of the genera Diphyllobothrium) occurs, surgical removal may be required. Prevention of infection includes avoiding raw or undercooked fish and

MICROSCOPIC DIAGNOSTIC FEATURE

General Classification—Cestode (fish tapeworm)

Organism	*Diphyllobothrium latum* "worm"
Specimen Required	Stool specimen
Stage	Scolex and proglottids are detected; although the egg is most commonly detected
Size	Worm may reach a length of up to 10 meters
Shape	Scolex has two sucking grooves (bothria); proglottid has prominent rosette-shaped uterus
Motility	Not demonstrated in *D. latum* larvae
Other Features	Proglottid wider than it is long, with a rosette-shaped uterus
	Scolex is 2–3 mm long and is elongated with two sucking grooves opposite each other dorsally and ventrally

D. latum

Delmar/Cengage Learning

MICROSCOPIC DIAGNOSTIC FEATURE

General Classification—Cestode (fish tapeworm egg)

Organism	*Diphyllobothrium latum*
Specimen Required	Feces
Stage	Egg
Size	The egg ranges from 58–76 μm × 40–50 μm
Shape	Broad and oval fertilized egg
	Infertile eggs are longer, 80–90 μm in length
Shell	Thick, yellow-brown, and mammillated
Other Features	Unfertilized eggs show disorganized internal contents
	Egg is unembryonated when passed and is operculated
	Egg has small, knoblike protuberance opposite the operculum at times, but size and lack of "shoulders" is used to differentiate the egg from that of *P. westermanni*

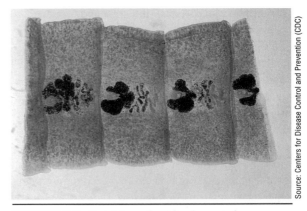

FIGURE 7-8 Gravid proglottids of a cestode

Source: Centers for Disease Control and Prevention (CDC)

proper disposal of human wastes, which might contaminate the waters and provide eggs to infect the copepods.

TAENIA SAGINATA/TAENIA SOLIUM

The adult tapeworm has three distinct regions. Following the scolex, there is a short "neck" region followed by any number of segments, called *proglottids* (Figure 7-8). Another characteristic feature of an adult tapeworm is the absence of a digestive tract, which is ironic because the adult worms inhabit the small intestine, a principal digestive system of the human host. This lack of an alimentary tract requires nutritive substances to enter the tapeworm across the *tegument* (membranous structure resembling skin that covers the segments). This structural arrangement is well adapted for transport functions because it is covered with numerous *microvilli* (hair-like projections) resembling those lining the *lumen* (open area of a tube-like structure) of the mammalian intestine. These villi serve to increase the surface area of the lumen and provide for better absorption. The excretory system is a specialized excretory cell type called a flame cell that functions in a similar manner to both kidneys and anus in mammals.

Of the two species in humans, *Taenia saginata*, or the beef tapeworm, is the larger of the two and *T. solium,* the pork tapeworm, use cattle and pigs as their respective intermediate hosts. The scientific study of the **taeniid** tapeworms of humans can be traced to the late seventeenth century and the observations of Edward Tyson, a British physician and scientist of anatomy who studied the tapeworms of humans, dogs, and other animals. Tyson was apparently the first person to recognize the "head" (scolex) of a tapeworm, and descriptions of the anatomy and physiology of the adult tapeworms led to the current body of knowledge regarding the biological life cycle of the taeniid tapeworms of humans (Cox, 2002). By the time of Tyson's contributions, it was quite evident that there were basic differences between the broad fish tapeworm and other tapeworms now categorized as taeniids, but the differentiation between *T. solium* and *T. saginata* was not fully discovered until later.

It was not until some years later that observations led to the belief that there were actually two species of *Taenia* responsible for infections by what was originally thought to be a single organism. The life cycles of the two species, *T. solium* and *T. saginata*, are practically the same. However, humans are capable of acting as the intermediate host for *T. solium* but not as an intermediate host for *T. saginata*. In the mid-nineteenth century, a Hebrew scholar and theologian named Gottlob Friedrich Heinrich Küchenmeister fed the pork tapeworm to others who became infected. He has been credited with recognizing the differences between *T. solium* and *T. saginata* based on the morphology of the scolex of the two tapeworms, which are now named after their primary hosts (pig and the cow) (Cox, 2002).

Morphology

The morphology of a *Taenia solium* tapeworm scolex reveals four suckers and two rows of hooks, making it almost impossible to dislodge the scolex from the tissue where it is attached (Figure 7-9). In the human intestine the cysticercus, or larval stage, for the organism develops over approximately a 2-month period into an adult tapeworm. These adults can survive for years by attaching to and residing in the small intestine by using the suckers and hooks located on its scolex.

    Taenia saginata can grow to a length of up to 4 to 6 m long and 12 mm broad, but *Taenia solium* is slightly smaller than *T. saginata*. *T. saginata* has a pear-shaped scolex with 4 suckers but no hooks and no neck, whereas *T. solium* has a neck. *T. saginata* has a long, flat body with several hundred proglottids; *T. solium* is only about 0.1 m long, which translates to approximately 3 in long. Each segment of the *T. saginata* is about 18 x 6 mm, with a branched uterus containing 15 to 30 branches; *T. solium* has proglottids that are 5 x 10 mm with 7 to 12 branches in the uterus. The eggs for both of the *Taenia* species exhibit the same appearance as mentioned earlier (Figure 7-10). They measure 35 x 45 micrometers and are roundish and yellow-brown. Peripheral radial striations appear and a visible embryo with 3 hooklets.

    The scolex at the anterior end of the organism contains a poorly organized and developed brain, called the "cephalic ganglion," comprising the simple nervous system typical of the tapeworm. When viewed externally, the scolex is characterized by organs that enable the parasites to hold fast to the tissues where they are feeding by attaching to certain organs of the host body. Depending on the species, these organs consist of a rostellum, bothria, or acetabula. A rostellum is a

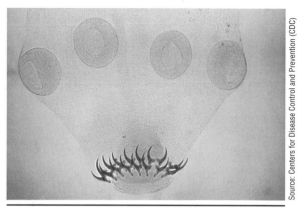

FIGURE 7-9 *Taenia solium* tapeworm scolex with its 4 suckers, and 2 rows of hooks

Source: Centers for Disease Control and Prevention (CDC)

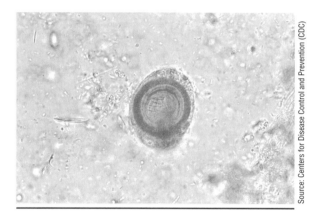

FIGURE 7-10 Egg of *Taenia* sp. with hooklets visible

Source: Centers for Disease Control and Prevention (CDC)

retractable, conelike structure that is located on the anterior end of the scolex and, in some species, is armed with hooks. Bothria are long, narrow, and weakly muscular grooves characteristic of the **pseudophyllidean** (order that includes *D. latum*) tapeworms, of which *Diphyllobothrium* and *Schistosoma* spp. are members. Acetabula (suckers like those of digenetic trematodes) are characteristic of **cyclophyllidean** tapeworms, of which *Taenia* spp. and *Echinococcus* are members (Figure 7-11). Please note that the majority of human tapeworms are cyclophyllideans.

Symptoms

Most cases of taeniasis result in the individuals being asymptomatic. If any symptoms occur, they usually include mild diarrhea, abdominal discomfort, indigestion, and mild fever may ensue. Slight increases in the

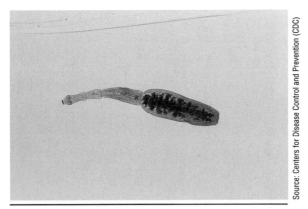

Source: Centers for Disease Control and Prevention (CDC)

FIGURE 7-11 Structural morphology of an adult cestode, *Echinococcus granulosus*

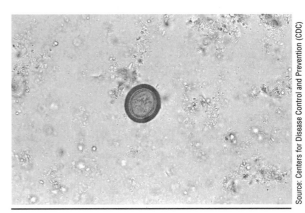

Source: Centers for Disease Control and Prevention (CDC)

FIGURE 7-12 Structural details of a *Taenia* sp. ovum

percentages of eosinophils may also occur, a condition that is not in itself diagnostic of any particular parasite. If the cysticerci migrate to the brain, however, headaches and seizures may result, and will possibly lead to a life-threatening medical condition.

Life Cycle

Cestodes are hermaphroditic, with each proglottid possessing both male and female reproductive systems similar to those found in flukes. Proglottids nearest the scolex are immature but the proglottids near the caudal end are called *gravid* (pregnant) *proglottids* and may contain numerous eggs in the uterus of each segment. However, tapeworms also differ from flukes in the manner by which eggs are deposited. Eggs of pseudophyllidean tapeworms exit through a uterine pore in the center of the ventral surface rather than through a genital atrium, a structure also found in flukes. In the cyclophyllidean tapeworm the female system includes a uterus without a uterine pore. Therefore, the cyclophyllidean eggs are released only when the tapeworms shed gravid proglottids into the intestine. Some proglottids disintegrate and release eggs that are evacuated in the feces, whereas other proglottids are passed intact.

The eggs of pseudophyllidean tapeworms are operculated (lid or covering), but those of cyclophyllidean species are not, so this is a valuable characteristic for identifying eggs of cestodal species. All tapeworm eggs contain at some stage of development an embryo or oncosphere. The oncosphere of pseudophyllidean tapeworms is ciliated externally and is called a **coracidium**.

The coracidium develops into a procercoid stage in its micro-crustacean copepod, which serves as its first immediate host. Later development resulting in a plerocercoid larva occurs in its next intermediate host, which is a vertebrate. The plerocercoid larva develops into an adult worm in the definitive or final host. The oncosphere of cyclophyllidean tapeworms, depending on the species, develops into a cysticercus larva, cysticercoid larva, coenurus larva, or hydatid larva (cyst) in specific intermediate hosts. These larvae, in turn, become adults in the definitive host. Remember that the eggs of the two *Taenia* spp. species of *T. solium* and *T. saginata* are not possible to differentiate from each other, or from other members of the taeniid family, Taeniidae. The eggs measure 30 to 35 μm in diameter and are radially striated. The internal oncosphere reveals 6 hooks (Figure 7-12).

Disease Transmission

Human infection with either *T. saginata* or *T. solium* results from eating uncooked or poorly cooked beef or pork, in the order presented. The cysticercus larvae of the parasite are contained in the meat. Cows and pigs as intermediate hosts eat contaminated food containing eggs, and become infected when the oncosphere hatches from the egg and develops into a cysticercus larva in the tissues of the animal.

Laboratory Diagnosis

The recovery of gravid proglottids and/or eggs from human fecal specimens following the rupture of the proglottids is the most effective method of identification.

MICROSCOPIC DIAGNOSTIC FEATURE

General Classification—Cestode "Worms"

Organism	*Taenia solium* and *Taenia saginata* differentiation
Specimen Required	Fecal specimen
Stage	Diagnostic stages include the ova, scolex (head), or proglottids (contains both male and female reproductive organs); the embryonated egg is the most common stage where *Taenia* species are diagnosed. The egg is yellow-brown and contains a thick wall with radial striations.
	Species differentiation is based on characteristics of proglottids, which are used to differentiate between the *Taenia* sp. (*T. saginata* has 15–20 uterine branches on each side of the uterine trunk, whereas *T. solium* has only 7–13 uterine branches).
Size	*T. saginata* adults reach a length of 10 m and *T. solium* is most often 7 m or less.
Shape	Segmented; both species are similar in shape in that they contain a scolex and proglottids with slight differences in internal structures.
Motility	Proglottids are motile; may actively move outside of the anus.
Other Features	Scolex may also be useful in addition to proglottid differences for identifying the species; the scolex of *T. saginata* contains 4 suckers for attachment and that of *T. solium* includes a rostellum with 25–30 hooklets along with 4 suckers.

T. solium

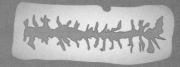

7–14 uterine branches

T. saginata

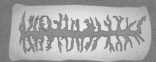

15–25 lateral uterine branches

Delmar/Cengage Learning

Eggs are normally not numerous and the scolex is seldom recovered. Radiological procedures including radiographs, computerized tomography (CT scans), and magnetic resonance imaging (MRI) and other procedures are required for diagnosing cysticercosis, where fluid-filled cysts contain the scolex. Serological studies may also be used to identify and confirm the diagnosis.

Challenges abound in the diagnosis of taeniasis. Gravid proglottids from human fecal specimens release their eggs after the proglottids rupture and are an effective method of identification, because eggs are not numerous and may be difficult to recover. In addition, the scolex is seldom recovered.

Treatment and Prevention

Taeniasis is effectively treated by the drugs praziquantel and niclosamide. Even if the infections are controlled in parenchymal lesions clinically associated with cysticercosis, it is often necessary to surgically remove the cysticercus larvae. Even when the cysts in the brain are destroyed by medication, serious inflammatory processes may occur after the cysts are destroyed in the brain and may require surgery for removal.

Prevention of infection by *Taenia* spp. is primarily achieved by thorough cooking of both beef and swine meat before ingestion. Good sanitary practices and

MICROSCOPIC DIAGNOSTIC FEATURE

General Classification—*Taenia* spp. (Cestode egg)

Organism	*Taenia solium* and *Taenia saginata*
Specimen Required	Feces
Stage	Egg
Size	30–43 µm for both species when passed in feces
Shape	Concentric or almost completely round
Shell	Yellow-brown
Other Features	Shells of ova are radially striated and have a 6-hooked oncosphere in the embryonated egg

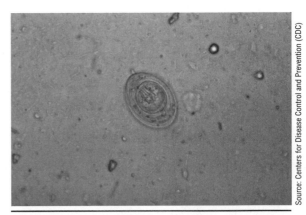

FIGURE 7-13 *Hymenolepsis diminuta* egg should be compared with *Taenia* spp.

avoiding the feeding of animals with foods that may be contaminated (i.e., raw meat mixed with the food) are effective. It has been reported that a vaccine is currently being developed to protect humans against *T. solium*.

HYMENOLEPSIS NANA

Hymenolepsis nana is called the dwarf tapeworm and is the smallest tapeworm known to infect humans. The term may also be used somewhat synonymously with *Hymenolepsis diminuta* but minor differences between the two species exist. It is the most frequently encountered tapeworm in some areas, including the United States. The *H. nana* species is parasitic for both birds and mammals such as mice and rats. Rodents are known to harbor the organism and are capable of transmitting the disease, although no intermediate host is required during its life cycle, unlike a number of the other tapeworms that infect humans.

Morphology

Two inner membranes surround the interior of the *Hymenolepis nana* egg (30 to 47 µm) and two thickened poles or areas of attachment are found from which 4 to 8 polar filaments spread through the spaces between the two membranes. The oncosphere or larval stage possesses 6 hooks (Figure 7-13). The adult worm ranges from 25 to 40 mm in length and are 1 mm wide. Remember that *T. saginata* does not have hooks, a fact which provides a valuable tool for differentiation between *H. nana* and *T. saginata*. *H. nana* has a scolex that contains a retractable rostellum with one single circle of between 20 and 30 hooks and has a tetrad (4) of suckers. The proglottids are visible macroscopically, being approximately 2 mm wide and 1 mm long. The gravid or pregnant uterus of *H. diminuta* when filled with eggs will almost completely fill the uterine cavity of the proglottid. The uterus is usually not visible; however, as it disintegrates to spill the ova into the area surrounding it.

Symptoms

Mild gastrointestinal distress may be encountered but the infected individuals are primarily asymptomatic. Mild diarrhea, weight loss, and abdominal cramps and mild pain may be experienced by some. *H. nana* infections can grow worse over time because, unlike in most tapeworms, eggs of this species can hatch and develop without ever leaving the definitive host.

Life Cycle

Ingestion of *H. nana* eggs is the most common manner in which the infection is contracted. Larvae most often develop in beetles and fleas where grains are contaminated by rat feces, although no intermediate host is required in the life cycle of *H. nana*. The cysticercoid larvae mature in the small intestine where the scolex attaches itself to the intestinal mucosa; there the adult tapeworm thrives and reproduces. Gravid proglottids are passed from the body following disintegration and the infective eggs may contaminate foodstuffs and work areas. The infective eggs may then be ingested by animals, including humans, which develop into cysticercoid larvae and the infectious cycle begins. It is possible for the eggs to hatch in the intestine and in this case cysticercoid larvae develop into adult forms without leaving the intestine of the host, resulting in a process called *autoinfection*.

Disease Transmission

Infection usually begins by ingesting infectious eggs, except in the cases of autoinfection where the eggs "hatch" in the intestine. As for most parasites, prevention is the best method for controlling the infection. A study in one northeastern state revealed that possibly one-third of the rats sold in pet stores in that state were infected by *H. nana*.

Laboratory Diagnosis

Adult worms and proglottids are seldom recovered from stool specimens. The usual process of diagnosis involves the recovery of eggs from fecal specimens.

H. nana is the most prevalent tapeworm found in the United States. It is unusual in the fact that it is a tapeworm that requires no intermediate host, as mice, other rodents, and humans may all be infected by ingestion of the eggs. The scolex is similar to that of *Taenia saginata* and must be differentiated between the two species of tapeworm.

Treatment and Prevention

Treatment for *H. nana* infections is usually the administration of praziquantel. Prevention entails cleaning of the areas of food storage, rodent control, and sanitary practices in food handling and personal practices. Control of beetles and fleas where grains and cereals are stored will also contribute greatly toward the prevention of infections with *H. nana*.

HYMENOLEPSIS DIMINUTA

Hymenolepsis diminuta resembles that of *H. nana*. *Hymenolepis* worms are often found in rat intestines. Because the organism is common in warmer climates, infections are common in the southeastern United States.

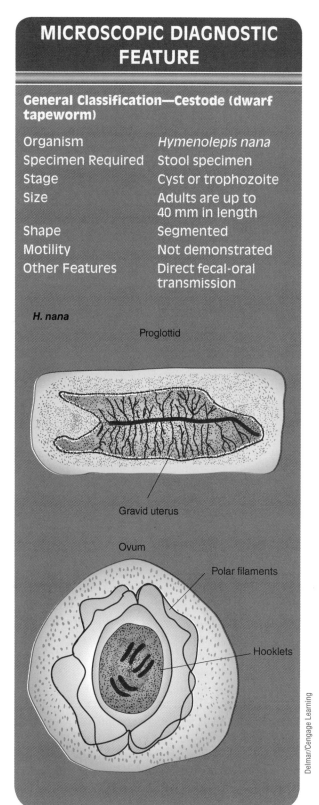

MICROSCOPIC DIAGNOSTIC FEATURE

General Classification—Cestode (dwarf tapeworm)

Organism	*Hymenolepis nana*
Specimen Required	Stool specimen
Stage	Cyst or trophozoite
Size	Adults are up to 40 mm in length
Shape	Segmented
Motility	Not demonstrated
Other Features	Direct fecal-oral transmission

H. nana

Proglottid

Gravid uterus

Ovum

Polar filaments

Hooklets

Delmar/Cengage Learning

MICROSCOPIC DIAGNOSTIC FEATURE

General Classification—Cestode (dwarf tapeworm egg)

Organism	*Hymenolepis nana*
Specimen Required	Feces
Stage	Egg
Size	Eggs are grayish and may range from 30–47 µm
Shape	Round to oval
Shell	Contains an envelope-like center with two thickenings at opposite ends of the structure
Other Features	Four to eight filaments extending from the polar thickenings; three pairs of hooklets are also visible

The secondary host is the beetle, particularly those who consume rat feces.

Morphology

One difference between the two species lies in the fact that the adult worms are slightly larger on average than *H. nana,* averaging 20 to 60 mm in length. The rostellum of *Hymenolepis diminuta* is small and resembles that of *H. nana* except it lacks the hooks found in *H. nana*. Proglottids of both *H. diminuta* and *H. nana* are similar in all aspects of morphology and cannot be differentiated by the proglottids alone, as the proglottids of each contain a uterus consisting of a saclike structure virtually full of eggs. Again, the uterus, when fully gravid, will disintegrate and spill the ova. The eggs of *H. diminuta* and *H. nana* are similar in appearance except that the polar filaments are absent in *H. dimunita*. In addition, the eggs of *H. diminuta* at 50 to 75 µm

are significantly larger than those of *H. nana* at 30 to 47 µm. Eggs of *H. diminuta* should be compared with those of the *Taenia* spp. when identifying the ova of *H. diminuta* (refer to Figure 7-13).

Symptoms

Mild gastrointestinal distress may be encountered but the infected individuals are most often asymptomatic. Symptoms are generally mild with occasional bouts of nausea. Minimal abdominal cramps and pain may be experienced by some.

Life Cycle

Rats are the definitive hosts for *H. diminuta*. Eggs are passed in rat or mouse (sometimes other rodents are involved) feces that may contaminate food sources. The organisms are perhaps eaten by insects such as grain beetles and fleas, among others, and therefore become the intermediate host. The chance ingestion of these insects by man from cereals and grains may lead to human infections as well as infections of other rats that ingest a beetle or flea containing the infective stage of the organism. The adult worm inhabits the human intestine and the life cycle is similar to that of *H. nana*, where the cysticercoid larvae mature and develop in the small intestine and the scolex attaches to the intestinal mucosa. The scolex grows and reproduces, and then discharges gravid proglottids that rupture and are evacuated in the feces. Humans and other hosts that feed on contaminated food products or contaminated household items become infected when cysticercoid larvae again develop and eggs are discharged. In addition to the eggs being defecated, the eggs may hatch inside the intestine and reinfect the host, a process that is termed *autoinfection*.

Laboratory Diagnosis

Adult worms and proglottids are seldom observed in stool specimens. Diagnosis is made by the recovery of the characteristic eggs from fecal specimens.

H. diminuta larvae develop in the definitive host, the rat, and an intermediate host may be the grain beetle or flea. Cysticercoid larvae may mature in the intermediate host and are then ingested by rats or humans who are eating the cereal grains.

MICROSCOPIC DIAGNOSTIC FEATURE

General Classification—Cestode (rat tapeworm)

Organism	*Hymenolepsis diminuta*
Specimen Required	Stool specimen
Stage	Eggs may be found; rarely scolex or proglottids
Size	The adult tapeworm may reach 20–60 cm
Shape	Segmented
Motility	Not demonstrated
Other Features	Direct fecal-oral transmission *H. diminuta* lacks the hooks of the rostellum that *H. nana* exhibits

H. diminuta

Ovum   Proglottids

Delmar/Cengage Learning

MICROSCOPIC DIAGNOSTIC FEATURE

General Classification—Cestode (rat tapeworm egg)

Organism	*Hymenolepsis diminuta*
Specimen Required	Feces
Stage	Egg
Size	Eggs are differentiated from *H. nana* by size, and are gray- to straw-colored and 50–75 µm
Shape	Eggs possess an inner membrane but have no polar filaments surrounding the oncosphere as does *H. nana*
Shell	Contains an envelope-like center with two thickenings at opposite ends of the structure similar to those of *H. nana*
Other Features	Proglottids of *H. diminuta* indistinguishable from those of *H. nana*

Treatment and Prevention

Treatment for *H. diminuta* infections is usually the administration of niclosamide, but praziquantel is also a drug of choice. Prevention entails cleaning areas of food storage, rodent control, and sanitary practices in food handling and personal hygiene. These practices, however, are greatly curtailed in low socioeconomic settings and in poor countries.

DIPYLIDIUM CANINUM

The *Dipylidium caninum* species of tapeworm sometimes infect humans as an accidental host when fleas are ingested, a route of infection found mostly in children. The organism is also called the *cucumber* tapeworm or the *double-pore tapeworm* as the adult proglottids have genital pores on both sides of the tapeworm. *D. caninum* is a cyclophyllid cestode, an important order that infects mammals afflicted with fleas, including dogs, cats, and the owners of pets, especially children. Proglottids are pumpkin-shaped and can reach a length of about 18 in. Eggs are found in characteristic "egg clusters" or "egg balls" of 15 to 25 eggs that are passed

Dipylidium caninum Infection
(*Dipylidium caninum*)

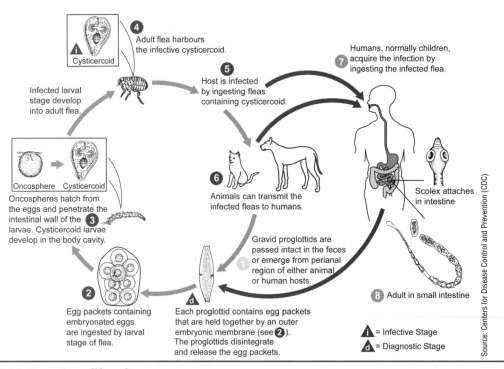

4 Adult flea harbours the infective cysticercoid.

i Cysticercoid

Infected larval stage develop into adult flea.

5 Host is infected by ingesting fleas containing cysticercoid.

Humans, normally children, acquire the infection by ingesting the infected flea. **7**

Oncosphere   Cysticercoid

Oncospheres hatch from the eggs and penetrate the intestinal wall of the larvae. Cysticercoid larvae develop in the body cavity. **3**

6 Animals can transmit the infected fleas to humans.

Scolex attaches in intestine

2 Egg packets containing embryonated eggs are ingested by larval stage of flea.

1 Gravid proglottids are passed intact in the feces or emerge from perianal region of either animal or human hosts.

d Each proglottid contains egg packets that are held together by an outer embryonic membrane (see **2**). The proglottids disintegrate and release the egg packets.

8 Adult in small intestine

i = Infective Stage
d = Diagnostic Stage

Source: Centers for Disease Control and Prevention (CDC)

FIGURE 7-14 *D. caninum* life cycle

in the host's feces and ingested by fleas that may be accidentally ingested by another mammal after the tapeworm larvae have partially developed (Figure 7-14). The species of fleas found on dogs and cats, *Ctenocephalides canis* and *C. felis*, respectively, may both be implicated in transmitting *D. caninum* to humans and other animals.

As in all members of family Dipylididae, proglottids of the adult have genital pores on both sides (hence the name *double-pore tapeworm*). Each side has a set of male and female reproductive organs. In cats, sometimes proglottids are visible hanging out of a cat's anus. When inside fleas, the eggs hatch and form oncosphere larvae that move through the wall of the flea's intestine into the body cavity where they develop into cysticercoid larvae and become infective to mammal hosts. As with most tapeworm infections, control of flea populations on pets is the best way to prevent human infection.

Morphology

The adult tapeworm may range from 10 to 50 cm in length. The scolex has a rostellum with four rows of small hooklet-like spines on a cone-shaped rostellum, along with the 4 suckers typical of all cyclophyllid cestodes. The uterus in a gravid proglottid will contain a large number of packets of eggs with as many as 5 to 20 eggs in each packet. The eggs of *D. caninum* are somewhat colorless and are roughly 30 to 60 μm in diameter with a 6-hooked arrangement of the oncosphere present in each egg. Eggs are enclosed in membranous packets.

Symptoms

Although some individuals with a heavy worm infection will experience mild symptoms of gastrointestinal distress, such as nausea and vomiting, diarrhea, and indigestion accompanied with stomach pain, most infected persons are asymptomatic.

Life Cycle

The definitive host is generally a cat or dog. Gravid proglottids are passed in the animal's feces and the intermediate host, the dog or cat flea, ingests the eggs, which continues the life cycle. Eggs may occur as clusters called *egg balls* and are eliminated in the host's feces and are then ingested by fleas. When the fleas are ingested accidentally by another mammal after the tapeworm larvae partially develop, the cysticercoid larvae that developed in the flea are swallowed. Humans, particularly children, become infected after accidentally ingesting the fleas containing larvae. The larvae from the fleas then mature to adulthood in the host.

Disease Transmission

Transmission of the *D. caninum* cestode occurs predominantly as a result of hand-to-mouth ingestion of fleas from infected domestic animals in which the developing cysticercoid larvae are found. Transmission of the infection also results not only from fleas but from ingestion of beetles and other arthropods that may be in contact with domestic animals.

Laboratory Diagnosis

Characteristic gravid proglottids and egg packets found following disintegration of proglottids in human feces

---

MICROSCOPIC DIAGNOSTIC FEATURE

General Classification—Cestode (cucumber or double-pore tapeworm)

Organism	*Diphylidium caninum*
Specimen Required	Stool specimen
Stage	Adult
Size	Worm may reach a length of up to 10–50 cm
Shape	Segmented
Motility	Not demonstrated
Other Features	The larvae mature to adulthood in the intestine
	Scolex has 4 suckers as do most cestodes, and contains several rows of small hook-like spines on a cone-shaped rostellum of the scolex

D. caninum

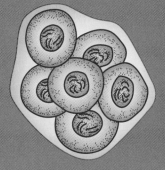

Delmar/Cengage Learning

MICROSCOPIC DIAGNOSTIC FEATURE

General Classification—Cestode egg

Organism	*Diphylidium caninum*
Specimen Required	Feces
Stage	Egg packet
Size	The eggs range from 30–60 μm
Shape	Almost completely concentric
Shell	Thin and colorless
Other Features	Colorless eggs have 6-hooked oncosphere present in each egg and are enclosed in a membrane-bound packet of usually 5–20 eggs per packet

is the major diagnostic procedure for *D. caninum*. However, neither the scolex nor the proglottids are found in many cases of the infection when examining stool specimens. Therefore, finding eggs is the most frequent manner of diagnosis.

Larvae mature in the intestine but are not the chief stage in which *D. caninum* is identified. The egg packets and gravid proglottids are the most diagnostic stages found in the laboratory.

Treatment and Prevention

Although praziquantel has been found to be somewhat effective, niclosamide is the drug of choice. Good veterinary care of cats and dogs by keeping the animals free of parasites and fleas (ectoparasites) is essential. Control of other insects such as beetles may aid greatly in the prevention of infections by *D. caninum*. Personal hygiene is also paramount in preventing hand-to-mouth ingestion of infected fleas.

SUMMARY

Cestodiasis, a term used for tapeworm infections, may occur from infections with up to 40 species of adult worms and perhaps 15 larval forms. Humans are most often incidental or accidental hosts, meaning that they are not definitive hosts. Disease from tapeworm infections usually results from eating uncooked meat from definitive hosts infected with the various cestodes.

Cysticercosis is another term for an infection by cestodes, contracted mainly by the eating of contaminated meat and its by-products and wastes. After ingestion of the eggs, they hatch in the stomach of the host. The resulting larvae penetrate the intestinal wall and circulate throughout the body systems of the host, frequently involving the brain. Neurocysticercosis, of which there are four types, occurs in larval death, which results in a strong immune response to inflammation. Sizes of lesions vary from 1 cm up to 7 cm in diameter, and are viewed via radiological procedures such as magnetic resonance (MR) and computerized tomography (CT).

Taeniid and diphyllobothriid tapeworms are among the most important cestodes implicated in human disease. The adult tapeworm has no digestive tract, and nutritive substances enter the tapeworm across the membranes structure covering the segments and excretion of digestive wastes is accomplished through a specialized structure called a "flame cell." The proglottids or segments of the tapeworm, are attached to a scolex or head, on which mechanisms for attachment to the intestinal wall are found. Mature proglottids contain numerous eggs, which are passed into soil or water through defecation. Eggs consumed by the intermediate host hatch in the intestine, releasing larval stages, or oncospheres that burrow through the gut wall to reach various tissues of the host. Here they develop into encysted cysticerci or bladderworms and when infected meat of the intermediate host is eaten, cysticerci are released and attach to the gut wall of the final host where they develop into adult tapeworms.

Cestodes are **hermaphroditic**, with both male and female reproductive systems in each segment. The proglottids nearest the scolex are immature, but the proglottids near the caudal end are called *gravid* (pregnant) *proglottids* and contain many eggs.

Taenia tapeworms include two human species, *Taenia saginata* (beef) and *T. solium* (pork). These two taeniid tapeworms were originally thought to be one species, until research proved otherwise. The *T. solium* variety of the taeniid tapeworm is the cause of a major complication called *cysticercosis*. *T. solium* is both an intestinal as well as a tissue-infective organism. The cysticercus resembles a bladder, giving rise to the term *bladderworms*.

These cysticerci are known to encyst the heart, brain, or eye, and muscles. The adult stages of *T. solium* and *T. saginata* rarely cause any overt signs or symptoms. Another cyst-forming organism is *Echinococcus granulosus*. *E. granulosus* may form cysts in the tissues of the central nervous system of dogs, causing seizures in the canine similar to those of the species of cestodes that may infect the human brain.

It is evident that most of the cestodal infections relate to eating various types of meats. *Diphyllobothrium latum* is an organism called the *fish tapeworm*, which humans harbor as adult parasites in the intestine. Human eat infected fish, and the plerocercoid develops into an adult tapeworm in the gut, and the cycle is repeated.

Early descriptions of the tapeworm were unreliable due to confusion with the two common species of *Taenia*. In the 1600s it became apparent that there were two very different kinds of tapeworms (broad and taeniid) in humans. *Diphyllobothrium* was first recognized as being distinct from *Taenia* by a Swiss physician, Felix Plater, who contributed the first descriptions of the disease. The first accurate description of the proglottids was by another Swiss biologist, Charles Bonnet. By the mid-1700s, it was apparent that infections with *D. latum* occurred in humans whose diet was mainly fish.

CASE STUDIES

1. A tourist from the midwestern area of North America traveled to coastal Washington State and in areas of western Canada. Taking advantage of the rich source of marine foods, the main dishes at both lunch and dinner consisted of some type of fish. Upon returning home, the traveler suffered from vague digestive upset along with considerable abdominal pain. His physician requested a stool examination, which was negative for pathological bacterial but contained large operculated eggs. What would be the probable causative organism that was the origin of these eggs?

2. An elderly Navaho Indian who raised sheep in northern Utah was forced to chase coyotes and wild dogs from the land where his sheep typically grazed. He had always been in good health but for the past year he had recurring bouts of pain in the stomach. When he visited his physician, palpation of the liver revealed hardening and rounding of the lobes of the liver. In addition, he complained of increased bouts of coughing, with chest pain and sometimes small flecks of blood in the sputum. Given his vocation as a sheep herder, and the fact that he spent a great deal of time outdoors and prepared his food in the wild, what would be a likely parasite from which the man is suffering?

STUDY QUESTIONS

1. Name the two cestode groups that contribute most often to infection of humans.

2. How do the eggs of the *Taeniid* species reach the intermediate host?

3. Which of the tapeworms, *T. saginata* or *T. solium*, become the largest, and what are their approximate lengths?

4. Are both male and female organisms found in the cestodes?

5. What is a valuable characteristic used in differentiating the eggs of pseudophyllidean tapeworms and cyclophyllidean species?

6. With what animals are the cestodes called *T. saginata* and *T. solium* associated?

7. How did Aristotle describe the appearance of the cysticercus structure?

8. What animal is affected by the *Echinococcus granulosus* organism, and how does it manifest itself?

9. Why do Jewish and Muslim religions have certain prohibitions on the eating of certain meats, particularly pork? Why must some of these foods be ritualistically prepared?

10. In your own thinking, how did observations of meat conditions lead to official offices responsible for food safety?

11. Dogs eating sheep meat led to the development of hydatid cysts. Who determined this in 1853?

12. What is the common name for *Diphyllobothrium latum,* and how is it normally contracted?

Intestinal Trematodes

LEARNING OBJECTIVES

Upon completion of this chapter, the learner will be expected to:

■ Outline the reproductive cycle of trematodes that primarily infect humans
■ Describe the clinical impact of trematodes on a worldwide basis
■ Discuss the relationship between flukes and their intermediate and definitive hosts
■ Associate the three major flukes with the organs they infect

KEY TERMS

Asexual	Hematuria	Peritoneal
Bilharzia	Intestinal fluke	Redia
Blood fluke	Katayama disease	Rice paddy itch
Cercaria	Liver fluke	Schistosomes
Cestodes	Lung fluke	Schistosomiasis
Clonorchiasis	Mesenteric	Schistosomula
Crabs	Metacercariae	Semisulcospira
Crayfish	Miracidia	Siberian liver fluke
Dermatitis	Mollusks	Snails
Digenetic	Nematode	Sporocyst
Duckworms	Opisthorchiasis	Swimmer's itch
Duodenum	Palaeoparasitology	Trematodes
Feline	Paragonimiasis	
Flukes	Pelvic	

INTRODUCTION

Trematodes were broadly discussed, along with some specifics, in Chapter Five, where the three types of "worms"—trematodes, nematodes, and cestodes—were compared. Flukes, or flatworms, are parasitic members of the class Trematoda, and to the phylum Platyhelminthes. The order Digenetica, to which the schistosomes belong, also have a complex life cycle. The term digenetic refers to two stages in trematodes where an asexual phase of reproduction—a sexual generation living in a vertebrate host as the final or definitive host—occurs in mollusks. Stages of a typical fluke include the adult, the ova, a miracidium, a sporocyst, a redia, a cercaria, and finally a metacercaria, which is similar in the trematode life cycle.

Trematode Life Cycle

The original symptoms of a condition technically known as cercarial dermatitis occur upon penetration by metacercaria. A number of terms are used to refer to infections by trematodes, including "swimmer's itch," as commonly used in some developing countries. Swimmer's itch translates into "rice paddy itch" and other descriptive terms in areas where rice is a staple food, as well as other terms reflected by the widespread geographic regions in which these organisms are found. Even in the United States, where intestinal trematodes are somewhat common as in coastal New Jersey, the malady is commonly called "duckworms" and is apparently due to water fowl ingesting waste products and then fouling the water by eating the intermediate hosts, or by another similar mechanism. This order, Digenetica, includes all four groups of flukes that are parasitic in humans. These four groups are found in the following table (Table 8-1).

Flukes are characteristically complex in their life cycles and most often require two intermediate hosts, where snails are most often the first intermediate host. Most trematodes are hermaphroditic, meaning that they contain both male and female organs responsible for reproduction. Fluke eggs might or might not contain a miracidium, depending upon the species of fluke involved. The miracidium is a ciliated larval form of the fluke, and some unembryonated eggs require a period of development in the water before the development of the miracidium is complete. The miracidium infects a snail living in a body of fresh water. The miracidium reproduces inside the snail and produces a large number of cercariae, a free-swimming stage of the fluke's life cycle.

The cercariae from some fluke species infect a host by penetrating the skin when the susceptible organisms, including humans, are exposed to fresh water. Other species infect (encyst) a second intermediate host, such as vertebrate (possess a backbone) fish and invertebrates, such as crayfish that possess an exoskeleton rather than bones to provide strength and structure to the organism. In addition, some cercariae cling to or encyst vegetation, which may be eaten by vertebrates, whereupon the life cycle continues. The encysted cercariae in the animals or vegetation evolve into a form

TABLE 8-1 Human Flukes		
COMMON NAME	**REPRESENTATIVE ORGANISMS**	**ANATOMIC REGION INHABITED**
Blood Fluke	*Schistosoma haematobium, S. mansoni, and S. japonicum*	**Mesenteric** and **pelvic** veins
Intestinal Fluke	*Gastroidiscoides hominis, Fasciolopsis buski, Heterophyes heterophyes,* and *Metagonimus yokogawai*	Human intestine
Liver Fluke	*Clonorchis sinensis, Fasciola hepatica, Dicrocoelium dendriticum,* and *Opisthorchis felineus*	Liver, biliary, and pancreatic ducts
Lung Fluke	*Paragonimus westermani*	Lung tissue exclusively

called *metacercariae*, which can infect a host who feeds on the animals or plants.

Liver and Lung Fluke Diseases

More than 80 other species of flukes other than *Schistosoma* are considered capable of infecting humans. Humans may be infected either during the adult stage or larval stage, but only the most common species that routinely impact human health are considered in this section: *Paragonimus westermani,* the lung fluke that causes **paragonimiasis;** *Clonorchis sinensis,* the liver fluke that causes **clonorchiasis**; and *Opisthorchis* spp., which causes **opisthorchiasis.**

Virtually all the important discoveries and advances regarding these parasites were made during the period from 1874 to 1918. Discoveries of these medically important parasite life cycles and other biological data often occurred as a result of observations of other parasitic flukes such as *Fasciola hepatica* in sheep and several other agricultural or zoological flukes rather than medical interest in humans. The life cycles of these other flukes are essentially the same as those described for each of the *Schistosoma* spp. discussed previously. However, there is an added complexity because some species require an additional intermediate or secondary host during development. Whereas snails are secondary hosts, humans become infected both internally (diet) or externally (skin penetration) when the cercariae encyst. Humans become infected only when they ingest the infected second intermediate host.

These various discoveries were made by a large number of people and often in independent and specialized reports that were initially shared with only a few biologists who had an interest in the topic. No attempt is made here by the author to list these individual achievements. The learner is encouraged to refer to a multitude of resources provided by Internet sources. Significant knowledge of the pathological effects of clonorchiasis and opisthorchiasis has emerged slowly and over quite a period of time. Few startling and interesting discoveries have occurred recently, except for finding an association with bile duct cancer called *cholangiocarcinoma* when clonorchiasis or opisthorchiasis infections are present. The basic flukes that cause human disease are described as follows, with the exception of the schistosomes, which are of such importance as to deserve a separate section for the organisms causing **schistosomiasis.**

FASCIOLOPSIS BUSKI

The correct handling, concentrating, and preserving of specimens as well as the competence of the laboratory worker and the timeliness of the specimen collection is vital in the detection and subsequent accurate identification of parasites and their eggs. An example of easily identifiable eggs (ova) is that of the giant intestinal fluke *Faciolopsis buski* (Figure 8-1). Different life stages of a number of parasites may require that several samples be collected and even pooled before steps toward identification of the parasite begins. This is particularly true for some of the protozoan diseases where certain stages of infection are only visible during a critical period when collection should be accomplished. This will be fully discussed during the presentations regarding specific species. *F. buski* is prevalent in Vietnam, Thailand, and all of Southeast Asia.

Morphology

F. buski is an organism known as the giant intestinal fluke. This species is the largest fluke known to inhabit the human body and lives in the small intestine of infected individuals. The adult fluke itself ranges from 2 to 7 cm in length. The egg is broad, ellipsoid, and contains a small operculum, or lid, at the more pointed end of the egg, which has a transparent eggshell and is unembryonated when passed. The egg measures 130 to 140 μm in length and 80 to 85 μm in width.

Symptoms

Bowel obstruction may occur in heavy infections and diarrhea and abdominal pain and cramping may be

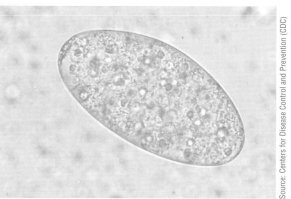

Source: Centers for Disease Control and Prevention (CDC)

FIGURE 8-1 Egg (ova) from the intestinal fluke *Fasciolopsis buski*

present. Local inflammation occurs when the worms attach to the intestinal mucosa, and eosinophilia is common as an allergic response to the invasion of this parasite.

Life Cycle

All trematodes have a similar lifestyle but differ as to the intermediate hosts utilized and the stage of development reached by eggs as they are passed in the feces. The primary reservoir for the intestinal fluke is the pig. Dogs may also harbor the parasite, which bolsters the position by some investigators that there is a close correlation between human parasites and those found in domesticated animals. Following the passing of unembryonated eggs in the stool, micacidia develop in the water within approximately a month. As is characteristic of flukes, the snail acts as the first intermediate host and is penetrated by the **miracidia**. Cercariae are then produced from these miracidia and are released from the snail where they encyst on freshwater vegetation, a life form that is considered the second intermediate host. Water chestnuts and bamboo shoots are the primary second intermediate hosts, where the cercariae develop into metacercariae. These forms encyst in the vegetation and, after being ingested into the intestinal tract, the metacercariae excyst (hatch from the cyst). Further development, self-fertilization, occurs in the intestine to the adult form. The eggs are evacuated in the feces, where they again go through development into cercariae and infect snails. The life span of the worm is somewhat short, existing for a period of approximately 6 months.

Disease Transmission

Ingestion of uncooked or poorly cooked and encysted vegetation containing metacercariae provides transmission for the organism. Animals that feed on raw vegetation also may become infected.

Laboratory Diagnosis

F. buski infection is diagnosed by examination of fecal samples for both ova and parasites. Eggs are quite characteristic and are often passed in the feces, but may be confused with the eggs of *Fasciola hepatica*, due to similarities in both size and shape.

MICROSCOPIC DIAGNOSTIC FEATURE

General Classification—Egg of Liver Fluke

Organism	*Fasciolopsis buski*
Specimen Required	Feces
Stage	Ovum (egg) most commonly; indistinguishable from *F. hepatica*
Size	130 μm × 60–90 μm (average length slightly exceeds *F. hepatica*)
Shape	Ellipsoid
Shell	Transparent
Other Features	Ovum unembryonated when passed in feces

F. buski

Operculum

Delmar/Cengage Learning

Treatment and Prevention

Treatment with praziquantel or niclosamide is most common for *F. buski*. Prevention entails proper human waste disposal and control of snail populations. Eating raw vegetation from watery areas is discouraged.

HETEROPHYES HETEROPHYES

Heterophyes heterophyes and *Metagonimus yokogawai* are presented together as so many similarities exist between the two parasites. The two parasites are easily confused but a distinguishing factor is that they are found in different geographic locations of the world. *H. heterophyes,* an organism that causes a disease known as heterophyiasis, is found primarily in both the Near and Far East as well as parts of Africa. *M. yokogawai* is found in Asia and Siberia and is known as the causative agent for the disease metagonimiasis. The two organisms are predominantly found as cat and dog parasites, as well as other fish-eating mammals, so heterophyiasis and metagonimiasis are known as zoonoses (animal related) when they infect humans. Birds may also be reservoirs for these related organisms.

Morphology

The eggs of *H. heterophyes* and *M. yokogawai* are indistinguishable from each other. They are small flukes known jointly as *heterophyids* (from the genus comprising these two species) and are approximately 30 μm by 15 μm. The eggshells of *M. yokogawai* appear to be thinner than those of *H. heterophyes*, although this can only be determined by close microscopic attention. The mature flukes of both species are approximately 1 to 2 mm in length.

Symptoms

Individuals with light infections are generally asymptomatic, whereas those with heavier infections with either species may experience diarrhea, abdominal pain, and eosinophilia. In severe cases, granulomas may develop. A *granuloma* is a structure that forms during the process of inflammation, when large numbers of macrophages are drawn to an infected area, which then enclose the area. Granulomas also occur in tuberculosis, leprosy, and some fungal infections.

Life Cycle

The eggs of the species are ingested by a freshwater snail. The eggs contain a fully developed miracidium and, upon ingestion, the miracidium is released from the egg, upon which it penetrates the tissues of the snail and develops into the cercarial stage. Mature cercariae are released into the fresh water, and find fish that become second intermediate hosts when they are encysted. When cercariae encyst into the flesh of the fish, they form metacercariae. The definitive host then ingests the fish containing metacercariae, at which time they excyst and develop into adult worms in the small intestine. The adult worms are then able to produce eggs to continue the life cycle.

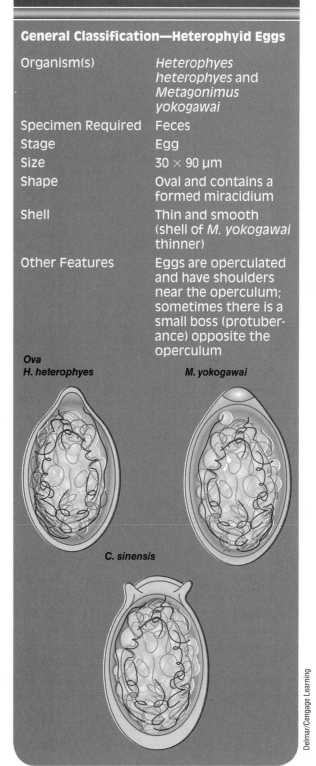

MICROSCOPIC DIAGNOSTIC FEATURE

General Classification—Heterophyid Eggs

Organism(s)	*Heterophyes heterophyes* and *Metagonimus yokogawai*
Specimen Required	Feces
Stage	Egg
Size	30 × 90 μm
Shape	Oval and contains a formed miracidium
Shell	Thin and smooth (shell of *M. yokogawai* thinner)
Other Features	Eggs are operculated and have shoulders near the operculum; sometimes there is a small boss (protuberance) opposite the operculum

Ova
H. heterophyes

M. yokogawai

C. sinensis

Delmar/Cengage Learning

Disease Transmission

Transmission of either of these two diseases happens when uncooked or inadequately cooked fish are eaten. The eggs of *H. heterophyes* and *M. yokogawai* may be confused with those of the liver fluke *Clonorchis sinensis*. Adult worms of these species are almost never detected in fecal waste.

Laboratory Diagnosis

Because the adult fluke is almost never seen in a fecal specimen, the presence of eggs provides the diagnostic tool for determining infection. When seen, the adult stages of both species are tiny, measuring 1 to 2 mm in length. The diagnosis of either heterophyiasis or metagonimiasis is most often accomplished by detecting the characteristic ova during a routine examination for ova and parasites in a stool specimen. The ova must be differentiated from those of *Clonorchis sinensis*, because the eggs of *H. heterophyes* and *M. yokogawai* are indistinguishable from each other. However, purported differences in the thicknesses of the egg shells of the two species may be possible, but differentiation of the two species is merely academic, as the treatment is the same for either species.

Treatment and Prevention

As for a number of other trematodes, praziquantel is the choice for treatment of infections from both *H. heterophyes* and *M. yokogawai*. Proper disposal of human wastes is paramount in preventing the diseases, where water runoff into bodies of water is controlled. Thoroughly cooking fish, especially those from endemic areas of the world, will also minimize the number of cases of infection by *H. heterophyes* and *M. yokogawai*.

FASCIOLA HEPATICA

F. hepatica is known either as the common liver fluke or sheep liver fluke and is a parasitic flatworm of the class Trematoda that infects the livers of various humans and other mammals. The term *hepatica* always refers to the liver, hence the common name of liver fluke. The disease is called *fascioliasis*, and the causative organism, *F. hepatica*, is distributed over a wide portion of the world. Besides infecting humans, the organism causes great economic losses in sheep and cattle. Eggs of *F. hepatica* are virtually indistinguishable from those of *F. buski*.

Morphology

Members of this family are large and leaf-shaped parasites of mammals including humans but mostly affect herbivores (cattle). The adult parasitic worm reaches a length of 2 to 3 cm. The eggs of *Fasciola hepatica* are operculated and can be as large as 130 to 150 µm by 63 to 90 µm. This parasite also has characteristically branched reproductive organs. The *Fasciola hepatica* organism also has oral suckers used to effectively anchor the parasite, as it frequently inhabits the bile duct. Adult flukes feed on the lining of the bile ducts and pass their eggs from the bile duct by which it reaches the intestines. It should be noted that the organism does not directly affect the liver, but the close proximity of the gallbladder and the bile ducts produces symptoms similar to those that directly impact the liver.

Symptoms

Abdominal cramps and pain, diarrhea, and indigestion are symptoms of this parasite. Migration through the liver may cause damage when the number of worms infecting the liver and the bile duct are excessive. Inflammation of the bile duct may mimic other diseases of the biliary system, and complete obstruction of the common bile duct may occur, leading to serious consequences.

Life Cycle

F. hepatica has a similar lifestyle to that of *F. buski*, with the passage of unembryonated eggs in the feces. Following the passage of the unembryonated eggs in the stool, micacidia develop within 2 weeks, escape from the eggs, and infect the snail, which acts as the first intermediate host penetrated by the miracidia. Cercaria are produced in the snail from these miracidia and are released into fresh water where feces is dumped or runs into the water. There they encyst and form metacercariae on freshwater vegetation, which is considered the second intermediate host. Humans and other mammals are infected after eating the contaminated vegetation. The metacercariae excyst in the duodenal portion of the intestine and the larvae penetrate the intestinal wall and enter the gallbladder and bile ducts of the human host. The adult worms attach themselves in the large bile ducts and the gallbladder of humans rather than in the intestines as other parasites do, but eggs are passed from the bile duct into the intestine and are excreted in feces.

Disease Transmission

Ingestion of uncooked or poorly cooked and encysted vegetation such as watercress that harbor infective metacercariae are capable of transmitting the infection. These practices greatly contribute to the transmission of the organism to another host.

Laboratory Diagnosis

The characteristic eggs of *F. hepatica,* which must be differentiated from *F. buski,* is the best mode of identification of the causative organism. Clinical history is essential in this differentiation and the Entero-test string procedure may also be helpful. The Entero-test string procedure is a simple and non-invasive method useful in sampling duodenal fluid. If eggs are recovered from duodenal aspirates containing bile fluid, differentiation between the two species may be made as *F. hepatica* resides exclusively in the bile duct and the gallbladder. Serological methodology is also available for early diagnosis of the liver fluke infection. The prognosis for an infected patient may also be tested serologically to determine if a cure has been effected.

Treatment and Prevention

Bithinol, which is a halogenated phenol, is used for treatment of the infection. Triclabendazole is also effective as treatment for this parasite. Prevention of infection is accomplished by avoiding raw vegetation growing in watery environments in endemic regions. Adherence to good sanitary practices where raw human sewage is properly treated and disposed of will also prevent infection.

CLONORCHIS SINENSIS

The human liver fluke, or *Clonorchis sinensis,* is a liver fluke that is a member of the class Trematoda and is sometimes called the Chinese liver fluke. It is also a flatworm of the phylum Platyhelminthes. The liver fluke was initially identified in 1875, but it was not until 1914 that the snail host was first recognized by a Japanese scientist. In 1915 a second intermediate host was discovered, which further complicated the issue. The first records of *Opisthorchis* infections in humans were made by Konstantin Wingradoff in 1892 and the snail and fish hosts and their roles in the life cycle were discovered by Hans Vogel in 1934. This second intermediate host was an important food fish from which human infections

are acquired (Figure 8-2). This discovery by Kobayashi had the greatest impact on our knowledge of and gave a means for control of this infection (Cox, 2002).

Morphology

The Chinese liver fluke, *C. sinensis,* produces eggs that look somewhat delicate in design, contain a thick browning shell, and prominent shoulders abutting the operculum. The egg is shaped much like a flask with a lid and is similar to that of *H. heterophyes* and *M. yokogawai.* The eggs measure 30 μm by 15 μm and contain a fully developed miracidium. An adult fluke ranges from 1 to 2.5 cm in length.

Symptoms

Except in the cases of heavy infections by *C. sinensis,* the patient is ordinarily asymptomatic and no liver damage is evident, but heavier infections may exhibit inflammatory changes in the biliary epithelial tissues. Abdominal pain with fever and eosinophilia may occur, along with obstructive jaundice due to liver involvement and bile duct involvement.

Life Cycle

This parasite lives almost exclusively in the liver of humans and may also be found in large numbers in the gallbladder and bile duct and feeds on bile produced by the liver. Such an infection can lead to complete obstruction of the common bile duct in extreme cases. This parasite is perhaps one of the most prevalent worm parasites in the world and is estimated to infect up to 30,000,000 persons. The life cycle of *Clonorchis sinensis* is somewhat similar to that of the other flukes. The egg, which contains the miracidium, will float in fresh water; fresh water is also required for the other flukes. No further development occurs until the egg is ingested by a snail—several species are capable of acting as the first intermediate host for *C. sinensis.* Upon reaching the digestive system of the snail, the egg hatches, and the resultant miracidium grows as a parasite of the snail. This miracidium develops into a sporocyst, which encompasses the redia, an asexual reproductive stage. Because mating is not required, this greatly facilitates a significant increase in the number of cercariae from each miracidium.

Upon maturation inside the snail, the redia burrow out of the snail's body and inhabit the fresh water

Clonorchiasis

(Clonorchis sinensis)

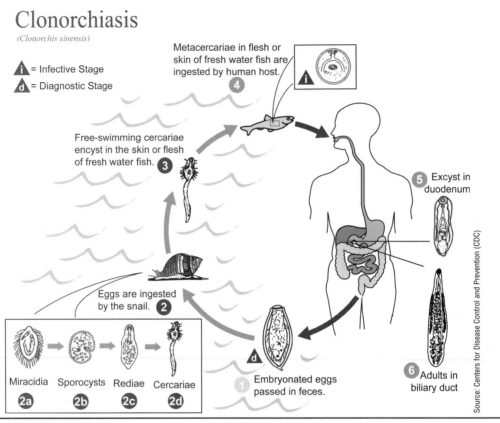

FIGURE 8-2 Life cycle of *Clonorchis sinensis*, the causal agent of clonorchiasis

surrounding them. They no longer require ingestion, but actively seek out a fish as a new host, where they bore into the fish's body and become parasites in their host. These redia are now cercariae and form a protective cyst in the fish muscle before becoming known as metacercariae. This cyst is resistant to stomach acids of the human host so the metacercariae are able to reach the small intestine after the fish is eaten. From there they travel to the liver where they feed on bile produced by the liver and reach sexual maturity. These organisms are hermaphroditic adults, as are other flukes, and are able to produce eggs at a rapid pace leading to a quick saturation of the liver with adults producing eggs.

Disease Transmission

The ingestion of raw or undercooked fish containing metacercariae is the most likely cause of a *C. sinensis* infection. Those with light infections are sometimes asymptomatic, but are still able to transmit the organism to others. These metacercariae are not released into the water where they can invade the skin of people entering the water, as is the case with some species of metacercariae.

Laboratory Diagnosis

Using the oil immersion objective providing a microscopic power of 1000×, structural features are somewhat easily visualized in a *Clonorchis sinensis* egg. *C. sinensis* is a trematode known as the Chinese or oriental liver fluke. The eggs of this organism are relatively small and range from 25 μm to 35 μm by 10 μm to 20 μm. The eggs are oval shaped with a sharply curved and convex operculum that rests on a rounded rim at the smaller end of the egg. At the larger end, a stem-shaped knob is usually visible (Figure 8-3). A miracidium is visible inside the eggs of *C. sinensis,* which are capable of floating in fresh water.

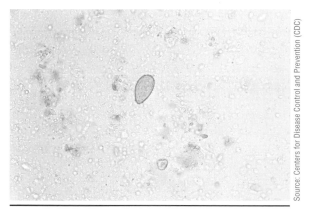

FIGURE 8-3 Structural features of a *Clonorchis sinensis* egg

Treatment and Prevention

The administration of praziquantel is the basic drug used for this infection. Prevention, as in most parasitic infections, requires good personal and food preparation sanitation, and the ingestion of only thoroughly cooked fish.

OPISTHORCHIS FELINEUS

This organism is known as a "cat liver fluke," hence the name of "felineus" from the word *feline*. The disease does frequently infect humans and is spread largely around the world. It was not until 1931 that the life cycle of this organism was defined but it was first discovered in 1884 by Sebastiano Rivolta of Italy (Figure 8-4). K. N. Vinogradov, a Russian scientist, in 1891 found the disease in a human victim and named the parasite after the region where he was performing his work by giving it the common name of "**Siberian liver fluke**." *O. felineus* is found mainly in Europe and Asia, including the former Soviet Union.

Morphology

Opisthorchis felineus adult flukes are 5.5 to 10 mm in length and 0.8 to 1.5 mm in width, and the testes of this species are not as deeply branched as those of *C sinensis*. The ova of *Opisthorchis* spp. range from 19 to 30 μm in length by 10 to 20 μm in width. They are often indistinguishable from the eggs of *Clonorchis sinensis*.

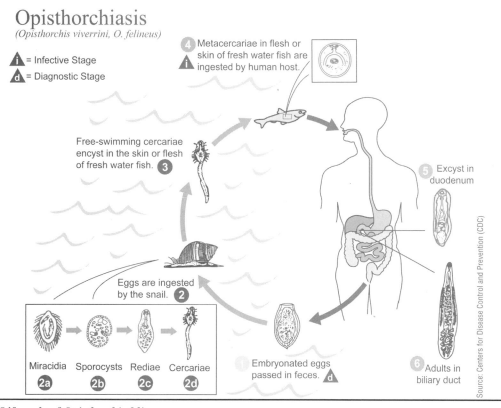

Opisthorchiasis
(Opisthorchis viverrini, O. felineus)

i = Infective Stage
d = Diagnostic Stage

FIGURE 8-4 Life cycle of *Opisthorchis felineus*

Geographic location and clinical data assist in differentiation between the eggs of *C. sinensis* and *O. felineus*. The eggs are operculated and possess prominent opercular 'shoulders' and abopercular (opposite the operculum) knobs. The eggs are distinctly embryonated when passed in feces.

Symptoms

Opisthorchiasis, the disease caused by *Opisthorchis felineus*, is quite variable in severity, ranging from asymptomatic infection to severe illness. Human cases of opisthorchiasis may affect the liver, pancreas, and gallbladder and, if not treated, cirrhosis of the liver may result. Cirrhosis from this infection leads to an increased statistical prevalence of liver cancer even years later. Approximately 2 weeks after flukes enter the body of the host, the parasites infect the biliary tract and produce symptoms of infection that include fever, general malaise, skin rash, and gastrointestinal discomfort. Severe anemia and liver damage may severely incapacitate an individual for up to 2 months.

Severity of the disease ranges from an asymptomatic state to severe medical conditions. Early detection and treatment are of the essence in preventing unwarranted suffering, and the resulting consequences of a long-standing infection. Opisthorchiasis in humans may result in damage to the liver, the pancreas, and the gallbladder. An increased risk exists in the development of liver cancer in chronic cases, as well as cirrhosis of the liver. Treatment with a single dose of an effective medication is most often sufficient, but again, prevention is the best course of action.

Life Cycle

The adult flukes deposit fully developed eggs that are passed in the feces. After ingestion by a snail of an acceptable species as the first intermediate host, the eggs release miracidia, which undergo several developmental stages in a snail's body, developing from sporocysts, to rediae, and then to cercariae. The cercariae are then released from the snail upon which they penetrate the flesh of freshwater fish as the second intermediate host. There they encyst as metacercariae in the muscles or under the scales of the fish. Mammalian definitive hosts that include cats, dogs, and various other fish-eating mammals including humans become infected by ingesting raw or undercooked fish containing metacercariae. After ingestion by the definitive host, the metacercariae excyst in the duodenum and migrate into the bile duct and gallbladder where they attach and develop into adults, which are capable of laying eggs after 3 to 4 weeks.

Disease Transmission

It is estimated that up to 1.5 million people in Russia are infected with the Siberian liver fluke. Inhabitants of Siberia and perhaps other regions of the world acquire the infection by consuming raw or slightly salted and frozen fish.

Laboratory Diagnosis

Diagnosis is based on microscopic identification of eggs in stool specimens. However, the eggs of *Opisthorchis* are practically indistinguishable from those of *Clonorchis*, and differentiation is based on geography and clinical data such as the involvement of the biliary system. Using the oil immersion objective providing a microscopic power of 1000×, structural features are somewhat easily visualized in *Opisthorchis*.

Treatment and Prevention

Treatment of opisthorchiasis is generally with a single dose of praziquantel, the basic drug used for this infection. Prevention, as in most parasitic infections, requires good personal and food preparation sanitation, and the ingestion of only thoroughly cooked fish.

PARAGONIMUS WESTERMANI

This fluke is known primarily as the lung fluke and may be parasitic to a number of mammals other than humans, including dogs, cats, pigs, mink, and perhaps others. A diet of poorly cooked crabs or crayfish provide the basic way of contracting this disease, which is primarily found in parts of Asia. The history of these infections as diseases begins with the discovery of the worms and continues with the elaboration of the life cycles. *P. westermani* was discovered in the lungs of a human by B. S. Ringer in 1879, a finding that he subsequently shared with others. Eggs in the sputum were recognized independently by Manson and Erwin von Baelz in 1880. Manson also suggested that a snail might act as an intermediate host and a number of Japanese scientists reported on the whole life cycle in a species of snail, *Semisulcospira*, between 1916 and 1922 (Cox, 2002).

Morphology

This oval and brownish worm as an adult measures roughly 10 mm in length and 8 mm in width. The eggs of the oriental lung fluke are oval and measure, on average, 100 μm in length and 55 μm in width. The egg is unembryonated when passed in the feces and the operculated egg appears similar in size and shape to that of the *Diphyllobothrium latum* tapeworm with the exception that the lung fluke has opercular shoulders and a thickened shell at the opposite end of the operculum as a differentiating characteristic.

Symptoms

The disease is manifested clinically in a number of ways that range from the victims who appear perfectly healthy to those with severe clinical signs and symptoms. Peritoneal infections often lead to dysentery, masses in the abdominal region, and significant pain. Invasions of the central nervous system may lead to seizures, paralysis,

and even progress to epileptic-like signs. Pulmonary symptoms may include cough with chest pain, hemoptysis (blood in sputum), and bronchitis. Eosinophilia is often present and the larval stage may migrate to the brain and produce neurological signs and symptoms.

Life Cycle

The life cycle of the worm of the genus *Paragonimus* occurs widely in Asia and includes the countries of Japan, Korea, Taiwan, China, the Philippines, and Thailand (Figure 8-5). Eggs from the adult larvae are coughed up in the sputum from the lungs and swallowed. Upon reaching the intestines the eggs are passed in the stool and contamination of fresh water sources ensues in some cases. Upon hatching, miracidia are produced that invade certain species of snails. Large numbers of these stumpy-tailed cercariae leave the snail and crawl into the muscles and visceral (gut) tissue of water creatures, such as crayfish and crabs, which become the secondary or secondary intermediate hosts that inhabit fresh water. Humans eat

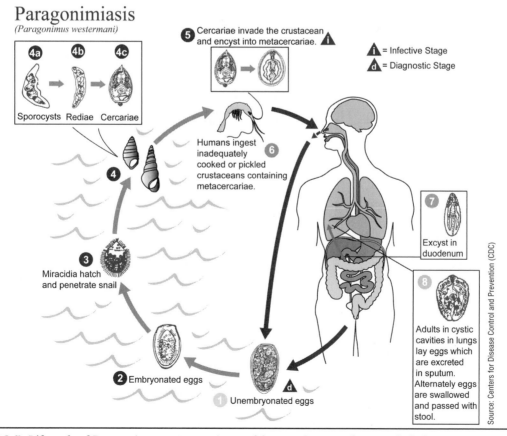

FIGURE 8-5 Life cycle of *Paragonimus westermani*, one of the causal agents of paragonimiasis

poorly cooked crabs and crayfish and become infected, upon which the infective larvae from the crabs or crayfish migrate from the **duodenum** to organs that include the intestinal wall, lymph system, genitourinary tract, central nervous system, and subcutaneous tissues of the body. Sometimes the respiratory system is affected and when the lungs become involved the victim develops a cough with hemoptysis. Flecks of blood in the sputum are often the first sign of paragonimiasis.

Disease Transmission

Infection occurs when encysted metacercariae are eaten, along with raw or undercooked crustaceans such as crabs and crayfish. The disease may progress to the lungs where pulmonary and extra-pulmonary infections become established.

Laboratory Diagnosis

Laboratory diagnosis is frequently based on the finding of eggs in either feces or sputum. The eggs measure roughly 100 by 50 μm, and are unembryonated when passed (Figure 8-6). Flecks of blood may appear in the sputum during infections with *P. westermani* whose eggs are easily

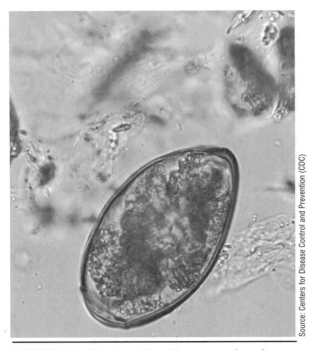

Source: Centers for Disease Control and Prevention (CDC)

FIGURE 8-6 Unstained, formalin-preserved stool specimen egg of *Paragonimus westermani* trematode

MICROSCOPIC DIAGNOSTIC FEATURE

General Classification—*Paragonimus westermani* ova

Organism	*Paragonimus westermani*
Specimen Required	Sputum specimens most commonly, less often in stool specimens
Stage	Eggs when coughed up and swallowed
Size	Range from 80–118 × 48–60 μm (average 100 × 50 μm)
Shape	Eggs are broadly oval
Shell	Shell of egg is thin but thickens toward the flattened operculum (lid)
Other Features	Must be differentiated from *Diphyllobothrium latum*
	Wet mount from sputum may reveal eggs in some patients

P. westermanni

Ovum

Delmar/Cengage Learning

confused with the eggs of the tapeworm *Diphyllobothrium latum,* as both are operculated and are essentially the same size. When seen, the adult worm is 10 by 8 mm and is brownish in color. Serological immunoassays for serum antibodies against the organism are available and pleural effusions are also used to detect the presence of the organism in both pulmonary and extra-pulmonary infections.

Paragonimus westermani infections are most frequently diagnosed by the presence of eggs in the sputum. Larvae may develop into adults in the bronchiolar area and may be seen there.

MICROSCOPIC DIAGNOSTIC FEATURE

General Classification—Flukes of the Lungs

Organism	*Paragonimus westermani*
Specimen Required	Sputum specimens most commonly, less often in stool specimens
Stage	Adults are reddish-brown and live in capsules of the bronchioles
Size	Adults are 10 × 8 mm (roughly 1 cm)
Shape	Adults of *Paragonimus* spp. are large, robust, ovoid flukes. They are hermaphroditic, with a lobed ovary located anterior to two branching testes. Like all members of the Trematoda, they possess oral and ventral suckers.
Motility	Motility in fresh water
Other Features	Shell of egg is thin but thickens toward the flattened operculum (lid)
	Must be differentiated from *Diphyllobothrium latum*
	Wet mount from sputum may reveal eggs in some patients

Treatment and Prevention

Praziquantel is available for treatment of the condition, as for many other trematodal infections. Cultural changes in attitude and practice and the undertaking of lifestyle changes to aid in the prevention of infection is the best method of control for *P. westermani*. These changes would include avoidance of poorly or undercooked crabs and crayfish, as well as personal hygiene and sanitary practices in disposing of human wastes and living conditions.

SCHISTOSOMES AND SCHISTOSOMIASIS

Schistosomiasis is a disease caused by the **blood fluke**, a significant **nematode**, and is a condition that has been recognized for hundreds if not thousands of years. Schistosomiasis is also known as **bilharzia**, particularly in Egypt and nearby regions, an endemic region for the disease today, is caused by trematode worms belonging to the genus *Schistosoma*. Three species of *Schistosoma* are important: *S. haematobium*, *S. mansoni*, and *S. japonicum*. In 1910 Marc Armand Ruffer apparently found *S. haematobium* eggs in two Egyptian mummies dating from at least 1000 BC. This finding that is widely accepted as the beginning of the subdiscipline of parasitology is called **palaeoparasitology**.

This disease, called schistosomiasis, is no doubt an ancient malady and is found in ancient written records and archaeological evidence exists that attests to this fact. Early medical practitioners documented the passage of bloody urine, a condition that is called **hematuria** and that today is associated with *S. haematobium* infections. The genus *Schistosoma*, when broken down, literally refers to a splitting of the body (*schisto-* refers to split, or cleft, and *soma-* means body). There was nothing exceptional in early medical records regarding the symptoms of schistosomiasis that might have attracted the attention of early victims. No recent evidence has emerged to lead to the belief that schistosomiasis is not an antique disease that has continued in importance epidemiologically for at least several thousand years. Thus, there is direct evidence that schistosomes were present in ancient Egypt where they are still prevalent and there have been numerous attempts to find descriptions of this condition in the medical writings of that era.

If explanations from the early Egyptian Ebers Papyrus are not accepted as documentation of the description of schistosomiasis in the earliest medical literature, the first definitive record would refer to that of an epidemic among soldiers in Napoleon's army in Egypt in 1798 by a French army surgeon. A. J. Renoult writes that "A most stubborn haematuria manifested itself amongst the soldiers of the French army . . . continual and very abundant sweats, diminished quantity of urine . . . becoming thick and bloody." Thereafter there are numerous reports of illnesses characterized by hematuria, particularly among armies involved in the Boer War (1899 to 1902) that occurred in South Africa. The worm *S. haematobium* was described by the German parasitologists Theodor Bilharz and Carl Theodor Ernst von Siebold in 1851. Bilharz, with Wilhelm Griesinger, made the connection with the urinary disease a year later. The common term *bilharzia* relating to schistosomiasis persists today in many parts of the world and is so named after Theordor Bilharz.

And in consideration of the knowledge of the history of intestinal schistosomiasis caused by *S. mansoni*, Sir Patrick Manson in 1902 first identified the species that now bears his name. Manson at that time concluded that there were only two species of *Schistosoma* in humans. Even though there had been similar suggestions by other investigators by that time, Manson's ideas were not accepted by everyone. It was R. T. Leiper who, in 1915, firmly established the existence of *S. mansoni* as a separate species. During the time that Manson and Leiper were performing investigations of the *Schistosoma* species, work independent of these two were ongoing in other areas.

The third important species which was undergoing study sometime before Manson and Leiper were working in other areas of the world is the Asian form of the disease that became known as *Schistosoma japonicum*. As early as 1847, Dairo Fujii was working with an ancient disease that had been known for many years but was not properly recorded in the Kwanami district of Japan. The report detailing **Katayama disease**, the disorder that is now recognized as *S. japonicum*, was not generally available for other investigators until 1909. Fujii was alerted to the malady when he found agricultural workers who had waded in watery fields. Cattle and horses were also affected by wasting and abdominal swelling, accompanied by severe rashes on the legs, but the cause was unknown to him at the time.

The actual parasitic worm of *S. japonicum* was not discovered and described until 1904 by Fujiro Katsurada. In 1913 the development of the organism during its time spent in the snail host was described by Keinosuke Miyairi and Masatsuga Suzuki (Cox, 2002). This work regarding the development of the infective form of the parasite occurred two years prior to Leiper's independent description of the life cycle of *S. haematobium*. More extensive discussions of the history of Katayama disease are available from a number of sources.

The twentieth century brought about the discovery of several other species of schistosomes: *S. intercalatum* and *S. mekongi*. *S. mekongi* is prevalent only in the Mekong river basin in Asia, which includes much of present-day Vietnam. *S. intercalatum* is found primarily in central Africa. Several other species of schistosomes have been identified and are known to infect birds and mammals but only cause an irritating dermatitis from the cercariae penetrating human skin. The history of such an important disease as schistosomiasis involves a great number of observations, events, and individuals. Today a detailed account of the history is given by David I. Grove as well as shorter accounts by W. D. Foster, L. G. Goodwin, and R. Hoeppli. Other accounts of the studies of schistosomiasis conducted during periods of American and British imperialism are provided by John Farley (Cox, 2002).

Morphology

The mature female blood fluke measures an average of 1.5 to 2.0 cm, the female being bigger than the male as in many parasites, ostensibly to carry and nurture eggs until they are ready for development into other stages. The single most prominent characteristic of *Schistosoma* ova is the presence of a spine, although it is not always recognizable for *S. japonicum*. The *S. japonicum* eggs are also rounder than those of the other two species, in addition to being the smallest of the three. Unlike the other trematodes, *Schistosoma* eggs are not operculated. The eggs of schistosomes are the most commonly used trait for identifying the species of organism to be identified (Table 8-2).

Symptoms

Symptoms for most cases of schistosomiasis when symptomatic are more than in most of the infections by other trematodes. Repercussions of schistosomiasis infections

TABLE 8-2 Characteristics of *Schistosoma* spp. Ova

	SCHISTOSOMA MANSONI	*SCHISTOSOMA HEMATOBIUM*	*SCHISTOSOMA JAPONICUM*
Size	115–180 × 40–80 μm	110–170 × 40–70 μm	50–80 × 40–60 μm
Appearance	Spine located laterally	Spine located terminally	*Spine small and lateral

*Frequently not recognizable

MICROSCOPIC DIAGNOSTIC FEATURE

General Classification—Blood Flukes

Organism	*Schistosoma* sp.
Specimen Required	Adult blood flukes are worms that parasitize chiefly the mesenteric blood vessels
Stage	May be found in blood vessels, although the diagnostic stages involve chiefly the finding of ova for differentiation of species
Size	Adult schistosomes range from 7–20 mm for males and 7–26 mm for females
Shape	Varies by species
Motility	Cercariae swim in water where hatched and penetrate skin
Other Features	Adults live in blood vessels of viscera of mammals; eggs enter bladder or intestine and are evacuated into water where the eggs hatch into miracidia that enter snails. Sporocysts develop from these miracidia and evolve into cercariae that are capable of penetrating the skin of a suitable host, where they develop into adults.

Schistoma sp. ova

S. mansoni S. japonicum S. hematobium

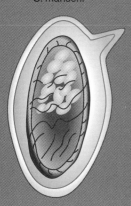
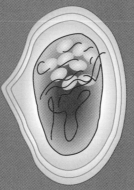
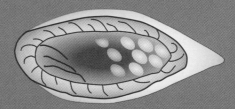

include the initial inflammatory reaction at the site where the metacercariae penetrate the skin and is commonly called swimmer's itch. Abdominal pain and weight loss are common and bloody diarrhea may occur along with eosinophilia and hepatosplenomegaly (enlargement of the liver and spleen). Painful urination with the excretion of bloody urine may develop in infections by *S. hematobium*.

Life Cycle

The adult worms live in blood vessels associated with the intestine or bladder depending upon the species. After the male and female worms mate, the ova produced migrate to the intestine or to the lumen of the urinary bladder and the females produce eggs that are passed out with feces or urine. When the eggs of *S. hematobium* enter the water, the larval stages of the organism, called miracidia, are released from the eggs. These potentially invasive forms then begin the search for a suitable snail host. When they find this intermediate host, the snail, they bore into the tissues of the snail and a period of multiplication commences.

In the next larval stage, the cercariae produced in the snail are released into the water to infect new hosts. These cercariae contaminate the water and penetrate the skin of humans exposed to the water. Following entry through the skin of the humans, the cercariae lose their tails and become known as **schistosomula**. These tailless forms enter the blood circulation (hence the name blood flukes) and migrate through the body until they reach their final position in blood vessels, where they mature into the metacercariae that are encysted in the host. They inhabit the blood vessels near the intestinal tract and the liver in the cases of *S. mansoni* and *S. japonicum*, and near the urinary bladder for *S. hematobium*. At this point they are now ready to leave the body in either urine (*S. hematobium*) or in feces (*S. mansoni* and *M. japonicum*) by being discharged into the water.

Disease Transmission

Humans enter the water where snails have become infected by the miracidia of one species of *Schistosoma*. The miracidia, which develop into cercariae, are released from the snail and penetrate the skin of the human host.

MICROSCOPIC DIAGNOSTIC FEATURE

General Classification—Schistosome Ova

Organism	*Schsitosoma* spp.	
Specimen Required	Feces and urine, depending on species	
Stage	Egg	
Size	By species	
	S. japonicum	50–80 by 40–60 µm
	S. mansoni	115–180 by 40–80 µm
	S. hematobium	110–170 by 40–70 µm
Shape	*S. japonicum*	Contains small lateral spine
	S. mansoni	Contains large lateral spine
	S. hematobium	Contains large terminal spine
Shell	Layered and lack an operculum	
Other Features	*S. japonicum* eggs are rounder, less oval than *S. mansoni* and *S. hematobium*	

Laboratory Diagnosis

Proposed serological methods of diagnosis are limited due to numerous instances of cross-reactions with infections by other helminthes. When travel history suggests visits to an endemic area and symptoms are present, the likelihood of schistosomiasis is probable. The recovery of eggs from feces and urine will enable diagnosis of the appropriate species based on the characteristics of the three species' eggs.

Differentiation is through differing morphology of ova for the three species affecting humans.

Treatment and Prevention

Praziquantel is an effective drug for treating the three species causing schistosomiasis, but oxamniquine is an economic drug for treating infections by *S. mansoni* only. Control of snail species that are capable of transmitting the organisms for schistosomiasis and the practice of good sanitation practices prevent infections effectively. Avoiding exposure to bodies of water in endemic areas are perhaps the most efficient way to control the infection rates as well as the application of a protective barrier on the skin that poses a barrier to penetration by the schistosome cercariae.

SUMMARY

The life cycles of the major trematodes, of which some are commonly known as flukes, are complex. The class of the phylum Nemathelminthes includes the parasites that are commonly known as flatworms. Many of these are parasitic, and either cylindrically shaped or shaped as a spindle. The most common genus found as the causative agent in nematodal infections is that of the schistosomes. Similar stages of a typical fluke occur in the life cycle of all trematodes. These stages include: the adult, the ova, a miracidium, a sporocyst, a redia, a cercaria, and finally a metacercaria.

Cercarial dermatitis, also known by various names, including swimmer's itch, occurs upon penetration of the skin by the metacercaria. This order, Digenetica, includes all four groups of flukes that are parasitic in humans. These four groups are blood flukes, intestinal flukes, liver flukes, and lung flukes, of which only a few organisms that are pathogenic to humans are included in human parasitology, although some of these also infect other mammals.

Intermediate hosts most often include the copecod and the snail, a gastropod. Archaeological evidence for many of these organisms exists, providing evidence that humans were infected thousands of years ago, particularly with those of the schistosomes. Schistosomes are also notorious for causing cancer of various organs due to immunological responses to eggs and to the embedded larvae.

Liver and lung fluke diseases are the next group in the number of worldwide cases, following schistosomiasis. *Paragonimus westermani* is the lung fluke that causes paragonimiasis, where eggs are coughed up into the sputum and swallowed to start the reproductive cycle in the intestines. *Clonorchis sinensis,* also called the Chinese liver fluke, causes clonorchiasis. This fluke is also responsible for numerous cases of biliary disease, particularly in Asia. *Opisthorchis* spp., and in particular *Opisthrochis felineus* and *O. sinensis,* are found in raw and partially cooked fish. These organisms are also commonly found in cats and other mammals, humans included.

Many important discoveries about flukes were made during the period of the late 1800s to the early 1900s. Observations from other parasitic flukes such as *Fasciola hepatica* in sheep and several others that infect mammals other than humans have provided much of the information regarding the life cycles. The life cycles of these other flukes are essentially the same as those described for each of the *Schistosoma* spp. But in a few species an additional intermediate host is present between the snail and the human in or upon which the cercariae encyst. Humans may become infected when they eat the infected second intermediate host.

CASE STUDIES

1. A young man from southeast Japan became alarmed when he developed a cough, which grew more severe over a period of several weeks, and then he noted flecks of blood in his sputum. He knew that a number of species of parasites were often present in raw or poorly cooked crabs and other seafood. The treating physician suspected pneumonia and obtained a chest X-ray as well as a sputum culture for pathogenic bacteria. The sputum culture was negative for bacterial pathogens and the chest X-ray did not reveal infiltrates suggestive of pneumonia. The physician conferred with a particularly astute microbiologist, who suggested a wet mount of a repeat sputum specimen and, upon examination, found helminth eggs. What is the probable causative condition and species of the eggs of the organism represented in the sputum?

2. A business entrepreneur from the United States spent a year teaching business practices at a university in Vietnam. For several months before returning to his home, he had been experiencing vague abdominal pain punctuated with periods of diarrhea. Upon his return home, he began to become jaundiced and suffered from indigestion. Alarmed, he visited his family physician who found that he had an obstruction of the bile duct and as well as eosinophilia. What would be the most likely parasite or parasites from which he is suffering?

3. A group of university students from North America embarked on an archaeological expedition to enhance their studies of ancient history. They traveled to a number of countries in the Mideast and Far East over a 2-week period. During a break from their travels they stopped along the Nile River in Egypt, near the Aswan Dam. Several of the students waded into the water near the shore. After returning home, Samuel noted small reddened areas on his feet but ignored them at the time. A short time later, he began to experience stomach pain along with bloody diarrhea and urine, accompanied by a tender abdomen. Upon a visit to his physician, he was questioned about any travels in the recent past. What parasitic organism was the physician suspecting?

STUDY QUESTIONS

1. Tissue flukes are known to infect human organs. Name these organs.

2. Name the range of size in parasitic flatworms.

3. What is a limiting factor in the spread of flukes over a geographic area?

4. How do the infective cercariae move about to find a host?

5. How do fasciola and schistosoma organisms cause tissue damage?

6. What were the first prevalent symptoms that led early medics to suspect schistosomiasis?

7. At what period in history were entire armies affected by what is believed to be schistosomiasis?

8. What are the seven stages in the life cycle of the flukes?

9. List the three species of *Schistosoma* that are implicated most frequently in human infections.

10. Break down the word *schistosoma*, and give the literal meaning of the word.

11. List the steps in the development of a human infection by *P. westermani*.

Invasive Tissue Parasites

LEARNING OBJECTIVES

Upon completion of this chapter, the learner will be expected to:

- Explain the invasion of tissue by the *T. spiralis* organism
- List the signs and symptoms of the trichinosis
- Discuss the role of carnivores in transmitting *E. granulosus*
- Understand reasons for difficulty in differentiating between *E. granulosus* and *E. multilocularis*
- Describe ways in which tissue-invading and cyst-forming parasites can be controlled

KEY TERMS

Acellular	Eosinophil	Osteitis deformans
Anaphylaxis	Feces	Paget's disease
Antigens	Fomites	Proglottids
Calcifies	Herbivores	Protoscolices
Canid species	Hydatid	Rostellum
CT scans	Hydatid cysts	Scolex
Dead-end hosts	Hydatid sand	Striated skeletal muscle
Definitive hosts	Hydatiform	Suckers
Deworming	Intermediate hosts	Talmud
Dissected	Intraperitoneal	Trichina
Echinococcus	Intrapleural	Trichinellosis
Edema	Metastasis	Trichinosis
Embryos	Multivesicular	Unilocular
Encapsulated	Nematodes	
Encysted	Oncospheres	

INTRODUCTION

Three major parasitic infections invade the major tissues and organs of the human body. One infection is trichinosis, caused by the roundworm *Trichinella spiralis*, which was discussed in Chapter Five of this book. The other two major species, *Echinococcus granulosus* and *Echinococcus multilocularis*, are organisms that cause a major disease called *echinococcosis*. Both similarities and differences exist between the trichinella organism and those of the genus *Echinococcus*. Both *E. granulosus* and *E. multilocularis* cause a serious disease where hydatiform cysts form, whereas *T. spiralis* causes single cyst forms in muscles, and is a self-limiting condition. *E. granulosus* and *E. multilocularis* are cestodal organisms, but unlike the cestodal diseases discussed earlier, these species are found only as organisms with only a few proglottids. The entire echinococcal organism may consist of only three segments, whereas other cestode species may grow to perhaps several meters.

One major difference that exists between the diseases of trichinosis and echinococcosis relates to the differing genera of the two, where the organism causing trichinosis, *T. spiralis,* is a roundworm, and the other two echinococcal organisms are classified as cestodes. Echinococcal infections begin initially as a tapeworm in the digestive system, and cysts may form in vital organs as a result of this primary infection. Therefore, for these reasons this disease is also treated as a tissue-invasive disease and is discussed along with trichinosis. The two genera of these parasites are similar in that they may be contracted through eating infected or poorly cooked meat. Another difference is that *T. spiralis* is found in pork primarily, although other meats have been implicated, and *E. granulosus* and *E. multilocularis* may be found in a variety of meats.

TRICHINOSIS, AN INFECTION OF *TRICHINELLA SPIRALIS*

Trichinosis is also known as trichinellosis or as a trichina infection and is caused by the intestinal nematode worm *Trichinella spiralis.* This organism requires two hosts in its life cycle. The female worms produce larvae that encyst in muscle upon which the new host becomes infected when the encysted muscle is eaten. Because human infections are usually acquired by eating pork containing the encysted larvae, this might have initially given rise to the Mosaic and Islamic traditions of avoiding pork. Eating pork is a practice that has also been attributed to tapeworm infection (see following sections of this chapter). Five species of *Trichinella*, a nematode characterized by its invasive larval stages, exist, including *T. spiralis, T. native, T. nelsoni, T. britoui,* and *T. pseudospiralis.* Of these five species, *T. spiralis* is most important as a parasite of humans as it does not have specific hosts that it infects, and the disease is distributed throughout the world.

The association between trichina infections and pigs has been long recognized but the encysted larvae in the muscle were not seen until 1821. Even after the cysts in the infected muscle were observed, the condition was not associated with disease in humans. The discovery of the worm in humans was made in 1835 by James Paget, who was then a medical student at St. Bartholomew's Hospital in London. Sir James Paget was later knighted for his accomplishments in this and other areas of medicine. Another important medical finding attributed to this observant physician is the bone disease osteitis deformans, or softening of the bones, which is a condition called Paget's disease. The definitive report of trichinellosis was written by Richard Owen who attempted to minimize Paget's role, although he failed to associate that the wormlike organism embedded in human muscle was the larval stage of a nematode.

Religious proscriptions relating to eating pork by Muslims and Jews perhaps stem from basic knowledge of cestodal infections and well as *Trichinella spiralis.* Certain ritualistic practices in food preparation in some religions and cultures almost certainly relate to avoiding the eating of meat contaminated by microorganisms. Many centuries ago the Jewish rabbis were known to inspect meat and other foods before they were pronounced edible, as evidenced by writings of that era. It could reasonably be concluded that some of these practices led eventually to the establishment of governmental offices responsible for ensuring food safety.

Morphology

The adult worms were discovered by Rudolf Virchow in 1859 and Friedrich Zenker in 1860. Zenker finally recognized the clinical significance of the infection and concluded that humans became infected by eating raw pork. The importance of these studies lies not only in the field of human parasitology but also in the more general field of parasitology concerned with the transmission of parasites between different animal species and the importance of predator–prey relationships in such transmissions. A number of good accounts by many investigators from more than a century ago relating to the history of trichinosis exist, as trichinosis is one of the oldest and most documented parasitic infections found in humans.

The condition where the muscle tissues are infested by the larval form of *T. spiralis* is not identifiable in general by examination of stool specimens, as is the case for a number of other species of parasites. The most specific identification for the infection is examination of biopsies of the muscles in which the larvae are encysted. It appears that the only way the organism is transmitted to humans is through ingestion of raw or undercooked meat, primarily pork, but several other types of animal meat are also be capable of causing the contraction of the disease.

Symptoms

The first stage of the infection is the intestinal phase, where the ingested larvae invade the intestinal mucosal tissues. The first symptoms develop within a day and the dose of worms ingested relates directly to the severity of these initial symptoms. The victim may experience symptoms similar to influenza or a similar viral illness. Some mistakenly believe they are suffering from acute food poisoning as nausea and vomiting, diarrhea, general malaise, acute edema of upper eyelids, abdominal cramps and pain, and fever soon emerge as major complaints.

More serious symptoms may ensue for heavy infections but often occur after the initial crisis when only vague muscular pains arise that may persist for weeks. The prognosis for the patient is positive and the severity and length of illness depends on the number of worms ingested. There may also be a generalized appearance of poor health during the initial phase of the illness.

Life Cycle

The development of the *T. spiralis* organism appears to be quite simple but the life cycle of *T. spiralis* includes several different stages. Once larvae are ingested through the eating of infected meat, the adult organism lives in the intestinal lining of such meat-eating animals. Following the mating of a pair of *T. spiralis* organisms, the male worm dies while the female proceeds to produce the offspring.

These roundworms or nematodes have a stage of development called the *embryonic stage*, which occurs in many species of parasites and other biological organisms. In trichinae, however, this stage occurs within the uterus of the female. The offspring are then released in the larva's second stage of life into the host's intestinal lining. Up to 1500 larvae may be produced from each female worm and these travel through the circulatory system to the heart, and from there to striated skeletal muscle. Those larvae that reach striated muscle will grow to a length of about 1 mm before coiling themselves into a cyst (encysting) for protection. Encysted worms may live up to 10 years in this stage. Humans are considered a dead-end host, as few animals have the opportunity to feed on humans.

In order to reproduce, larvae are released from the encapsulated cysts of the muscle tissue that was eaten and mature to the adult stage in the intestines. Females then produce larvae that are able to penetrate the intestinal mucosa and then enter into the blood circulatory system. These organisms have an affinity for striated skeletal muscle and form multiple cysts in the fibers of skeletal muscle. They grow and mature, reaching adulthood in approximately a month. As the encysted larvae grow they coil into the cavity in the muscle and may remain alive for a number of years before the cyst calcifies and the larvae within die (Figure 9-1). The encysted larvae may cause a great deal of pain but during the intestinal phase of development few if any symptoms are experienced, except for vague abdominal discomfort and perhaps slight diarrhea. After producing larvae, the adult dies, so reinfection is required for a continuous cycle of reproduction.

Disease Transmission

The contracting of trichinosis requires ingesting raw or uncooked meat containing *Trichinella* larvae, leading to human infection. The most common type of meat containing the *Trichinella* parasites that infect humans is pork and, in the past, feeding scraps of meat and other foods to pigs provided a ready source of the larvae that infected the animals. The larvae are released from the muscles of the food source where they go on to mature and reproduce in order to encyst in the host's muscle tissues.

Laboratory Diagnosis

Trichinella organisms are rarely found in a patient's stool, blood, or cerebrospinal fluids. Clinical chemistry tests

LIFE CYCLE of—

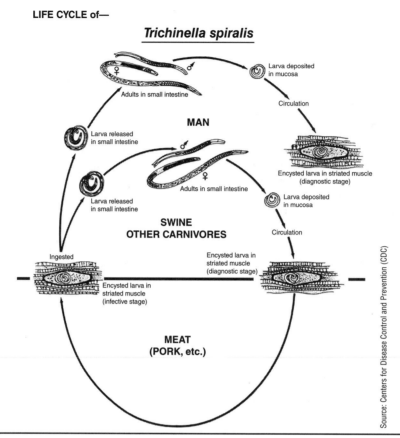

FIGURE 9-1 Various stages in the nematode life cycle of *Trichinella spiralis*

such as creatinine kinase reveal muscle damage through the encysting larvae, providing indirect evidence that a *Trichinella* infection has likely occurred. The assumption that an individual is suffering from trichinosis is bolstered when accompanied by a patient's history of eating certain meats, particularly pork. Serological testing has been somewhat unreliable as a substantial percentage of falsely negative results occur with the use of current testing methods. The most definitive diagnosis entails a muscle biopsy, which is prepared for a microscopic examination, and shows the presence of encysted larvae. Laboratory tests, such as a complete blood count to evaluate the number of white blood cells and a differentiation of the various types may reveal an elevated **eosinophil** count.

Encysting of Trichinella spiralis

This infection occurs after eating pork from pigs that have often been fed contaminated waste products rather than safe, commercially prepared food. Some other animals may be infected by *T. spiralis*, but meat from a pig is the general cause of the disease where humans are concerned. Cysts that have formed in the muscles of the meat may not be killed if inadequate cooking has occurred or if it has been eaten raw. Larvae encyst in the duodenum and invade the mucous lining of the small intestine where adulthood is reached by the end of 1 week. After exposure to gastric acid and pepsin in the stomach, the larvae are released from the cysts and invade the small bowel mucosa where they develop into adult worms. These male and female organisms proceed to mate and, after approximately 1 week, the females release up to 1500 or more larvae that may enter the blood or the lymphatic system. These larvae then circulate to the various organs of the body where they encyst within the tissues, but the preference for *T. spiralis* is that of skeletal muscle (Figure 9-2). Diagnosis may be made on the basis of muscle biopsy and symptoms and signs because no ova are produced in the life cycle to be passed in the **feces**.

The severity of the disease is dependent upon the number of muscles involved and the number of cysts that form. When symptoms occur they are usually most evident during the encysting and encapsulating

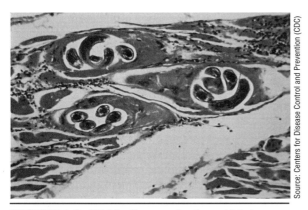

FIGURE 9-2 *Trichinella* cysts develop within human muscle tissue

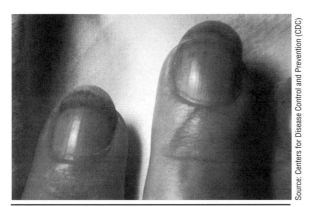

FIGURE 9-3 Splinter hemorrhages under fingernails in trichinosis

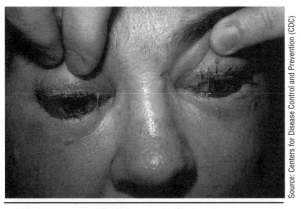

FIGURE 9-4 Clinical appearance of eyes, periorbital swelling, muscle pain, diarrhea, and increased eosinophil count

MICROSCOPIC DIAGNOSTIC FEATURE

General Classification—Nematode (roundworm)

Organism	*Trichinella spiralis*
Specimen Required	Muscle biopsy; hard to recover adults or larvae from fecal sample
Stage	Larvae in muscles; adults in stool samples
Size	In adults, F = 4.0 mm × 150 µm; M = 1.4–1.6 mm × 40–60 µm
Shape	Worm-shaped
Motility	Migration through walls of intestine, circulation in blood to muscle tissue
Other Features	Calcified larvae are found by radiographic exam; stained with hematoxylin and eosin

T. spiralis

Encysted larvae form

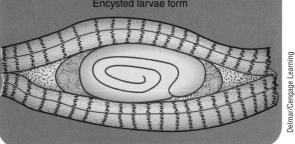

near the orbital bones of the eyes, muscular pain, and tenderness, accompanied by generalized weakness (Figure 9-4).

Treatment and Prevention

For heavy and symptomatic infections, anti-parasite medication is recommended. Anti-parasite (antihelminthic) medication is the first line of treatment

period. Increased allergic responses to parasitic infections and hemorrhages beneath the fingernails may be evident (Figure 9-3). Other symptoms and signs may occur including headaches and edema

against trichinosis. If the *Trichinella* parasite is discovered early, in the intestinal phase, albendazole (Albenza) or mebendazole is usually effective in eliminating the intestinal worms and larvae before considerable damage to skeletal muscles occurs.

The adult trichina also lives in the intestinal lining of many meat-eating animals as wild swine, bears, walruses, horses, rodents, and a number of other animal species including humans. The best defense against contracting trichinosis is accomplished through proper food preparation. Humans should avoid undercooked meat by ensuring that the meat is cooked to an internal temperature of 170°F (77°C) before eating it. A food thermometer is preferable to ensure that meat is thoroughly cooked. Other methods exist for ensuring meat is safe by storing the meat for at least 3 weeks or by the process of irradiation. Irradiation will kill parasites in wild-animal meat, and deep-freezing for 3 weeks kills *Trichinella* in some meats; however, *Trichinella* organisms in bear meat do not ordinarily die by freezing. Neither irradiation nor freezing is necessary if you ensure that the meat is thoroughly cooked. Smoking or pickling of meat will not always kill *Trichinella* in infected meat.

ECHINOCOCCOSIS

The causative organism for echinococcosis is the *Echinococcus granulosus* tapeworm. This is one of the most serious of human diseases that is caused by a larval cestode. This condition may also be known as hydatid disease, and frequently results from accidental infection with the larval stages found in the canid species (originating from a dog ancestor) tapeworm called *Echinococcus granulosus*. The disease most often occurs in adult dogs and as a larval cyst(s) particularly in sheep but also in other species of both wild and domesticated animals. The potential for echinococcosis to become more prevalent in the United States certainly exists. The canid species, includes carnivores such as wolves and coyotes, which hunt and eat both domesticated and wild animals, and could potentially aid in the spread of the organisms from sheep-raising country in the western United States and into other areas of the country where cattle are raised.

The massive bladder-like hydatid cysts, particularly those found in the liver, were well known in ancient times. References to such cysts in animals that were slaughtered in religious rituals are found in the Babylonian Talmud. Approximately 400 years before the birth of Christ, Hippocrates mentioned these phenomena in animals butchered for food, and subsequently by several other investigators over the next several centuries. Other ancient medical practitioners have also made references to cystlike structures in food animals.

Descriptions of hydatid cysts in humans are found in European medical texts, where references are made of structures described as enlarged glands or bags of mucus, accompanied by blood vessels with abnormal growth patterns, lymphatic varices (dilated veins), and accumulations of body fluids. A number of observant scientists appeared to associate these cysts as products of parasites, and more specifically as damage caused by larval tapeworms. Although not credited with the theory that *E. granulosus* was responsible for the formation of hydatid cysts, Francisco Redi in the 1600s proposed this initial framework for the formation of the cysts.

The German clinician and natural historian Pierre Simon Pallas showed a parasitic link to the cysts in 1766 (Cox, 2002). Carl von Siebold demonstrated in 1853 that *Echinococcus* cysts from infected sheep were the origin of adult tapeworms when raw meat was fed to dogs (Cox, 2002). A demonstration by Bernhard Naunyn in 1863 definitively proved that adult tapeworms developed in dogs fed with hydatid cysts (Figure 9-5), which were obtained from a human (Cox, 2002). The history of hydatid disease and the transmission of

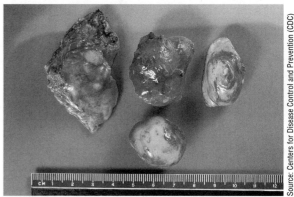

Source: Centers for Disease Control and Prevention (CDC)

FIGURE 9-5 Membrane and hydatid daughter cysts from human lung

cysts by eating meat infected by *E. granulosus* is well researched and accepted.

Morphology

E. granulosus is well established as a hydatid tapeworm of dogs, and the infection commonly causes neurological disorders in dogs whose nervous systems contain hydatid cysts. One old definition associated with the presence of hydatid cysts in dogs described the dogs as suffering from "running fits." The eggs of *E. granulosus* are almost never found in fecal specimens but when they are recovered they appear almost identical to those of the *Taenia* spp. (described earlier). The worm of *E. granulosus* is only about 4 mm in length and consists of a **scolex** with four **suckers**, numerous hooks, and only three proglottids, unlike other cestodes; for example, *T. solium*, as well as a number of other tapeworm species, may include up to 1000 proglottids.

Symptoms

Humans are not **definitive hosts**, so the adult tapeworm does not infect humans but does inhabit the intestines of members of the canid family (dogs, foxes, wolves, etc.). In humans a hydatid cyst may develop in one or more tissues and organs of the body, producing symptoms related to the organ affected. Cysts may develop in any area of the body but the lungs and liver are most frequently impacted, followed by organs of the central nervous system. Pulmonary symptoms may also arise, with coughing accompanied by chest pain and lung infection. The presence of hydatid cyst disease is also capable of eliciting anaphylactic shock if the cyst ruptures.

Life Cycle

Herbivores such as sheep and other cattle act as **intermediate hosts** after ingesting ova from pastures where the ground and the pasture grass are contaminated by feces from dogs or other canids. When carnivores ingest the tissues of these animals, which contain the infective cysts, they in turn become infected. Each cyst contains a scolex that can develop into an adult tapeworm. The tapeworm itself resides in the small intestines of dogs and related species, but does not primarily infect humans. A hydatid cyst can become the

size of a large orange and has a laminated outer layer and an inner germinal layer of tissue capable of nourishing and supporting the daughter cysts and brood capsules. These smaller cysts bud from the germinal layer and contain loose pieces of germinal tissues as well as scolices, which are known as hydatid sand. The cyst is also filled with fluid. Humans become infected when *E. granulosus* eggs are ingested accidentally, chiefly by hand-to-mouth contact with infected dog feces. The human is a dead-end host, so the life cycle is halted at this stage. Therefore, humans who suffer from this disease do not spread the organisms to other mammals.

Disease Transmission

Transmission of the disease to humans, a dead-end host, occurs when the eggs of *E. granulosus* are ingested by humans from contact with infected dog feces. These eggs then are transported to body tissues throughout the body, where they produce hydatid cysts. Those who work with herds or flocks of animals and where herd dogs are used are especially vulnerable to infection with this organism. Hand-to-mouth contact while eating in the field and while working with animals lends itself greatly to transmission of the infection.

Laboratory Diagnosis

Since *E. granulosus* eggs are not often found in humans, radiographic and serological studies are primarily used for diagnosis of echinococcosis. A demonstration of the presence of hydatid sand in the cyst(s) is also a diagnostic laboratory tool that may be employed for a definitive diagnosis and to ensure eradication of the parasite when no more cysts are present in the body.

Treatment and Prevention

Surgical removal of hydatid cysts may be necessary, and several anti-helminthic medications are also available for treatment. Good personal hygiene is effective in preventing hand-to-mouth transmission of eggs from dog feces to humans. But the most effective manner for controlling the transmission of the disease can be accomplished by preventing dogs and other carnivorous animals from eating sheep viscera and other organs. Routine and regular treatment of working dogs for parasites is quite effective.

OTHER COMMON TISSUE-INVASIVE PARASITES

Echinococcal Organisms

The second species of the genus *Echinococcus* that forms hydatid cysts that invade and reproduce in various tissues of the human body is *E. multilocularis*. As with so many other parasite infections, the course of an *Echinococcus* infection is complex. This worm has a life cycle that requires two types of hosts: a definitive host and an intermediate host. Typically the definitive host is a carnivore such as a dog or a wolf. The intermediate host is usually an herbivore such as sheep or cattle, but the disease is most prevalent in sheep. As in infections with *E. granulosus*, humans function as accidental hosts and are usually known as a *dead-end host*, because humans do not pass the organisms to other species or individuals during the infection and reproductive cycles. This is primarily due to the fact that most humans who are infected seldom or never defecate in the woods or fields but in restroom facilities.

Echinococcus granulosus is tapeworm that chiefly infests dogs and other carnivores. The larval form of this organism is called a *hydatid* and develops in other mammals. The disease cycle begins when the adult tapeworm gains entry and attaches to the gut of the definitive hosts. The definitive host is usually a carnivore and can either be of the canine (dog) or the feline (cat) lineage. The adult tapeworm then produces eggs in the fecal waste from the host and the eggs are eliminated from the body of the host into the soil. Then an intermediate host such as a cow, goat, or sheep becomes infected by eating the grass where the eggs of the parasite may be found. Prepared foods contaminated by feces containing the *E. granulosus* eggs may, on rare occasions, also be a source of infection for a human. The following illustration reveals the typical structural morphology found in an adult cestode, *Echinococcus granulosus*, which was recovered from the bodies of dogs (Figure 9-6).

Morphology

E. granulosus causes the disease known as *cystic echinococcosis*. As dogs and other canids are the only definitive hosts for *Echinococcus*, adult forms of the organism are not expected to be found in the human host. Adult worms range from 3 to 6 mm in length and usually

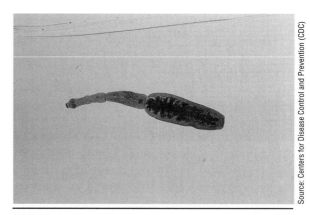

FIGURE 9-6 Morphology of an adult cestode, *Echinococcus granulosus*

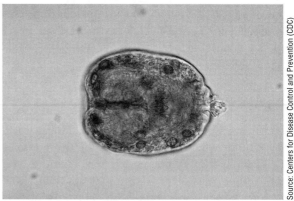

FIGURE 9-7 Scolex of *Echinococcus granulosus* from hydatid cyst

consist of a scolex and only three proglottids, unlike the lengthy number of proglottids exhibited by other species of cestodes. The third (terminal) proglottid is the only gravid link and is longer than it is wide as can be seen in the following image. The scolex contains four suckers and a rostellum with 25–50 hooks (Figure 9-7).

Life Cycle

Because dogs and other canids such as foxes and wolves are definitive hosts for *Echinococcus* spp., humans are only infected by the larvae after ingesting either food containing these larvae or by drinking contaminated water or contact with fomites (something to which feces may cling), which is also contaminated with dog feces. After the human host ingests the eggs, the oncospheres move from the intestinal lumen to other areas of the body, where development begins into hydatid cysts. These cysts may be found in many parts of the body but are frequently found in the liver, lung, and particularly in the central nervous system.

Inside the intermediate host of an herbivore, or typical grass eater, which has eaten infected vegetation, eggs hatch and release very small embryonic forms called *oncospheres* that contain hooks and travel through the circulatory system. These oncospheres eventually gain a hold in the organs of the body, and are chiefly found in the liver, kidneys, and lungs, where they develop into hydatid cysts. These cysts are a hollow bladder-like structures where brood (breeding) capsules are formed, and are sometimes attached to a mother cyst, sometimes called a unilocular type of hydatid (Figure 9-8).

The scolex (plural is scolices) is the headlike structure of tapeworm organisms, and these newly formed organisms grow inside the brood capsules. Inside these cysts grow thousands of tapeworm larvae called hydatid sand, which is the next stage in the life cycle of the parasite. When a predator eats the intermediate host, the larvae that are eaten develop into adult tapeworms in the intestine and the infection cycle restarts. Again, because humans do not ordinarily eat carnivores, humans do not spread the tapeworm for this species in the way that meat-eating animals do. During their life cycle within the host, these tapeworms pass through an egg stage followed by an oncosphere stage. The next step of the life cycle is the formation of a cystic stage which undergoes enlargement, thereby producing protoscolices and daughter cysts. Rupture of these cysts releases the larval

protoscolices, producing hydatid sand, which is what is depicted in Figure 9-9.

The second echinococcal organism, *Echinococcus multilocularis*, invades the tissues of humans who serve as dead-end hosts. It produces an alveolar-type cyst, which contains an inner, nucleated germinal layer that gives rise to brood capsules. As *Echinococcus multilocularis* infections progress, larger and larger cysts develop in intermediate hosts. Symptoms of infection with *E. multilocularis* arise as the cysts progressively grow larger and begin eroding the surrounding tissue and perhaps placing pressure on blood vessels and other organs. Small secondary parasitic cysts, usually a derivative of a hydatid cyst called a *mother cyst*, contain brood chambers which increase the number of organisms (Figure 9-10). Large cysts may eventually induce anaphylactic shock, which may be fatal if the cysts do rupture.

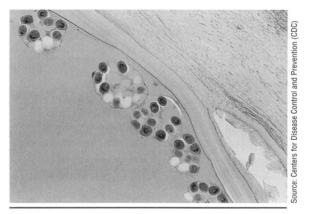

Source: Centers for Disease Control and Prevention (CDC)

FIGURE 9-9 Rupture of cysts release larval protoscolices, resulting in hydatid sand

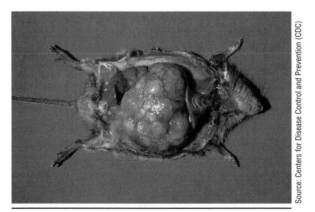

Source: Centers for Disease Control and Prevention (CDC)

FIGURE 9-8 Dissected (pronounced *dis*– sected, not *di*– sected, as there are two s's) rat showing evidence of echinococcosis due to *Echinococcus multilocularis* in organs at 45 days

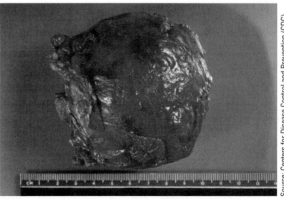

Source: Centers for Disease Control and Prevention (CDC)

FIGURE 9-10 Membrane and hydatid excised cyst

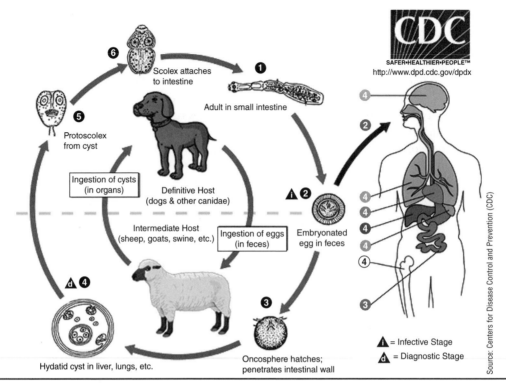

FIGURE 9-11 Life cycle of *Echincococcus* spp., with intermediate and definitive hosts

The definitive or primary hosts of *E. multilocularis* are dogs and foxes occasionally domesticated cats who hunt rodents, similar to that of *E. granulosus*. This organism may be found farther north and in colder climates than *E. granulosus*, as the eggs are somewhat resistant to cold weather. Field mice, muskrats, ground squirrels, and several other species are the intermediate hosts (Figure 9-11). The primary site of infection is the liver but protoscoleces (precursors to the head of a tapeworm) from cysts may invade a number of other organs and tissues. In humans, protoscoleces are rarely produced in those who are infected. Infiltration into the blood vessels may cause metastatic formations primarily in the lung and brain. As in most parasitic infections an increased eosinophil count is also found with this disease.

Differentiation between *E. granulosus* and *E. multilocularis*

Adult worms of *E. granulosus* are larger than those of *E. multilocularis*. Eggs of the taeniid-type organisms are practically indistinguishable from those of both *E. granulosus* and *E. multilocularis*. In addition,

E. granulosus organisms are confined to an **acellular** membranous vesicle, whereas *E. multilocularis* in its intermediate rodent hosts is of an invasive, **multivesicular** arrangement with no limiting layer around it. Remember that *T. solium* and *T. saginata*, respectively, known as taeniids, are the pork and beef tapeworms found earlier in this publication that are also capable of causing these cyst-like structures in the organs of the body. Although serological testing for the presence of specific **antigens** is usually reliable, the practice may lead to erroneous conclusions and misdiagnosis. Basic microscopic morphology, when possible, is the best and most accurate way in which to diagnose current infections.

Laboratory Diagnosis and Disease Progression of Hydatid Disease

Visualization of the organisms causing echinococcosis may be accomplished through the use of various imaging and serological procedures, an indirect means of testing where antibodies to the organism may be determined. Cysts may be detected by ultrasonography, with

CT scans (computerized tomography), and in some advanced cases by routine radiographic pictures. The appearance of these structures can be similar to tumor metastasis (spreading to distant sites from the original infection site). In the liver the hydatid disease appears as a dense fluid cyst that often includes areas of calcification. Hydatid disease of either the lung or liver may be asymptomatic, but the condition can cause serious complications if the cyst ruptures.

Prevention of shock associated with a rupture of these hydatid cysts as well as the risk of intrapleural or intraperitoneal requires early medical intervention. Dissemination of the organisms released by a rupture of a cyst may result in a secondary infection and may be accompanied by an abscess of the lung or liver. In these life-threatening cases, surgical removal of the cysts becomes of primary importance. Medications may also be administered for a somewhat prolonged course of therapy that is sufficient to rid the body of the offending organisms. Other treatments that have been explored involve the direct infusion of a medication that will destroy scoleces by a needle insertion into the infected area, where the needle is guided by radiological imaging directly into the cysts.

Infection with *E. multilocularis* may result in the growth of dense parasitic structures that appear as tumors in the liver, lungs, brain, or other tissues. Unlike intermediate hosts, definitive hosts are usually not harmed to a great extent by an infection with *E. multilocularis*. A number of intestinal parasites that primarily dwell in the intestines of humans will sometimes result in a lack of certain nutrients, including vitamins, minerals, and proteins. Rapid growth of parasitic organisms exacts a high toll on the nutrient intake of the host in whom the organisms flourishing.

Transmission and Prevention

As one can see from the life cycles illustrated previously, all disease-causing species of *Echinococcus* are transmitted to intermediate hosts via the ingestion of eggs and are transmitted to definitive hosts by eating infected, cyst-containing organs. When thinking about transmission, it is important to remember that humans are accidental intermediate hosts that become infected by handling soil, dirt, or animal hair that contains eggs and seldom or never in the woods and fields where animals would be exposed to the organisms.

MICROSCOPIC DIAGNOSTIC FEATURE

General Classification—Tissue Cestode

Organism	*Echinococcus granulosus*
Specimen Required	Tissues (*eggs are not often recovered*)
Stage	Adult
Size	3–6 mm in length
Shape	Scolex with only three proglottids
Motility	Not indicated
Other Features	Scolex contains 4 suckers, rostellum with 25–50 hooks, enabling differentiation from other cestodes

E. granulosus
Ovum

Delmar/Cengage Learning

A number of methods will prevent echinococcosis in humans, most of which involve breaking up the parasite's life cycle. For instance, feeding raw meat that includes entrails and organ meat to work dogs should be avoided as a sure means for minimizing the risk of infection on a farm or ranch. Regular **deworming** of farm dogs with the appropriate drugs will aid in killing a number of tapeworms, including those of the *Echinococcus* genus. For humans, basic hygiene practices will prevent infections by both parasites and pathogenic bacteria and thoroughly cooking food and effective hand washing before preparing and eating meals can prevent the eggs from entering the human digestive tract. Employing these simple practices in some areas has practically rid the populations of hydatids such as *Echinococcus* infections in both humans and domestic animals, even when the disease was prevalent at one time.

GENERALIZED LIFE CYCLE OF THE TAPEWORM

The tapeworm needs two hosts to complete its life cycle:

1. **Intermediate host**—these hosts vary depending upon the region of the world and the intermediate hosts available there, but which typically include the grazing animals. In some areas, grazing animals such as pigs, cattle, goats, and horses most commonly are hosts. In Australia, dingoes (wild dogs), wallabies, and kangaroos are the animals most commonly infected with tapeworms. The normal fauna of the various geographic regions of the world that graze in areas where canids also exist provide the conditions that may lead to infections with species of the *Echinococcus* genus. Infection begins when the grazing animal eats grass infected with the feces from a dog or other canid species that is infected with tapeworm eggs. The eggs hatch in the animal's gut into embryos (called oncospheres). These embryos penetrate the wall of the intestine and are carried in the bloodstream to vital organs such as the liver, lungs, or brain where they can develop into hydatid cysts. These cysts contain around 30 to 40 tapeworm heads (the first segment of the tapeworm). A mature fertile cyst may contain several million such heads.

2. **Definitive host**—such as dogs and other canine species. Infection begins when the animal eats wastes that contain hydatid cysts. The swallowed cysts burst and the tapeworm heads travel to the gut and attach themselves to the intestine wall. The tapeworms are mature after about 6 weeks. An adult *E. granulosis* tapeworm is only 6 mm, or about 1/4 in., in length. Thousands can inhabit the gut of an infected animal. Each mature worm grows and sheds the last segment of its body about every 2 weeks. This last segment contains immature eggs. The eggs are passed from the animal's body in fecal material and may stick to the animal's hair or contaminate the vegetable garden. The eggs are highly resistant to weather conditions and can remain viable for months. The eggs have to be swallowed by an animal (intermediate host) to form hydatid cysts.

INFECTION IN HUMANS

Human infection does not occur from eating infected meat that includes organs and entrails. People usually become infected by accidentally swallowing the tapeworm eggs passed in dog feces. This occurs from petting the animal without adequately washing hands and then eating or smoking and then making contact with the mouth using dirty hands. The human takes the role of the intermediate host by substituting for sheep, horses, or cattle, and perhaps other herbivores. The organisms travel through the blood vessels before lodging in organs where they form watery hydatid cysts full of tapeworm heads (scoleces). This is known as hydatid disease or echinococcosis. Hydatid disease is not contagious and is not passed by person-to-person contact, which is why a human is considered a dead-end host.

Symptoms of Hydatid Disease

Typical symptoms of hydatid disease will depend on the severity of the disease and which organs are affected. For *E. multilocularis*, the most commonly affected organ is the liver. The kidneys, brain, and lungs are sometimes affected. In rare cases, hydatid cysts may form in the thyroid gland or heart or within bone. *E. granulosus* is found in more diverse tissues and organs than *E. multilocularis*. Signs and symptoms may not occur for considerable lengths of time following the contraction of an infection, possibly even up to months or several years later. In some cases, no symptoms are ever experienced and presence of the disease may be purely accidental. When symptoms do occur, they may include any or all of the items from the following list:

- Stomach upset frequently accompanied with diarrhea
- Unexplained weight loss that in many cases includes anemia
- Distended abdomen
- Extreme fatigue and feelings of weakness

- Racking cough with blood that is sometimes diagnosed as tuberculosis
- Jaundice as a result of pressure by an enlarged cyst that might obstruct bile drainage

Treatment and Prevention

Remember that hydatid disease can lead to eventual death without adequate medical treatment. Therefore, an accurate diagnosis is important, as a number of symptoms and signs can be attributed to other medical conditions. A life-threatening allergic reaction (**anaphylaxis**) resulting from a heavily infested organ that may fail or a cyst may rupture and cause a serious consequences. Both phases of the tapeworm's life cycle, the definitive and the intermediate host infections, must be broken in order to prevent infection since the life cycle is a complex sequence. Guidelines that will help to prevent infection include:

- **Personal Safety**

  The most important facet of preventing infection includes washing hands before eating, drinking, and smoking and after gardening or handling animals. Wash hands thoroughly, particularly after cleaning dog pens, after which the waste is most often buried or burned. Even after handling or being in contact with a dog or its feeding containers, wash hands thoroughly with warm water and soap. Children should be taught the dangers of failing to wash their hands effectively and very small children should be supervised when they wash their hands. Home vegetable gardens should be fenced to make sure that both pets and wild animals can't defecate on the soil where the plants are grown. As added insurance against becoming infected, personal protective equipment, particularly disposable gloves, is mandatory when gardening or removing droppings and disinfecting the kennel.

- **Prevention of Animal Infections**

  Controlling tapeworm infections in domestic dogs, working dogs, and a number of pet species is paramount. Deworming dogs on a routine basis is important to prevent the spread of echinococcosis. The careful disposal of excrement, particularly for dogs being treated for tapeworm infection, is extremely important. It should be realized that infected dogs often have no symptoms while suffering from a tapeworm infection and infected dogs may show few or no signs of infection and may appear happy and healthy.

  In rural areas dogs may have exposure to wildlife and animal carcasses and this puts them at increased risk for contracting an infection. Make it a practice to feed dogs with only commercially prepared dog foods from reputable manufacturers. Do not feed raw or cooked waste meats that include organs and entrails to a dog. This precaution extends to animal products obtained from a butcher or supermarket. In addition, dogs should be restrained to prevent them from going into areas where feces from wild animals, sheep, and cattle may have contaminated the ground. If dogs are not free to roam, there is less likelihood of their coming into contact with animal feces.

SUMMARY

Both nematodes and cestodes are capable of invading tissues of the body, causing extensive immune responses and tissue damage. The trichinella species (*Trichinella spiralis*) chiefly is ingested with poorly cooked food and during the life cycle of the organism; the muscles are invaded and the larval forms encyst in the muscles, causing pain to the infected victim. Hydatifiorm diseases are caused by a cestode, or tapeworm, contracted through contaminated materials and may invade the body of a human, including the nervous system. These are caused by *Echinococcus granulosus* and *Echinococcus multilocularis*.

Trichinosis may also be known as **trichinellosis** and trichina infection. The causative organism is the intestinal nematode worm *Trichinella spiralis,* and it requires two hosts in the life cycle. Infection occurs when **encysted** muscle, particularly from pork, is eaten and the infected meat breaks down to release the organisms that then infect the muscle tissue. The relationship between pork and associated disease in humans was established by James Paget in 1821. Adult worms were observed in 1859 and 1860, where a positive link between eating raw port and the development of trichinellosis was established. Stool specimens are not used to determine infection by *T. spiralis*, but when necessary a muscle biopsy may be performed. As in other parasitic infections, the white blood cells called eosinophils may be a valuable indicator of an invasive disease.

CASE STUDIES

1. A group of factory workers from the Southeast had been planning a hunting trip to Wisconsin for years. Finally, they were able to arrange time off and had secured a hunting cabin deep in a rural area. It was the dream of several of them to kill a bear, eat the meat, and take the skin and the head for curing and mounting. After a successful hunt in which two bears were dispatched, the friends roasted and ate the meat over a large camp fire. The hunt concluded, they salted the skins with the heads attached, and travelled back to their homes. Several weeks later, most of the men complained of nausea, vomiting, epigastric pain, coughs, and blurred vision. Each person with these symptoms visited their family physician. Blood tests revealed eosinophilia, and a physical exam showed edema about the eyes, rash, and breathing difficulties. What would be the most likely parasite from which the men are suffering?

2. Julian, a college student in western Canada, obtained a summer job working at a local animal shelter. Part of his duties entailed picking up stray dogs, cleaning the pens where the dogs live, and disposing of the fecal materials by burying them. Some of the dogs were involved with herding sheep, but have become old and physically unable to continue their duties, or were abandoned by their owners. A year after completing this summer job, Julian begins to suffer from severe coughs and chest pain, and seeks medical attention from the student health center at the university he attends. What would be a possible parasite from which Julian is suffering?

STUDY QUESTIONS

1. Name the two cestode groups that contribute most often to human infection.

2. How do the eggs of the taeniid species reach the intermediate host?

3. Which of the tapeworms, *T. saginata* or *T. solium*, become the largest, and what are their approximate lengths?

4. Are both male and female organisms found in the cestodes? If not, what is the form of reproduction called for these organisms?

5. What is a valuable characteristic used in differentiating the eggs of pseudophyllidean tapeworms and cyclophyllidean species?

6. With what animals are the cestodes called *T. saginata* and *T. solium* associated?

7. How did Aristotle describe the appearance of the cysticercus structure?

8. What animal is affected by the *Echinococcus granulosus* organism and how does it manifest itself?

9. Why do Jewish and Muslim religions have certain prohibitions on eating certain meats, particularly pork?

10. In your own thinking, how did observations of meat conditions lead to official offices responsible for food safety?

11. Eating sheep meat by dogs led to the development of hydatid cysts, which was determined by whom, in 1853?

12. What is the common name for *Diphyllobothrium latum*, and how is it normally contracted?

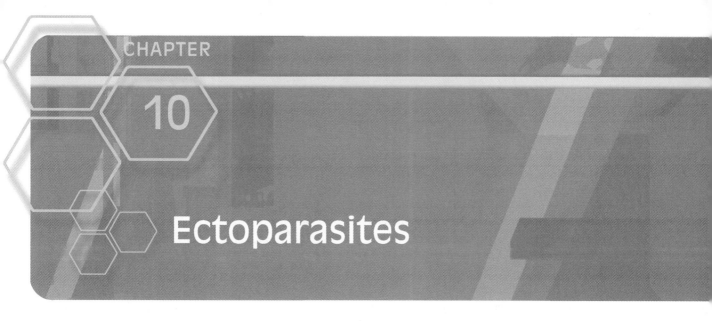

CHAPTER

10

Ectoparasites

LEARNING OBJECTIVES

Upon completion of this chapter, the learner will be expected to:

- List the major characteristics of an ectoparasite
- Name the four major genera of ectoparasites that infect the human body
- Relate some diseases that are commonly transmitted by the dog tick
- List the steps required for ridding an area of bedbugs
- Discuss a reason that bedbugs are so prevalent when living in abandoned buildings

KEY TERMS

Acarida
Acarina
Amputation
Annelids
Anoplura
Apterygotes
Arboviruses
Babesiosis
Bacillus
Bedbug
Borrelia
Brucellosis
Bubo
Bubonic plague
Chiggers

Chigo
Ehrlichiosis
Guillain-Barre syndrome
Hard ticks
Hemimetabolous
Hirudinea
Jigger
Leech
Lyme disease
Mange
Molt
Nit
Nymphal stage
Parthenogenetic
Pediculosis

Prophylactic
Pupa
Q fever
Redbugs
Relapsing fever
Rocky Mountain spotted fever
Scabies
Scavengers
Soft ticks
Spirochete
Tularemia
Typhus
Ulcerations
Vectors

INTRODUCTION

A large number of ectoparasites feed upon the skin cells of the human body. Some survive by embedding themselves into the skin of the body and feeding upon the body's blood supply, whereas others actually feed upon the bacteria and oils of the body, in at least one case. Ectoparasites are differentiated from endoparasites in that they thrive outside of the human body. Therefore, those known as endoparasites live inside the body, some of which have already been described and that include amoebae, worms, and flukes. Three major ectoparasites plague human beings and these have apparently been in existence for possibly as long as humanity has inhabited the world. Lice and mites are the two major groups that include four common genera, three of which are lice and one of which is classified as a mite. Besides lice and mites, ticks are also classified as ectoparasites, and these three are commonly encountered in human diseases. Several other groups that may cause considerable discomfort will also be discussed in this chapter. The term used for those on whom ectoparasites are living is called an *infestation* rather than the term *infection* used for those who have parasites dwelling within.

LICE

Infestations of lice, of which *Pediculus humanus* and *Pthirus pubis* are the best-known parasites known as lice, have infested entire armies, villages, and cities. A common name for *P. pubis* is that of *crabs*, a term based on the physical appearance of the organism with its stout crablike appearance. These organisms are transmitted sexually as well as through common contact with others that are infested, or by use of clothing and bedding in which the organisms are found. Lice must spend their entire lives on their host, undergoing metabolic and morphologic changes, and gaining all of their nourishment from their host (Figure 10-1). They have developed adaptations which enable them to stay in close contact with a host and the various species may occupy different regions of the body depending on their physical needs.

Lice are extremely small, some less than 1 mm long. Both *P. humanus* and *P. pubis* are species possess stout legs with claws. These claws allow them to cling tightly to hair, fur, and feathers because some species also afflict animals and birds as well as humans. Some species are equipped to live on plant leaves and pose no medical

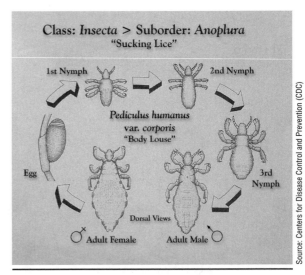

FIGURE 10-1 Life cycle of a "sucking louse," *Pediculus humanus* var. *corporis*, and the morphologic changes that take place during development

threat to humans but are of agricultural and horticultural importance. Lice are **apterygotes**, which means that they are wingless and they are dorsoventrally (backs and abdomens) flattened.

Lice, the singular form of which is louse, belong to the suborder **Anoplura** for those that infect humans. They are usually found in crowded areas where sanitation and hygiene are poor. The control of these infections will require a significant change in hygienic practices and control of living conditions for those infested, to avoid infestations of those who come in contact with them. Infestations are called *pediculosis* and the bites of these organisms allow obtaining of blood meals by piercing the skin and sucking the blood through their mouth parts. The areas where bites have occurred become itchy and inflamed and frequently become infected from scratching the areas with fingernails that may also contain other organisms, such as bacteria, resulting in a secondary infection. Another important role of some lice is one in which they play the role of a vector that is able to transmit diseases through their bites. Typhus is one such disease that is spread through the bites of lice.

Some species of lice have no eyes but do possess short sensory antennae as a substitute for eyes and the bodies are not well defined between the thoracic and the abdominal portions of their bodies. Most lice have relatively simple chewing mouthparts, but in some these organs may be highly adapted for piercing and sucking.

MACROSCOPIC DIAGNOSTIC FEATURE (REQUIRES MAGNIFYING GLASS IN SOME CASES)

General Classification—Louse

Organism	*Pediculus humanus* var. *corporis*
Specimen Required	Epidermal tissue or individual organism
Stage	Organism and its **nit**, or egg, on hair
Color & Appearance	White-gray to brown
Size	Egg is 0.8 mm, adult slightly larger (1.5 mm)
Shape	Elongated, crablike
Motility	No wings or ability to jump; move by crawling

P. humanus corporis organism

Delmar/Cengage Learning

Close contact with an infected person is required for transfer of the organism between humans and other mammals because lice cannot jump or fly to other victims. The human body louse, called *Pediculus humanus corporis,* lives on the body and clothes of humans. The head louse, which is called *Pediculus humanus capitis,* attaches itself to the hairs of the head and is best known for causing outbreaks in schoolchildren. This is a common occurrence in some crowded schools and the organisms spread rapidly. Because the pubic, or crab, louse called *P.hthirus pubis* is most often sexually transmitted, it prefers the environment of the moist and dark areas found in regions of the body. The louse resembles a miniature crab and causes intense itching in pubic areas, but it can also infect the eyebrows, eyelashes, and beards.

The two species of lice that afflict humans are scavengers that feed on the skin and other debris found on the host's body. But some species will also feed on sebaceous (sweat gland) secretions and blood. Most are found only on specific types of animals, and in some cases, they are confined to only a specific part of the body. Some animals are known to host up to 15 different species simultaneously, although 1 to 3 is typical for mammals and often 2 to 6 may be commonly found on birds. For example, in humans most of the different species of the louse inhabit the scalp and pubic hair. Lice generally cannot survive for long if removed from their host as they are unable to live freely in the environment as is the case for some organisms. So cleaning living quarters would be quite effective in preventing infestations and reinfestations.

Because lice live chiefly in the head hair and in the pubic hair of the body, they are somewhat easy to control through sanitation and medication. The louse's color varies from pale beige to dark gray, but when feeding on blood the organism may become considerably darker and therefore blends in well with the hair of a human. This makes them all but invisible to the naked eye. Just keeping the hair clean is not a deterrent to these lice as they prefer clean hair to dirty hair. Female lice are usually more common than males in most species, but some species are even known to be parthenogenetic, which means that they may self-fertilize themselves for reproduction. A louse's egg is commonly called a nit, commonly attaches to a hair shaft, and is how most infestations are discovered as nits are easily seen (Figure 10-2).

As the nit is more readily visible, it is often the first sign that a child may be infected with head lice even before symptoms appear. Many lice attach their eggs to their host's hair with specialized saliva, which makes the bond very difficult to break without specialized products such as shampoos designed to sever this bond as well as to kill the organisms. More than one treatment is necessary as some of the reproductive stages

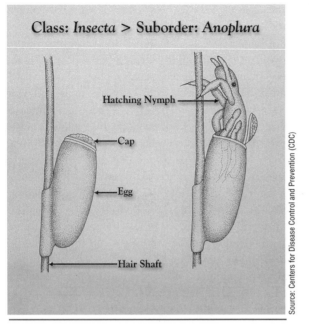

Class: *Insecta* > Suborder: *Anoplura*

Hatching Nymph

Cap

Egg

Hair Shaft

Source: Centers for Disease Control and Prevention (CDC)

FIGURE 10-2 The nit, or louse, eggs are glued to hairs of a host

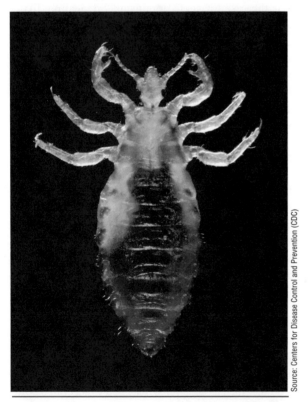

Source: Centers for Disease Control and Prevention (CDC)

FIGURE 10-3 Body lice are parasitic insects that live on the body and in the clothing or bedding of infested humans

are less sensitive to the special shampoo than others and repeat applications will kill the next stage as it matures. Lice inhabiting birds, however, may simply leave their eggs in parts of the body that are inaccessible to preening, such as the interior of feather shafts. Lice that almost exclusively inhabit birds may briefly infest humans but will not survive for a sufficient period of time for reproduction.

Living lice eggs tend to be pale white, whereas dead lice eggs are yellowish in color. Lice have a simple life cycle because they are born as small adults called *nymphs,* and as they molt, or shed, their skin they become larger in size as they progress toward adulthood. Organisms that reproduce in this manner are known as being hemimetabolous. After three sequences of molting, the lice are in the final adult form, which usually occurs within a month of hatching from the egg. Lice are transmitted through close contact and from infested bedding, clothing, and furniture (Figure 10-3).

OTHER COMMON ECTOPARASITES

Although not as common as the lice previously discussed, the following are some other common ectoparasites that may not be as common as the previous three. However, they may sometimes be found in endemic proportions.

Mites

A number of members of the order Acarina are called mites and are nuisances to both humans and animals in some cases. Mites are minute arthropods, some of which are parasitic and cause a variety of conditions in humans and in domestic animals (Figure 10-4). In addition, a few serve as vectors of disease organisms such as viruses and bacteria that contribute greatly to somewhat serious diseases. In some cases they may also serve as the intermediate host for some species of cestodes, commonly known as tapeworms, and therefore transmit other microorganisms. Asthma may be caused, or exacerbated, by mites.

Although similar to ticks, mites differ considerably in size as they are quite small and are difficult to see due to their minute size. The fact that they may be either almost clear (transparent) or they may be semi-transparent makes it more difficult to visualize them. Colloquially, they are sometimes called either chiggers or redbugs.

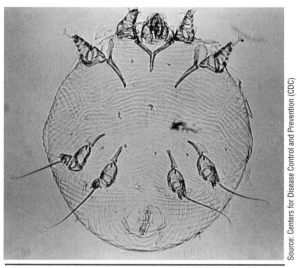

Source: Centers for Disease Control and Prevention (CDC)

FIGURE 10-4 Ventral view of a *Sarcoptes scabei* mite, prepared specimen

Mites usually burrow into the skin, in opposition to lice, and cause intense itching, resulting in inflamed areas of the skin. Mites that are prevalent as inhabitants of the human body may live for only a few days away from humans or other animals and birds that they typically infest. Discussions of some of the more common species that affect humans by order of prevalence and health impact include the following:

- Itch mites (*Sarcoptes scabiei*) cause a condition of the skin commonly known as *scabies* and undergo all of their developmental stages in the skin (Figure 10-5). This species of mite lays its eggs in tunnels in the skin, where it takes about 2 weeks for them to hatch.

- Diagnosis is often made by a medical professional who observes the skin tunneling prominently visible to the naked eye. Symptoms and signs include intense itching, especially at night, and usually accompanied by a rash (Figure 10-6). This rash may be seen most often on the hands and arms, but other common areas are in the armpits and genitalia of both males and females. Commonly, a person infected by the *S. scabiei* organism will harbor only around a dozen adult mites who can cause a great deal of torment for the victim. But a subspecies called the *Norwegian scabies*, which is rare and indistinguishable from the other type in morphology, presents a more severe form of the disease as it may

contribute up to two million organisms in a human infection. Both varieties of scabies will spread rapidly in households and among playmates as well as those who are intimate partners or have extremely close contact.

- Those with deficient immune systems or reduced consciousness such as senility or retardation frequently fall victim to a more severe form of scabies, but the same species of mite is responsible for both conditions. Treatment is a topical chlorinated hydrocarbon insecticide called "lindane," a benzene hexachloride toxic to both the blood and nervous systems. These medications should not used on children, pregnant women, or those with a history of seizure disorders where the central nervous system is affected. Recently, some resistance to lindane has been found in some populations of the "itch mite" called scabies.

- Another drug administered orally is "ivermectin," but this medication has been blamed for increased death rates in nursing home patients who have this medication prescribed. Fortunately there are less toxic treatments that include home remedies based upon plant extracts that have been found to be effective. Systemic antibiotics and steroidal preparations as well as antihistamines may be used to treat the symptoms and to prevent the secondary bacterial infections that almost invariably come from vigorous scratching. **Mange** in dogs and other animals are also caused by a mite belonging to two different families, *Sarcoptidae* and *Psoroptidae*. It is possible that humans have an inherited immunity against these two organisms.

- Two types of dust mites, *Dermatophagoides pteronyssinum* and *D. farinae,* ingest human skin cells that have been shed or dislodged by scratching. Face mites and follicle mites (*Demodex brevis* and *D. folliculorum*) are also found as a normal part of the normal flora (microorganisms) of the face. These organisms are quite small and can only be seen with a microscope or magnifying glass and reside in hair follicles, pores, or sebaceous glands. They may cause mild allergic reactions and also may contribute to or exacerbate an asthmatic condition in humans.

- Chiggers, caused most commonly by the *Trombicula autumnalis* variety, but sometimes by

Scabies
(Sarcoptes scabei)

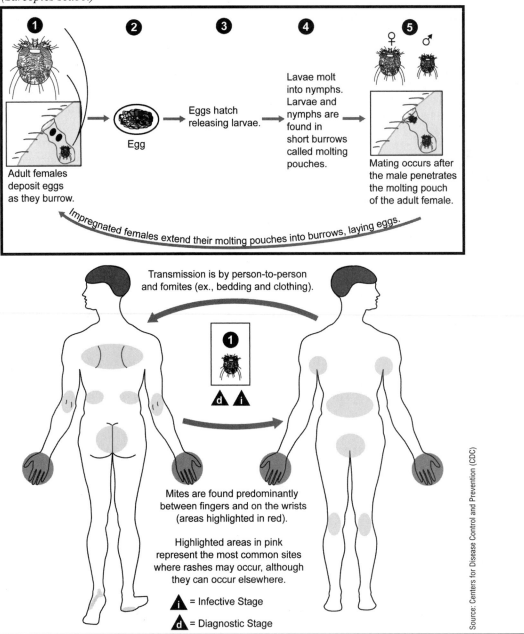

FIGURE 10-5 Life cycle of *Sarcoptes scabei*, causal agent of scabies

Eutrombicula alfreddugèsi and E. splendens), are six-legged red larvae of the mite family Trombiculidae, also known as the harvest mite. In some regions of the country these mites are commonly called the "redbug" and are usually contracted when working outside harvesting blackberries and other foods that grow wild. Chiggers attach to the skin of a host and bite the victim, causing a wheal (elevated area of the skin) accompanied by intense itching and severe dermatitis. These skin

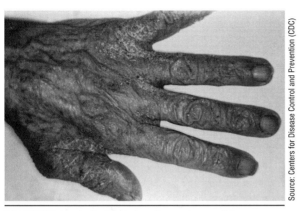

FIGURE 10-6 Patient's hand reveals a scabies infestation of the mite species *Sarcoptes scabiei* var. *hominis*

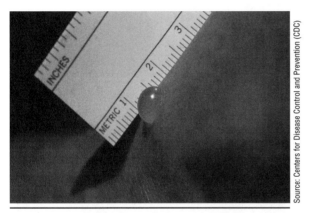

FIGURE 10-7 Chiggers (larvae of mites from the genus *Trombicula*) can cause intense itching and reddish welts on skin

rashes may be found where tight clothing is near the skin such as collars and cuffs of shirts and socks (Figure 10-7). Irritation of the skin appears to occur due to an allergic reaction to the saliva of the insect rather than to the mechanics of the bite and these organisms may also act as vectors for a number of infectious diseases. Currently these mites are not known to transmit any infectious diseases in the United States. However, in some Asian countries, they are vectors of scrub typhus, which is caused by a rickettsial (bacteria-like) organism.

Ticks

Ticks belong to the phylum Arthropoda, meaning that they move by use of jointed legs (arthro) and feet (poda).

In addition, they are a member of the class Arachnida because they possess eight legs and are not insects, which have six legs. Ticks are capable vectors for a number of infectious organisms that are termed arboviruses because they are transmitted by arthropods. Some of these diseases include Rocky Mountain spotted fever, caused by *Rickettsia rickettsii*; Lyme disease, caused by *Borrelia burgdorferi*, Tularemia (rabbit fever), caused by *Francisella tularensis*; and human granulocytic ehrlichiosis (HGE), caused by the *Ehrlichia chaffeensis* organism.

These organisms are bloodsucking arachnid parasites of the order Acarida. Unlike the mites of an associated group, adult ticks are relatively large and are easily seen by the naked eye and act as vectors for certain bacteria and viruses known to cause disease in humans. They are the only venomous creature that hunts down humans in some species of ticks. Fortunately, most insects and arachnids try to avoid human contact rather than actively seeking them. There are two kinds of ticks simply called "hard" and "soft" and each carry different diseases. Hard ticks, of the family Ixodidae, do not burrow into the skin. But soft ticks, of the family Argasidae, that primarily infest birds but sometimes will affect humans, do burrow into the skin and must be removed with great care, for otherwise their heads will possibly remain imbedded when the body is pulled away (Figure 10-8), resulting in infections in the bite area, and transmission of disease organisms.

The life cycle for ticks is relatively simple when compared with those of the endoparasites, as they exist in stages that do not remotely resemble the adult form (Figure 10-9). The nymphal stage is of particular interest because usually there is only a single nymphal stage through which a tick passes; however, some ticks pass through multiple nymphal transitions during the nymphal stage prior to becoming a mature adult organism.

Dog ticks may bring slow paralysis, similar to that of the Guillain-Barre Syndrome, and may be fatal to children. Interestingly, both the nymphal and adult stages of most species of ticks are capable of infecting a host organism with a variety of disease agents. Nymphal forms of ticks are more difficult to discover on the body, although they are perfectly capable as vectors for many infectious diseases that may result in acute or chronic disease with lasting effects in humans (Figure 10-10).

Fortunately ticks must remain embedded for at least 18 hours or more in order to transmit the various

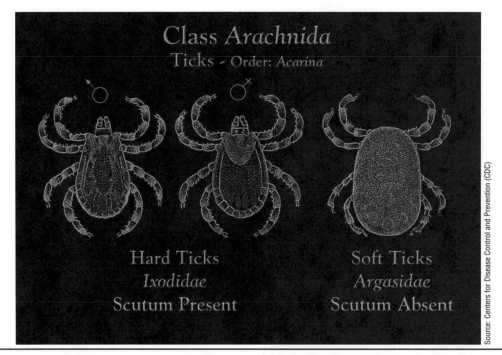

FIGURE 10-8 Image depicts the morphologic differences seen between the Ixodidae hard ticks, and the Argasidae soft ticks

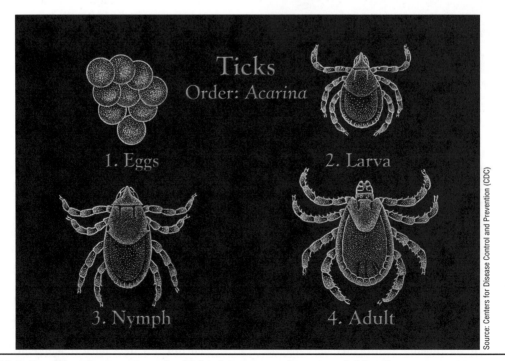

FIGURE 10-9 Four life cycle stages through which a tick passes on its way to adulthood

infections to humans. Some species of ticks are efficient vectors of more than one infectious agent. An example of this is found in the North American species of tick, *Dermacenter andersoni* vector, which is an efficient purveyor of both Rocky Mountain spotted fever and tularemia. Other important pathogens are rickettsial organisms, an obligate intracellular parasite that is spread by vectors such as fleas, ticks, mites, and lice.

Lyme disease is caused by a spirochete (Borrelia), which is spread by a tick vector called *Ixodes dammini*. A number of tick species may embed themselves into the skin of humans and animals, from which diseases may be transmitted from these vectors (Figure 10-11). The disease affects multiple organs and entire systems of the human body and after recovery often leaves residual complaints of arthritis of the large joints, along with myalgia and malaise, and in some instances neurologic and cardiac problems. The Borrelia are parasitic organisms responsible for several diseases (including relapsing fever) transmitted by ticks and the human body louse. Prophylactic treatment before exposure with antibiotics has not halted the development of the disease to any great extent. Australian paralysis ticks cause paralysis in humans but upon removing the tick, paralysis often becomes worse rather than improving. A number of tick species are capable of transmitting many diseases around the world, and avoiding the bites of these vectors is of utmost importance in preventing disease.

Fleas

Fleas are small, wingless, bloodsucking insects that act as vectors for the spread of such diseases as tularemia, typhus (rickettsial disease spread by lice, fleas, or mites), and brucellosis (a bacterial disease). Fleas are parasites that infest mostly warm-blooded animals including humans. Various species infect certain animals, with humans being chiefly infected by the bites from a human flea *Pulex irritans* (Figure 10-12). Throughout history, rats that flourish in large cities have harbored fleas capable of transmitting diseases to humans. The most prominent occurrence of a serious epidemic that killed

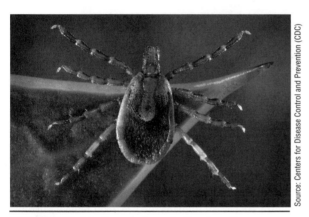

Source: Centers for Disease Control and Prevention (CDC)

FIGURE 10-10 Dorsal view of a female yellow dog tick, *Amblyomma aureolatum*, vector of Rocky Mountain spotted fever in Brazil

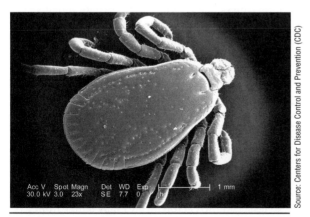

Acc V 30.0 kV   Spot Magn 3.0   23x   Det SE   WD 7.7   Exp 0   1 mm

Source: Centers for Disease Control and Prevention (CDC)

FIGURE 10-11 Dorsal view of an unidentified male *Dermacentor* sp. tick found upon a cat

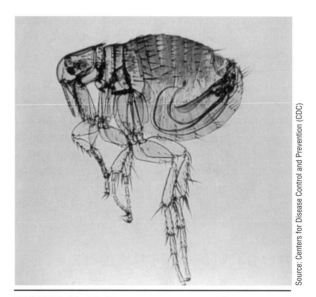

Source: Centers for Disease Control and Prevention (CDC)

FIGURE 10-12 Humans may contract plague, *Y. pestis*, when bitten by a rodent flea

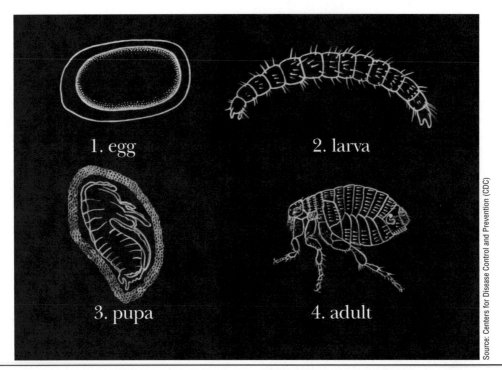

Source: Centers for Disease Control and Prevention (CDC)

FIGURE 10-13 Morphologic changes experienced by a flea during its life cycle, from an egg to an adult insect

hundreds of thousands of Europeans in the Middle Ages was simply called "the plague," which refers in general to bubonic plague. This disease is caused by a bacterial bacillus called *Yersinia pestis*, and was spread from rats to humans via the rat flea, although there is some argument regarding the link of flea bites and the development of bubonic plague. The term *bubonic* comes from the word *bubo*, which indicates swollen and enlarged lymph nodes, main sign of the disease.

Humans can allegedly contract plague, *Y. pestis*, when bitten by a rodent flea that is carrying the plague bacterium or by handling an infected animal. "Murine" typhus, due to *Rickettsia typhi* bacteria, can also be transmitted by rodent fleas to man. Four stages, with changing morphology in the flea's life cycle, include the egg, followed by a larva that becomes a pupa, and then finally metamorphoses into an adult organism (Figure 10-13).

Tropical Chigoes or Jiggers

The term jigger, or chigo, is the common name for a parasitic flea called *Tunga penetrans*. Parasitic infestations

by this vector usually involve pigs, dogs, and humans who traditionally go barefoot as the groups most susceptible to attacks by this organism. These fleas are found in the tropical and subtropical parts of America and Africa (Figure 10-14). In humans the pregnant female burrows into the spaces between the toes where she causes a painful and open sore. The gravid (pregnant) flea must be removed with a sterile needle and the wound treated with iodine to destroy any remaining fleas and eggs. This penetration causes intense itching and irritation that sometimes results in ulcerations and if left untreated, extreme cases may result in amputation of the affected limb as a medical necessity.

OTHER LESS COMMON ECTOPARASITES

Although they may be less common than many of the other organisms that infest the skin and hair of humans and other mammals, those who become infected by these lesser-known ectoparasites may suffer from irritating and exacerbated conditions. Serious infections

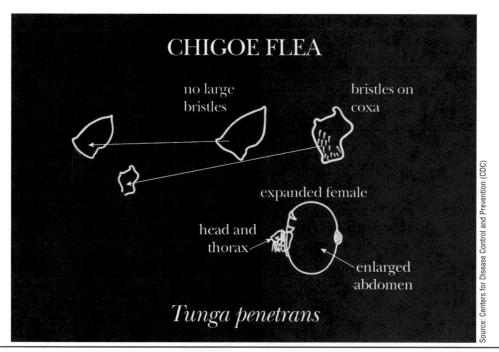

FIGURE 10-14 Identifying morphologic characteristics of the chigoe flea, *Tunga penetrans*

sometimes occur when the skin is broken by the following ectoparasites.

Common Bedbugs

The common bedbug, *Cimex lectularius*, contains an irritating chemical in its saliva that causes uncomfortable skin reactions. These insects are 4 to 5 mm in length, quite visible, and may survive at low temperatures for periods of up to a year without feeding. Therefore, bedding may be infected and remain so until the next victim arrives at some point in the future. On occasion, infestations of bedbugs will be publicized and will gain public attention. Often these organisms may be found in transient motels and homeless shelters where the personal hygiene of the residents may be suspect.

These insects are flat and oval in shape and may impart a reddish-brown color. They may inhabit the house and furniture, as well as beds that have not been cleaned and freshly made. They feed on humans, especially at night, causing bites that are extremely itchy and which may become infected if not properly cared for. Although the amount of blood ingested is quite small and

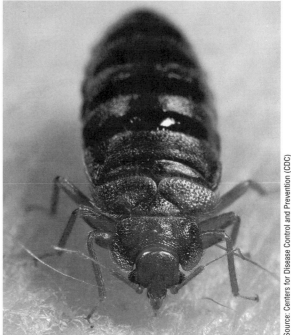

FIGURE 10-15 Adult bedbug, *Cimex lectularius*, as it was in the process of ingesting a blood meal from the arm of a "voluntary" human host

MACROSCOPIC DIAGNOSTIC FEATURE (REQUIRES MAGNIFYING GLASS IN SOME CASES)

General Classification—Insect

Organism	*Cimex lectularis*
Specimen Required	Individual organism, usually obtained from skin or bed linens
Stage	Adult
Color & Appearance	Reddish (newly hatched are translucent)
Size	Adult is 4–5 mm in length; 1.5–3 mm in width
Shape	Flat and oval
Motility	Nocturnal crawling

requires several days to use as much as 1 mL of blood from a victim, infants have been known to develop anemia from blood loss to these creatures (Figure 10-15). It is possible, but not proven, that the transmission of hepatitis B and perhaps some of the other strains of hepatitis have occurred through bedbug bites. Insecticides are required for ridding an area of these parasites and cleaning should include furniture, mattresses, bed frames, walls, and baseboards in order to remove nesting sites for these insects. Secondary infections may occur from scratching the bedbug bites.

Leeches

The term leech is applied to any of the annelids from the class Hirudinea, especially *Hirudo medicinalis*. Some species are bloodsuckers and were once used to draw blood out of those who were ill. These organisms are parasitic in that they require sustenance from a victim in the form of blood, so medical practice in the past has included the use of leeches for bleeding areas of the body. Even today leeches are used to remove blood from large bruises and are available from scientific supply houses. The leech has not been known to transmit any diseases to its human hosts.

Tooth Amoebae

The amoeba *Entameba gingivalis* is a microscopic parasite that hides in the tiny crevices where the teeth meet the gums. Brushing does not remove them because of their ability to assume different shapes that enable them to fit into minuscule hiding places. These organisms may be considered beneficial organisms because they ingest mouth bacteria that may cause inflammation. But with poor mouth hygiene, their numbers may proliferate and they may become harmful when the lack of hygiene forces them to multiply too quickly.

SUMMARY

Ectoparasites derive their nourishment from the outside of the body, primarily the skin, but also for some species, taking advantage of either the host's blood supply or debris on the skin of the host. Other ectoparasites exist by eating the bacteria on the skin of the host. There are several major types of ectoparasites that plague human beings. Lice and mites are the two major groups that include four common genera, three of which are lice and one of which is classified as a mite. Fleas and ticks are also considered ectoparasites.

Infestations of lice include *Pediculus humanus* and *Pthirus pubis* as the best-known representatives, and may infest large groups of people and even large cities. Lice are capable of infesting a variety of hosts, as they are adapted with structures that allow them to cling tightly to hair, fur, and feathers. The range of potential hosts for lice includes some aquatic creatures as well as land mammals, birds, and others.

Close contact with an infected person is required to transfer the organism because lice cannot jump or fly. Lice chiefly occupy crowded areas such as refugee camps and prisons due to the poor sanitation and hygiene that foster the growth of these infestations. Some lice may be vectors and transmit diseases through their bites. Typhus is a disease that may be spread by both lice bites or flea bites and is a rickettsial disease, which invades the lining of blood vessels and smooth muscles.

Two species of the human body louse—*Pediculus humanus corporis,* known as the body louse, and *Pediculus humanus capitis,* the head louse—attach themselves to the hairs of the head, and causes outbreaks in schools and daycare centers. The pubic or crab louse, *Phthirus pubis,* is usually sexually transmitted and can also infect any hairy areas such as the eyebrows, eyelashes, and beards.

Other common ectoparasites include a group called mites. Some members of the order Acarina are parasitic and may affect both humans and domestic animals and a few mites even transmit viruses and bacteria and at least a few species of tapeworms may be transmitted by mites. Other complications include allergic reactions to the infestation, which may exacerbate or cause respiratory problems such as asthma.

Mites are often called chiggers or redbugs and burrow into the skin, causing intense itching and skin irritation. Itch mites (*Sarcoptes scabiei*) cause a skin condition known as scabies. Symptoms include intense itching, which occurs mostly at night accompanied by a rash on the hands, arms, armpits, and genitalia. There are two varieties of *S. scabiei* organisms. Both varieties spread rapidly in households and among intimate partners.

Dust mites, including mostly *Dermatophagoides pteronyssinum* or *D. farinae,* ingest human skin cells that are shed or may be abraded by scratching. Face mites or follicle mites (*Demodex brevis* and *D. folliculorum*), are found as a normal organism of the face. These organisms can only be seen with the help of a microscope, and may cause mild allergic reactions and contribute to asthma in humans.

Three species of chiggers are commonly called the "redbug" in some areas of the country. Chiggers attach to the skin and bite the host, causing intense itching and severe dermatitis. Irritation of the skin may be due to allergic reactions to the saliva of the mite. These mites also act as vectors for scrub typhus.

Two kinds of ticks, "hard" and "soft," each carry different diseases. Soft ticks (family Ixodidae) do not burrow into the skin, but hard ticks (family Argasidae) do and require great care in removing them to avoid leaving the head imbedded in the skin. Dog ticks are known to cause paralysis similar to that of the Guillain-Barre syndrome, sometimes fatal to children. Both adult and nymphal forms of ticks may be vectors for transmitting infectious diseases and transmit a significant number of diseases including Rocky Mountain spotted fever, Q fever, borreliosis, ehrlichiosis, tularemia, babesiosis, and Lyme disease.

Fleas are mostly found on furry and hairy animals but humans may also be affected. They are vectors for several human diseases including tularemia, typhus, and brucellosis. Rats in large cities harbor fleas that transmit diseases to humans and apparently were responsible for the deaths of hundreds of thousands of Europeans with the plague several centuries ago.

Jigger is a common name for a parasitic flea called *Tunga penetrans.* Parasitic infestations of this organism typically involve pigs, dogs, and those humans who traditionally go barefoot. These fleas are found in the tropical and subtropical Americas and Africa. Complications of ulcerations and attendant infections sometimes require amputation if early treatment is not obtained.

Other common parasites include the bedbug *Cimex lectularius.* This "bug" contains an irritating chemical in its saliva that causes irritating skin reactions, and feeds on humans at night. Bedding may be infected and remain so until the next victim arrives at some point in the future so scrupulous cleaning is necessary to control the infestation of a dwelling. These organisms are prevalent and may be found in transient motels and homeless shelters where the personal hygiene of the residents may be poor. Blood loss leading to anemia in protracted cases and the transmission of hepatitis B are possible complications to infestations of this bug.

Leeches are not known to transmit any types of diseases to human hosts and they often infect other mammals that enter the water. The term *leech* is applied to any of the annelids from the class Hirudinea, especially *Hirudo medicinalis.* Some species are bloodsuckers and were once used to draw blood out of those who were ill.

Tooth amoebae, *Entamoeba gingivalis,* are microscopic parasites able to hide in the tiny crevices where the teeth meet the gums. Brushing does not remove them because of their ability to assume different shapes, enabling them to fit into minuscule hiding places. These organisms may be considered beneficial organisms, as they eat mouth bacteria that may cause inflammation. But with poor mouth hygiene, their numbers may proliferate and they may become harmful when the lack of hygiene forces them to multiply too quickly.

CASE STUDIES

1. Mary Beth is traveling across the country with a group of friends. They have always tried to find economical lodging, and many of the places where they have stayed have been dirty, musty, and somewhat old. One morning, after spending the night in a somewhat decrepit motel, Mary Beth awakes and experiences wheezing and difficulties in breathing. She has never been diagnosed with asthma, but a number of relatives have told her that they have a reactive type of asthma aggravated by certain environmental factors. Could the condition be precipitated, or aggravated, by a parasite? Explain how this could happen, the potential organism, and other factors that could become medical problems for Mary Beth.

2. During the Middle Ages in Europe, a serious epidemic took the lives of tens of thousands victims of a devastating infection. The organism was allegedly spread by rats and the fleas that inhabited their bodies in these large and crowded cities. What is the common name and causative organism that resulted in the epidemic? Provide the name of the insect vector that supposedly led to the widespread malady.

STUDY QUESTIONS

1. What are two ways that ectoparasites gain nourishment from the body of humans?

2. What is a common name for sexually transmitted body lice, and how did they acquire their name?

3. What is a serious disease that may be spread by lice?

4. What is the element of a louse that is called a nit?

5. What are some ways that mites can cause serious medical conditions?

6. What are some common names for mites that infest the skin of human?

7. What is a serious consequence of being bitten by dog ticks, and that may be fatal to children?

8. What are some serious infectious diseases that are transmitted by ticks?

9. What was once a medical treatment performed with leeches?

10. How can tooth amoebae be helpful?

Organisms Borne by Ticks and Other Vectors

LEARNING OBJECTIVES

Upon completion of this chapter, the learner will be expected to:

■ Explain the dual role of ticks as vectors and as parasites of warm-blooded mammals
■ Discuss the ways in which ticks are equipped to find hosts
■ Explain how the population of deer ticks is controlled by the white-tailed deer population
■ List steps one can take to avoid being bitten by a tick
■ Relate the ways ticks are attracted to their victims
■ Describe how DEET and similar insect repellents keep biting insects away
■ Define the localized symptoms and signs of Lyme disease
■ Describe in general the three stages of Lyme disease
■ List some medical conditions of a victim that may cause serious threats to their health when babesiosis is contracted

KEY TERMS

Acetone	Ehrlichiosis	Macrophages
Anaplasma	Erythema chronicum migrans	Malaise
Bioterrorism	Glandular	Mandibles
Black flies	Human granulocytic ehrlichiosis (HGE)	Methylene blue stain
Bull's eye rash	Hypostome	Mononucleosis
Chelicerae	Insect repellent	Neutrophil
Chloramphenicol	Intracellular	Nymphal ticks
Conjunctivitis	Jaundice	Oculoglandular
Deer flies	Leukopenia	Ohara's fever
Deer fly fever	Lone star tick	Permethrin
Deer tick	Lymphocyte	Rodents
DEET		Scutum

Sebaceous gland

Seed ticks

Southern Tick–associated
    Rash Illness

Spirochetal

Tachycardia

Thrombocytopenia

Tularemia

Turkey ticks

Ulceroglandular

Wright's-Giemsa

INTRODUCTION

Ticks are singularly well adapted to the role of the vector, both in the practice of feeding from warm-blooded animals with an infectious disease and in the process passing certain infective organisms into the subsequent host. Ticks as vectors are some of the most efficient transmitters of parasites and other bacterial and viral diseases in existence. A simple description of a parasite is an organism that lives in or upon an organism at the organism's expense without contributing to the host's survival in any way. Some bacterial infections transmitted by ticks also become intracellular, as do blood parasites from mosquitoes, and survive and reproduce while inside the blood cells, most often red blood cells but some organisms inhabit white blood cells. Some of these organisms must specifically inhabit blood cells in order to complete their life cycles. Therefore, several diseases

that are tick-borne are presented in this chapter, some of which are not considered strictly as being parasite based. Therefore, some overlap occurs between parasitic and bacterial infections. Both types of infections, of which some are strictly parasitic and some which are bacterial and that become intracellular inclusions infecting blood cells, will be presented in this section.

Ticks are blood-feeding parasites that are often found predominantly at the edges of woods and in tall grass and shrubs where they await the opportunity to attach themselves to a passing warm-blooded animal host. Ticks can be found in most wooded or forested regions throughout the world and are most common in areas where there are deer trails or human pathways. In these areas a tick attaches itself to its host by inserting its sharp mandibles, called chelicerae, and a hollow feeding tube for aspirating blood, called a hypostome, into the skin of its host (Figure 11-1). The tick can attach equally well

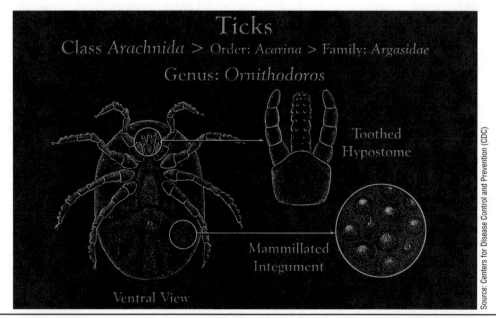

Source: Centers for Disease Control and Prevention (CDC)

FIGURE 11-1 Soft tick, ventral view, with its toothed hypostome and mammillated (possessing nipple-like protuberances) integument

to both hairy and smooth skin. There the tick becomes firmly anchored and feeds on the blood of the host. This practice provides an excellent mechanism through which ticks are quite proficient at transmitting parasites and other organisms into the bodies of their hosts while they are feeding on the host's blood.

Ticks do not have wings and are unable to jump as they have somewhat short legs that are not adapted for jumping, so physical contact is the only method of infestation. Ticks often fall onto their hosts from vegetation when the potential host walks under the tick's plant haven but some actually stalk the host on foot. They become aware of their prey due to heat and carbon dioxide emitted from their victims, and they become most active in the spring when the temperature rises and the days are longer. Ticks often take several days to complete a blood meal and the attachment must last for roughly a day in order to transmit the infective organisms to their hosts.

TICKS AND DISEASES COMMONLY TRANSMITTED BY THESE VECTORS

Fortunately not all tick bites result in the contraction of an infectious disease. Some of the more common illnesses that can be contracted from a tick bite include Lyme disease, babeosis, Rocky Mountain spotted fever (RMSF), ehrlichiosis, Southern Tick–associated Rash Illness (STARI), or tularemia, as well as some others that are not as common. Certain species of ticks are more likely to transmit these diseases based on the species found in certain geographic locations. Commonly encountered species by geographic location are listed throughout this section. For example, white-tailed deer, common throughout the southern United States, are frequently infested by "seed ticks," which are small forms of the deer tick called *Ixodes scapularis*, a species that is widely distributed along the eastern seaboard of the United States. Deer tick populations in the eastern United States are dependent almost entirely on the white-tailed deer herd as the number of ticks in a given area roughly correlates with the size of the deer population.

The life cycle of a tick is quite simple and undergoes similar stages in development as those of other ectoparasites. The nymphal stage as a smaller version of the adult stage, is rather diverse; however, for most there is often only one nymphal stage through which a tick passes. However, some species of ticks pass through several metamorphic changes during the nymphal stage before becoming a mature adult tick (Figure 11-2). And, dependent upon the species of the tick and the organisms with which the tick is infected, different stage(s) of the tick's life cycle may be required for transmission of a tick-borne pathogen. If these criteria as to species and

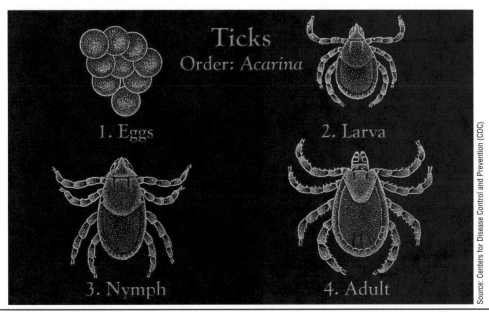

Source: Centers for Disease Control and Prevention (CDC)

FIGURE 11-2 Morphologic features associated with the four life cycle stages a tick experiences during its passage to adulthood

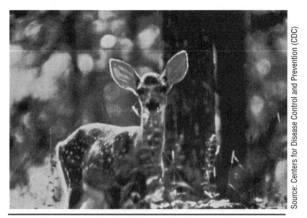

Source: Centers for Disease Control and Prevention (CDC)

FIGURE 11-3 White-tailed deer, *Odocoileus virginianus*, responsible for tick populations and transmission of disease

pathogenicity are met, the contraction of a disease may result when bitten by a tick.

A related species, *Ixodes pacificus*, is found in the western portion of the United States and is responsible for the majority of Rocky Mountain spotted fever cases in that region. Livestock, rather than deer, are the adult host of this species of tick found in the western states (Figure 11-3). Immature stages or nymphs of the *Ixodes scapularis* tick also feed on smaller mammals or birds until they are ready to infest deer or livestock. The female tick as an adult must have a blood meal for several days before reaching the point where she can be productive in laying eggs.

A considerable number of species of ticks are spread throughout the United States and around the world, and are responsible for spreading diseases worldwide. Discussions of these numerous species is beyond the scope of this publication, but those commonly associated with infectious diseases in the United States are discussed in this publication. A significant number of these species are also primarily important because they impact agricultural endeavors rather than spreading pathogens to humans. Many of these parasitic ticks attack cattle, sheep, goats, and horses, causing death and illness among these animals and thereby extracting a great economic toll. Ticks are divided into two general and basic groups called "hard" ticks and "soft" ticks.

Another "hard" tick of the *Ixodes* genus is the lone star tick (*Amblyomma americanum*), a member of

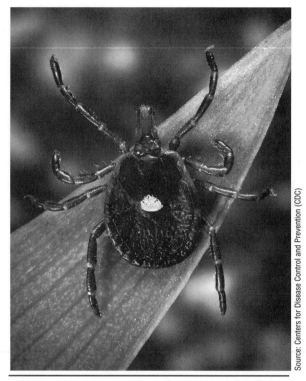

Source: Centers for Disease Control and Prevention (CDC)

FIGURE 11-4 Dorsal view of female lone star tick, *Amblyomma americanum*, with characteristic star marking on dorsal surface

the Ixodidae family (Figure 11-4). These female ticks have a white marking on their back resembling a star and are responsible for the transmission of Southern Tick–associated Rash Illness. The causative organism for this disease is the *Borrelia* species, the same genus as the organism that causes Lyme disease. These species will be considered when discussing specific diseases transmitted by each of them later in this section.

It should again be stressed that a tick must generally remain imbedded in the skin of its victim for at least 18 to 24 hours in order to transmit a pathogen to a human or other animal. Therefore it is important to remove the tick when it is still roaming about the body before it becomes embedded in the skin. Removal of the feeding tick must be performed carefully in order to avoid decapitating the tick and leaving the head in the skin, resulting in infections of various pathogens. Although almost a thousand species of ticks exist, around 80 species of Ixodidae (hard ticks) and perhaps 10 species of soft ticks are currently found in the United States. In addition to the lone star tick and the deer tick, two species of

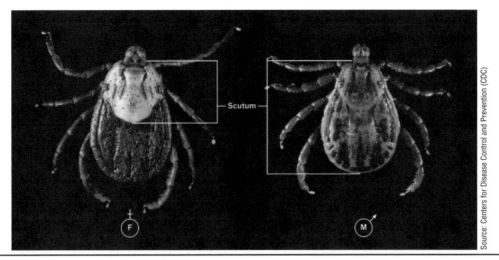

FIGURE 11-5 Dorsal view of both a female and male wood tick, *Dermacentor andersoni*; smaller female's scutum when compared to the male's larger scutum

dog ticks are important in North America: *Dermacentor variabilis*, commonly called the *American dog tick* or the *eastern wood tick* and the *Rhipicephalus sanguineus*, or the *brown dog tick,* which is seldom implicated in transmitting diseases to humans.

As mentioned previously, ticks are divided into two general groups called hard and soft ticks. Hard ticks are named due to a hard, shiny **scutum** that resembles a shield on their backs, also known as the dorsal region. The male tick is smaller than the female and the scutum covers the majority of the dorsal surface of the male. The female's scutum is not as large, an anatomical feature that equips her to expand in size as she feeds and becomes engorged with the host's blood. Common examples of hard tick species in the United States and over North America that are vectors of various diseases are the genera *Amblyomma, Ixodes, Dermacentor, Anocentor, Haemaphysalis, Hyalomma, Rhicephalus,* and *Boophilus*. The first three representatives of these genera are those most prominent in causing human diseases in the United States. Examples of soft ticks species that are not as medically important as hard ticks include the genera *Arga, Alectrobius, Alyeonasus, Cario, Ornithodoros,* and *Otobius*. The following figure of a female wood tick, *Dermacentor andersoni*, is a known vector of *Rickettsia rickettsii*, the causative agent for Rocky Mountain spotted fever (Figure 11-5). *D. andersoni* is sometimes considered the Rocky Mountain tick and is responsible for a portion of the tick-borne diseases contracted in, or at least attributed to, the Rocky Mountain region.

The *Ixodes pacificus* tick, found in the Pacific Northwest region of the United States, is responsible for the majority of Rocky Mountain spotted fever cases in that area, along with the previously mentioned *Dermacentor* species. Livestock are the primary adult hosts of this species of tick, whereas in the eastern United States, is the deer. Immature stages of the *Ixodes scapularis* ticks prefer the deer as their primary host but may spend their juvenile stage of life on small mammals and birds before they are able to infect a deer. The female adult tick is able to lay more than 2000 eggs, but must have a period of several days of ingesting blood before being able to lay her eggs (Figure 11-6). And to again emphasize a point, the North American *Ixodes* are hard ticks due to the

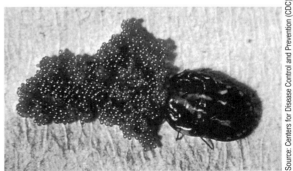

FIGURE 11-6 Upon laying eggs, this female *Ixodes* hard tick will die, whereas the soft tick female may lay many batches

presence of a dorsal plate, or scutum. There are over 200 member species of the genus *Ixodes* and a number of separate species are capable of transmitting Lyme disease to humans. Hard ticks die after producing a clutch of eggs, whereas soft ticks can produce eggs over a period of several years.

Avoiding the Contraction of Disease from Tick Bites

Several methods exist for avoiding tick bites and the possibility of becoming infected through contact with a tick, some of which will be practiced concurrently. First, and most important, avoiding habitats such as the edges of brushy fields frequented by ticks and proper body searches will eliminate many ticks. Staying away from certain habitats where ticks are prevalent during the peak of tick season is perhaps the best way to prevent tick bites and potential infections. In most areas of the country, this time period is usually from early April into early fall. But depending upon the temperature of the various latitudes, this period may vary by several weeks and starts earlier in the more southerly latitudes and will end a few weeks later than in the northern zones. Extremely cold weather in the early fall serves to lower a population of ticks that may overwinter in the larval stage and emerge to breed the following spring.

The second most important means of preventing tick bites and perhaps subsequent infections, is by wearing protective clothing. If it is necessary to enter a tick habitat, wearing light-colored clothing, including a long-sleeved shirt tucked into trousers and long-legged pants tucked into socks, is beneficial. This will not only help to prevent ticks from reaching your body, but as ticks roam the body they are easier to see against a light background. It is quite simple to remove these ticks before they find a way to reach the skin. DO NOT wear flea and tick collars around ankles to prevent ticks from attaching to the skin. This practice can be extremely dangerous, because the insecticide is absorbed through the skin and into the body. In addition, do not crush these ticks between unprotected fingers, as this may release infectious pathogenic organisms.

The third method of prevention of tick bites requires the help of a friend. Because both male and female adult ticks tend to explore the body of a host for sometimes up to several hours before they attach themselves to the skin, body searches are quite effective in avoiding attachment. Preventive practices such as body searches should be scrupulously performed for effectiveness. For this reason, a thorough body check should include special attention to hairy areas, including the head, chest, underarms, and pubic regions, in order to find adult ticks before they attach and begin to feed. Nymphs and larvae may not be as easily seen as adult ticks because they are quite small and practically transparent in some species, so extreme care should be exercised in searching for these forms. In addition, to further avoid the multitude of infections that may be contracted by pets from a tick bite, a daily examination of a pet's body is also necessary when the pet has visited an area in or near woods or fields.

When considering the use of an insect repellent, one of the best tick repellents is called DEET (N,N-diethyl-m-toluamide). Products containing 10 to 35 percent DEET, an effective and versatile insect repellent, will provide sufficient protection under normal conditions when used according to instructions. Insect repellents that contain DEET have stood the test of time, as they have been in existence for more than 40 years and are especially effective when used in conjunction with protective clothing. If these practices are followed, the chances of becoming bitten by ticks is greatly minimized (Figure 11-7). They have been used by people throughout the world in order to avoid a host of insects and other related organisms, which include not only ticks but other important vectors and pests that include flies, mosquitoes, fleas, and chiggers, to name a few. DEET preparations are available in many forms that

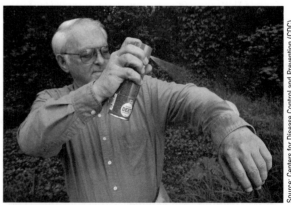

Source: Centers for Disease Control and Prevention (CDC)

FIGURE 11-7 Wear long sleeves with trousers tucked into socks during peak tick season. Spray DEET directly onto clothes

are designed to fit the environment, such as creams for wet environments, lotions, DEET-saturated towelettes, gels, aerosol and pump sprays. Although these repellents have proven to minimize the numbers of bites by most biting insects and related organisms, the products must be used as intended for optimum results.

Repellents containing DEET and permethrin serve to initially repel and, over a period of time, will actually kill ticks that contact the clothing. The Centers for Disease Control and Prevention can provide information pertinent to the safe use of repellents and their correct use. In addition, it is important to follow directions found printed on the product label. And it bears repeating that immediately upon concluding an outdoor outing in woods and fields and even when a repellent has been used, the clothing should be removed and a careful check of the entire body should be accomplished.

How do DEET and other similar repellents keep biting creatures at bay? Ticks are attracted by body heat of the intended victim and the carbon dioxide from the breath of humans and other animals. Some insects and flies, including black flies , deer flies , and mosquitoes, are also attracted by skin odors from oily sebaceous gland secretions and sweat. As a mosquito comes within a short distance of a host, DEET and some other repellents serve to confuse the insect's sensors, making it difficult for the insect to identify a desirable host and to successfully bite the host. Repellents are effective at only a short distance so flies and other insects may be flying near the intended victim but will be affected only upon close contact with the treated skin surfaces.

So, in summary, several steps are required to most effectively avoid bites by disease-carrying creatures. First of all, avoiding the habitats frequented by ticks is important in avoiding tick bites. The use of insect and arthropod repellents, along with obstructive clothing, will also assist greatly in avoiding diseases transmitted by ticks. Utilization of these three preventive practices will reduce and should practically eliminate the problems associated with tick bites. But it is impossible to always avoid all tick bites, so the final step would be to remove the embedded tick quickly and properly in order to avoid the possibility of infection.

Lyme disease

Lyme disease is a disorder that is capable of involving multiple systems of the body and is the most common tick-borne illness in the United States. Lyme disease is endemic in the northeastern United States but has been diagnosed over the past few decades in all 50 states. If Lyme disease is left untreated it has the potential to progress in stages from mild symptoms to serious, long-term disabilities. Three distinct stages of Lyme disease vary in intensity between victims. Most cases are manifested in the early and localized stage. The next stage is called the *early disseminated stage* and then is followed by the *late persistent stage.*

As a matter of academic interest, however, Lyme disease–like illnesses are found not only in the United States but also are somewhat prevalent in both Europe and Asia where etiologic disease agents and vectors may be more diverse than those seen in North America. Several related species of ticks common in Eastern Europe and Asia differ from those found in North America and transmit the *Borellia* species that cause human diseases on those continents (Figure 11-8). In North America, *Borrelia burgdorferi* is the only causative

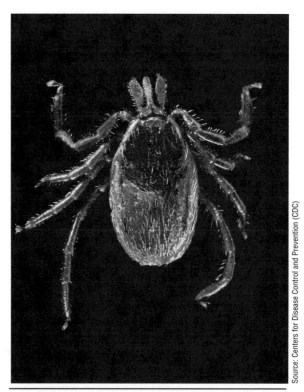

Source: Centers for Disease Control and Prevention (CDC)

FIGURE 11-8 Dorsal view of an adult female western blacklegged tick, *Ixodes pacificus*, which has been shown to transmit *Borrelia burgdorferi*, the causative agent of Lyme disease

organism of human Lyme disease but different causative species that cause similar diseases have been discovered on other continents. These spirochetal agents of human disease are transmitted by members of the *Ixodes* complex, which includes *I. dammini* in eastern North America and *I. pacificus* in western North America.

Symptoms of Lyme Disease

As previously listed, three distinct stages of Lyme disease exist. During the first stage, called the *localized phase*, symptoms and signs initially emerge. In approximately 80 percent of the cases the accompanying signs will eventually include a rash called *erythema migrans* at the site of the tick bite. It is estimated that about 50 percent of those who are infected with Lyme disease will rather quickly develop a rash within 4 weeks following the bite by an infective tick. This circular rash may grow progressively larger over a period of time. However, some who have contracted Lyme disease will have only mild symptoms and signs or perhaps none at all. Victims clinically diagnosed with a Lyme disease infection may not even recall receiving a tick bite or finding any ticks on themselves.

Those who live in endemic areas where Lyme disease occurs most frequently includes states along the Atlantic coast, the Midwest, and more recently some locations in Oregon and California. The circular or bull's eye rash appears especially during the warm months of the year and is frequently the only sign of a very early stage of Lyme disease (Figure 11-9). The disease progresses through three major stages:

■ **Stage One**

Some who become infected with the causative organism for Lyme disease will have flulike symptoms that may include a rash but in a considerable number of cases will not result in such symptoms. Symptoms may even mimic those of mononucleosis due to the swollen lymph nodes and other well-known maladies early in the disease process. Most often there will be general malaise and fatigue that may include a headache and stiff neck, which might become confused with meningitis. Fever and chills are somewhat common and in particular muscle and joint pain will appear.

■ **Stage Two**

After a month or more (sometimes up to 4 months) following the initial infection, the second stage, early

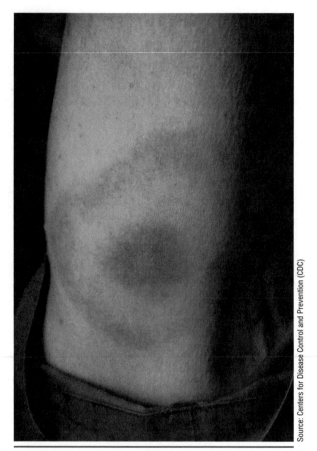

FIGURE 11-9 Erythematous rash in bull's-eye pattern at the site of a tick bite

Source: Centers for Disease Control and Prevention (CDC)

disseminated infection, will ensue if treatment has not been initiated during the early stage and when early symptoms first appeared. At this point the infection, which is multi-system in its attack, may affect the skin, skeletal joints, heart, and the nervous system within a relatively short period of a few weeks to a few months. Subjective symptoms and clinical signs at this point may include additional rashes over the body other than the area where the initial bite occurred. Considerable fatigue may be accompanied by pain, weakness, or numbness in the upper and lower extremities due to the nervous system involvement, and may even include partial paralysis of some facial nerves. Recurring headaches, problems with memory, and an inability to think clearly are further manifestations of disturbances of the central nervous system. Tachycardia (rapid heartbeat) may occur during this stage and in rare instances serious heart damage may occur. Mucous membranes may become inflamed, particularly the tissues around the eyes, a condition called conjunctivitis.

■ Stage Three

The third and final stage, called late, persistent infections, results in permanent damage to the joints of the body and the entire nervous system. Clinical signs will include swelling and inflammation of the joints, causing considerable pain. Numbness and tingling of the hands and feet and sometimes in the back will occur. Extreme feelings of tiredness are commonly experienced. These symptoms, due to damage to the tissues of the body, may not occur for months or years following the initial infection. When the condition has become chronic the signs and symptoms are extremely serious with a grave prognosis.

Nymphal stages of ticks transmit the majority of the disease agents through the injection of spirochetes contained in the saliva of the tick and into the victim, but some cases are known to have occurred from bites involving the adult stage of a particular species of tick. Lyme disease cases are more significant in some pockets of geography than in others with small areas of high prevalence. Lyme disease spirochetes may be found in roughly two-fifths of nymphal ticks in endemic areas and in almost all species of rodents, such as rats and ground-welling squirrels as well as other species of rodents, found in areas where the disease is prevalent (Figure 11-10). These small ground-dwelling animals are particularly vulnerable to tick bites as they also inhabit tall grasses along with the ticks. In the United States the majority of vector-borne cases of diseases may be attributed to the causative agent for Lyme disease.

The name for the disease is derived from an area of the northeastern United States, specifically from Old Lyme, Connecticut, where it was first described, although it most likely existed prior to this time. The Lyme disease spirochete, *B. burgdorferi,* employs the traditional pattern of other parasites where the vector is the deer tick (*I. dammini*) and the white-footed mouse serves as the reservoir host. White-tailed deer are not directly involved in this method of transmission but they are crucial in maintaining a large tick population as the primary host for the adult stage. Other rodents and at least one species of bird are also known to serve as hosts in the United States and to transmit disease organisms to the vectors, the *I. dammini* tick.

Rocky Mountain Spotted Fever

Why the name "Rocky Mountain spotted fever" was ascribed to the infection of the organism whose scientific name is *Rickettsia rickettsii* has apparently been lost to history, because it appears to be a misnomer. As early as the 1930s, it became clear that this disease occurred in many areas of the United States other than the Rocky Mountain region. In the 1980s the disease gained a great deal of publicity and it can now be shown that this disease is broadly distributed through almost all of the states, and even extends into Canada and to the south through Central America and parts of South America. Transmission of Rocky Mountain spotted fever from ticks mostly occurs when the tick vectors are most active and during warm weather when people tend to spend more time outdoors.

Rocky Mountain spotted fever, along with Lyme disease, are two of the most frequently reported rickettsial illnesses in the United States and are also among the most lethal diseases transmitted by ticks. Because it has been diagnosed on both of the American continents, there is an increasing potential for even more widespread outbreaks. Some synonyms for Rocky Mountain spotted fever used in other countries include "tick typhus" as well as a number of names used exclusively in certain regions and countries of Mexico and of South America. Rocky Mountain spotted fever, caused by a species of bacteria called *R. rickettsii*, is spread to humans by the Ixodid (hard) tick. This is a species involved in the

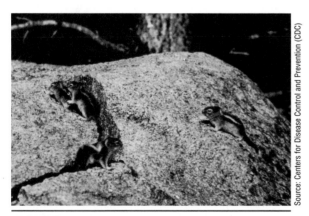

Source: Centers for Disease Control and Prevention (CDC)

FIGURE 11-10 Rodents, which also include prairie dogs, ground squirrels, mice, and other mammals, can transmit tick-borne illnesses, including Lyme disease

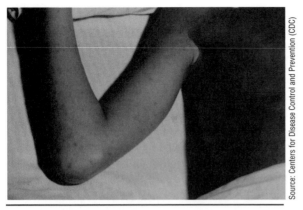

Source: Centers for Disease Control and Prevention (CDC)

FIGURE 11-11 Child's right arm depicts the characteristic spotted rash of Rocky Mountain spotted fever

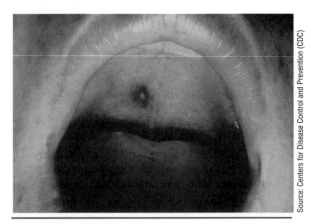

Source: Centers for Disease Control and Prevention (CDC)

FIGURE 11-12 Small, hard lump or lesion due to Rocky Mountain spotted fever, on hard palate of child's mouth

transmission of most of the diseases transmitted by tick vectors. Initial signs and symptoms are similar to other tick-borne infections, including sudden onset of fever, headache, and muscle pain, followed by development of a rash (Figure 11-11). This disease can be difficult to diagnose in the early stages. In a small percentage of cases, the bull's eye rash fails to develop and the symptoms and signs appear insignificant, but without quick and adequate treatment it can lead to death.

Despite effective treatment developed from experiences with treating the disease for at least the past 75 years, Rocky Mountain spotted fever still is a serious and potentially life-threatening infectious disease today. Up to 5 percent of those who contract Rocky Mountain spotted fever will still die from the infection even with the somewhat effective treatment available today. But dramatic progress has been made from the early days of the documentation of the disease and effective antibiotic therapy has greatly reduced the number of deaths caused by Rocky Mountain spotted fever. In the years before the development of two antibiotics called tetracycline and chloramphenicol in the late 1940s, perhaps as many as one-third of those infected who developed Rocky Mountain spotted fever died. These figures are only estimates because mortality records at that time period were sketchy at best in some areas of the country.

RMSF can be contracted in two ways, most commonly through the tick bites or through infectious organisms that enter the body through breaks in the skin. Ticks can quickly and painlessly attach themselves to the skin and proceed to feed on the blood of the host. They can lodge anywhere on the bodies of animals, including humans, but most often are found in the hair, around the ankles and in the genital area. Once embedded in the host's skin, ticks can cause a small, hard, itchy lump surrounded by a red ring or halo. Other than the red ring or halo, the organism may cause signs or symptoms in any area of the body (Figure 11-12). The longer an infected tick stays attached to the skin, the greater the chances grow for acquiring an infection by the host.

When the rickettsial organism enters through breaks in the skin including small wounds such as cuts or scrapes on the hands, fingers, or other exposed areas of the body, and even when going barefoot and perhaps stepping on an infected insect. But unlike some infective organisms that reside only in a certain area of an insect vector's body such as in the saliva, bacteria that cause Rocky Mountain spotted fever may circulate in all the fluids inside the tick vector's body. If the fluids are squeezed from or crushed from an infected tick when personally removing it from the body or from another person or a pet, an infection can occur if the fluid happens to come in direct contact with an area of broken skin. It is also possible to develop an infection when a mucous membrane or an eye is touched after coming in contact with the fluids from an infected tick.

Babesiosis

Babesiosis is the term for a somewhat rare infection of the blood caused by a parasite that lives in some species of ticks. The disease is caused by a malaria-like parasitic organism from the genus *Babesia*, an intracellular

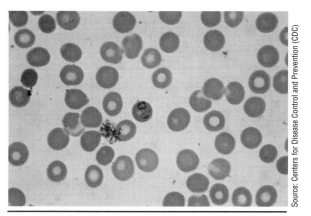

Source: Centers for Disease Control and Prevention (CDC)

FIGURE 11-13 *Babesia microti* in blood smear, an intracellular parasite of red blood cells; note the clump of platelets to the left of the infected RBC

parasite called a protozoan that is an intracellular parasite that infects the red blood cells, as does the organism *Plasmodium* that produces malaria (Figure 11-13). Following the infection called trypanosomiasis, also caused by a blood parasite, *Babesia* organisms are thought to be the second most common blood parasites of mammals. In addition, these organisms contribute to a major impact on the health of domestic animals in areas that do not experience a severe winter season.

Babesiosis infections are more common in animals than in humans but human cases have been reported in certain parts of the United States. And although human babesiosis is uncommon, reported cases have risen recently, presumably because of an expanded medical awareness. The locations in which babesiosis has been reported are approximately the same as those where Lyme disease is also endemic. For the transmission of babesiosis, a vector-borne illness usually transmitted by Ixodid ticks, the deer tick typically carries the parasite that causes this illness. *Babesia microti* is transmitted by the same tick vector, *Ixodes scapularis,* as are Lyme disease and ehrlichiosis, and may occur in conjunction with these other diseases. In endemic areas, *B. microti* may also be transmitted through blood transfusions as the organisms could possibly survive the testing and the storage required for preparing bags of blood for transfusion.

In North America, the illness is prevalent in the coastal areas of Connecticut, New Jersey, and on islands off the coasts of New York and Massachusetts including eastern Long Island and its barrier island, Fire Island. But the states of Wisconsin, Georgia, and California have also experienced significant numbers of cases of babesiosis in recent years. It is sometimes called the "malaria of the Northeast" because babesiosis and human malaria are both intra-erythrocytic parasites (dwell inside the red blood cells) and both may eventually cause the destruction of red blood cells and both are caused by a single-celled protozoan. And along with *Babesia microti*, other species of *Babesia* infect people on continents other than North America. These related species of *Babesia* cause similar illnesses in both humans and animals in a number of countries other than the United States.

But contrary to the *Plasmodium* genus of parasites that cause malaria, the *Babesia* species lack an exo-erythrocytic phase, one in which stages of the life cycle occur outside the red blood cells as occurs for malaria in the mosquito vector. Therefore, in the liver involvement found in malaria, of which there are four major human varieties, significant **jaundice** may exist due to destroyed red blood cells. Jaundice is usually not found in *B. microti* infections to the extent that malaria is. It has not been definitively documented that there are significant cases of *Babesia* species that occur in malaria-endemic areas. If this were the case the misdiagnosis of malaria, of the genus *Plasmodium*, could easily be made in cases of babesiosis. In addition, another major difference lies in the fact that malaria is spread exclusively by a particular species of mosquito, that of the *Anopheles* mosquito, rather than by a tick vector. The range of geographic regions where one species of organism is found might not be conducive to the requirements for survival of the other disease agent. However, Lyme disease and babesiosis could occur concurrently because the tick species known to be vectors of the two diseases may be found in close proximity.

Cases of babesiosis have also been reported over a wide area of Europe. Most countries of Europe have experienced at least some evidence of the illness. The disease in Europe, as is the case in North America, is due to infection of the *Babesia* genus of which *Babesia divergens* is the most common species found. In the United States, *B. microti* is the species most commonly associated with human disease but there are at least some cases in this country also attributed to *Babesia duncani*. Cases of babesiosis have also been observed in both North and South Korea.

Some people, especially healthy people younger than the age of 40, often may have few if any noticeable symptoms upon infection. Others may present with symptoms such as fever, headache, fatigue, and muscle and joint aches. Because the organisms infect red blood cells, anemia sometimes occurs as a result of the lysis (destruction) of red blood cells. This is a condition that frequently leads to enlargement of the liver and spleen (hepato- and splenomegaly), as these organs are in part responsible for removing infected blood cells from the body along with broken down and damaged red blood cells.

The risk of becoming severely ill and dying is increased in people who have had their spleen removed as well as those who take illicit or immunosuppressive drugs. For those who have accompanying disorders that tend to weaken the immune system, particularly for those suffering from AIDS, an increased risk of mortality appears. In this group of victims, babesiosis may also resemble malaria by causing episodes of cyclical high fever, accompanied by anemia, dark urine, and jaundice or yellowing of the skin from liver damage and kidney failure. The disease of babesiosis is transmitted by the same type of deer ticks of the family *Ixodidae* that also transmits the organism causing Lyme disease. Again, this infection is common among animals but is somewhat rare and may even be asymptomatic in humans except for those with immune system disorders.

Symptoms of Babesiosis

Most patients with *Babesia* infections are asymptomatic or only experience mild fevers and slight anemia that go virtually unnoticed. Babesiosis can afflict people of all ages, but most people who contract the disease are in their 40s or 50s. Some people who contract babesiosis may not have any symptoms and will later have no knowledge of having been infected. Most of these patients will recover spontaneously without treatment. However, in certain circumstances where the health of the individual is compromised, as in patients with an immunodeficiency such as HIV/AIDS, and in the elderly and the very young, the illness can quickly become serious. The disease can even cause death, especially in people who have had their spleen removed or who have weakened immune systems.

Symptoms in the more severe cases will include fever with temperatures rising as high as 104°F, accompanied with chills, sweating, weakness, tiredness, joint and muscle aches, poor appetite, and headaches. In extremely severe cases there are symptoms similar to malaria, with fevers rising to 105°F/40°C, shaking chills, and severe anemia from red blood cell destruction.

Organ failure may follow, including adult respiratory distress syndrome (ARDS).

Under what conditions is babesiosis most often discovered and when is it usually diagnosed? When an illness strikes with certain symptoms and signs in an endemic area of the country, the physician may suspect babesiosis and will request appropriate blood tests to determine if the patient has been exposed to this illness. Some people with babesiosis will sometimes suffer from an additional tick-borne illness such as Lyme disease. Sometimes the infection is discovered accidentally when the physician has asked to have other blood tests performed that are unrelated to tick-borne illnesses but to diagnose other medical conditions that exist or when other tick-borne illnesses are suspected. Remember that symptoms and signs of babesiosis may be so mild as to be unnoticed by the victim.

Diagnosis of Babesiosis

Babesia may not be observed in a blood smear unless the laboratory professional is particularly astute, or is looking for intracellular parasites of the blood. To diagnose babesiosis, a laboratory technician, technologist, or parasitologist will examine a stained blood sample as a stained smear using a microscope. Both thick and thin blood smears are stained with a special stain called Wright's-Giemsa for the microscopic examination (Figure 11-14). But frequently treatment is not necessary for a mild infection in healthy people with a functioning spleen and who do not have other predisposing factors, as the infection typically is resolved on its own.

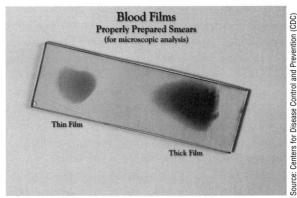

FIGURE 11-14 Giemsa-stained slide depicts an example of properly prepared thick and thin film blood smears to be examined

A thorough history of recent travels along with a high degree of suspicion may be necessary in order to diagnose babesiosis. Babesiosis may develop in patients who live in or travel to an endemic area, but also is possible for those who may have received a blood transfusion contaminated with the causative organism for babesiosis within the previous few weeks. This component of medical history is of utmost importance as a number of other infective diseases may be transmitted through blood transfusions and it is not uncommon for patients to suffer from more than one infective organism.

Babesiosis may be suspected when a person who has had exposure to an endemic area also develops persistent fever cycles accompanied by hemolytic anemia. The only definitive diagnostic test for babesiosis to date involves the identification of parasites on a Wrights-Giemsa-stained thin blood smear. An observation of "Maltese cross formations" on a stained blood film may be presumptively diagnostic of babesiosis and at the same time will rule out malaria when examining blood samples from a patient with symptoms and signs related to babesiosis.

The parasites of the *Babesia* species reproduce in red blood cells. There they can be seen as cross-shaped inclusions where four merozoites produce asexual budding but are attached together to form a figure similar to that of a "Maltese Cross." This structural formation results in hemolysis (destruction) of the red cells, resulting in anemia, in a similar manner to that of malaria. But careful scrutiny of multiple blood smears may be required, as *B. microti* may be easily overlooked because the organism typically infects fewer than 1 percent of the circulating red blood cells. A reported increase in babesiosis diagnoses in recent years is thought to be due to more widespread testing rather than to an actual increase in cases. In addition, due to better treatment and longer lives for those suffering from immunodeficiencies and a more active lifestyle by these patients may afford this group more opportunity for contact with ticks, the disease vector.

Treatment for Babesiosis

In people who have healthy immune systems and only mild cases of babesiosis, no treatment is typically needed. The body's immune system is able to effectively and successfully combat the infection when the general health of the infected person is adequate. However, in the event that shortness of breath occurs or if an allergic reaction begins after an initial dose of antibiotics, the physician should be consulted immediately. Because some patients may develop severe cases of babesiosis, especially when the immune system is weak, hospitalization may be required for advanced treatment. Those who have a more severe case of babesiosis are usually treated with one of two antibiotics that are administered orally, including clindamycin or azithromycin. Most people with symptoms of babesiosis may be treated with a drug called atovaquone, with oral antibiotics, or with an anti-malarial drug called quinine. Those patients without spleens and who develop substantial symptoms and signs may also require an exchange transfusion of blood in order to remove infected and damaged blood cells.

Prevention of Babesiosis

During the months of May through September and sometimes beginning in April and extending past September in the southern states of the United States, staying away from places where ticks are common, such as the edges of woods and fields can be rather effective in preventing infection with the *B. microti* organism. The elderly, the very young, and those who have had their spleen removed or have had an organ transplant should in particular avoid areas where ticks are likely to live. These groups are especially in danger of complications when babesiosis has been contracted.

The use of a safe and effective insect repellent when camping or working outdoors, especially in wooded or grassy places, will help to prevent most tick infestations. Early removal of both roaming and embedded ticks is important. A tick must remain attached to the body for at least 24 hours before it can transmit the parasite that causes babesiosis. For those who spend extended periods of time outdoors in areas where ticks live, the body should be carefully examined daily for ticks that may be moving about the body or those who have become embedded. Pets that enter the home should also be examined for both mobile and embedded ticks, as pets may also contract babesiosis. Because there are approximately 80 species of hard ticks and perhaps 10 species of soft ticks, it may be wise to save any ticks found on the body. These can be taken to a health care professional who may be able to identify the species and thus gauge the potential for insect's harboring of a disease agent.

To remove an attached tick, use fine forceps (tweezers) to obtain a secure grasp at the head or as close to the head as possible and gently pull or tease the tick from its attachment to the skin. It is not a wise

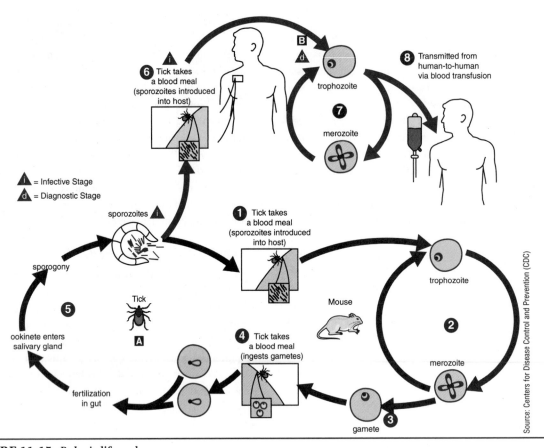

FIGURE 11-15 *Babesia* life cycle

practice to use heat such as a lighted match, acetone, petroleum jelly, or other methods to try to make the tick release its attachment. These latter methods are not often effective practices for removing an embedded tick and may even kill the tick while leaving its head imbedded in the skin.

Tick infestations and tick-borne diseases are economically important in many breeds of domestic animals. The development and production of innovative tick control methods included in the life cycle of babesiosis is directed primarily toward economically important tick-borne diseases of cattle and work animals (Figure 11-15). The tick-borne protozoan *Babesia* parasite remains a crucial consideration when cattle industries are being broadened around the globe. In animals, *Babesia canis rossi*, *Babesia bigemina*, and *Babesia bovis* cause particularly severe forms of the disease that may result in a severe hemolytic anemia. Effective control of *Babesia* and a considerable number

of other tick-borne diseases are usually focused on the eradication of the vectors by dusting the cattle and other domestic animals with an insecticide. In addition to the attempts to eradicate tick vectors that transmit the disease organisms, vaccination of animals is also possible against the *Babesia* parasites.

HUMAN EHRLICHIOSIS IN THE UNITED STATES

What is meant by the term *ehrlichiosis*? Ehrlichiosis is the general name used to describe any of several bacterial diseases capable of affecting both animals and humans. These diseases are caused by organisms of the genus *Ehrlichia*. On a global basis, four ehrlichial species of organisms are currently known to cause disease in humans. The causative organism included in the four *Ehrlichia* species typically infect two types of white blood cells that are classified as being of mononuclear and granulocytic series and are produced in bone marrow.

Five types of white cells circulate in the vascular systems of humans and of some other animals, although the percentages of each of the types may vary among the various animal species. Two types of white blood cells are required for the Ehrlichia organism to survive, one of which is a mononuclear cell called a lymphocyte and the other is a segmented neutrophil (a granulocyte) which are the most prevalent types of white blood cells useful in fighting viral and bacterial infections, respectively. The disease was first diagnosed in 1987 and is now considered an emerging disease that has the potential for perhaps explosive growth in the numbers of cases. Ehrlichiosis is found in the majority of the states within the United States.

Ehrlichiosis is characteristic of many other significant parasitic and bloodborne bacterial infections as it is a tick-borne bacterial infection caused by bacterial strains of *Anaplasmataceae*. This is a family of bacteria in the order *Rickettsiales*, which includes the genera *Ehrlichia*, *Anaplasma*, *Wolbachia*, and *Neorickettsia*. The genera of the causative bacterial organisms for ehrlichiosis include both *Ehrlichia* and *Anaplasma* (formerly known as *E. phagocytophila*). The disease is known to be transmitted by the *Ixodes* genus of tick vectors that include the western blacklegged tick called *I. pacificus* for the strain of bacteria called *Anaplasma phagocytophila* and by the lone star tick, *Amblyomma americanum*, for the strain of the disease called *Ehrichia chaffeensis* (Figure 11-16). These bacteria are called *obligate intracellular bacteria*, and are capable of infecting and killing the two types of white blood cells (mononuclear lymphocytes and neutrophils), as previously listed.

Five species have been shown to cause human infection, including the three discussed here. *Anaplasma phagocytophilum* causes human granulocytic anaplasmosis and was formerly known as human granulocytic ehrlichiosis (HGE). *Ehrlichia ewingii* causes a human disease known as ewingii ehrlichiosis, and *E. chafeensis* is responsible for an infection called human monocytic ehrlichiosis (HME) (Figure 11-17). *E. canus* and *Neorickettsia sennetsu* are not as well studied, and in addition, the latter is found in Japan. Recently, human infections have been traced to the newly discovered Panoloa Mountain Ehrlichia species, but still little is known of this species. Ehrlichiosis infections have been found to also affect dogs but to a lesser extent, apparently, than for humans.

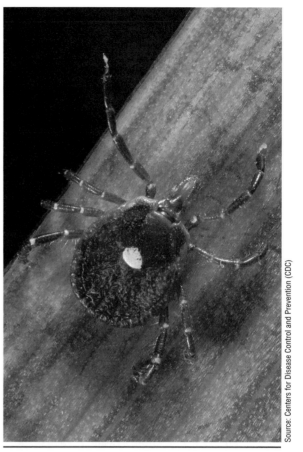

FIGURE 11-16 Obvious white dot, or lone star, identifies this organism as an adult female of the species *Amblyomma americanum*

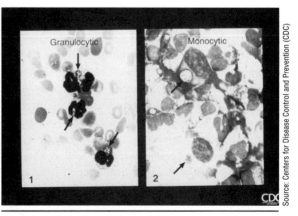

FIGURE 11-17 Human monocytic ehrlichiosis and human granulocytic ehrlichiosis

How Is Ehrlichiosis Contracted?

In the United States, Ehrlichiae organisms are transmitted via two different genera of hard ticks. As stated previously, the specific vector responsible for any of these tick-borne illnesses is based upon geographic location. There are two known vectors of the bacterial species capable of causing ehrlichiosis in the United States. The lone star tick (*Amblyomma americanum*), the blacklegged tick (*Ixodes scapularis*), and the western blacklegged tick (*Ixodes pacificus*) are both known vectors of ehrlichiosis in the United States. The bacterial species of the causative agent for ehrlichiosis may vary between the two major genera of *Anaplasma* and *Ehrlichia*.

Thirty states within the United States have reported the disease, whereas most of the southern states are responsible for the majority of the cases, as the climate supports a large tick population. On the European continent, *Ixodes ricinus* is the primary tick vector responsible for transmitting the disease. An Ixodid, or hard tick, *A. americanum* is found through the eastern and south-central states and can transmit a number of disease agents including ehrlichiosis that affects humans, dogs, goats, and white-tailed deer. Representatives from all three of its life stages may aggressively bite people in the southern United States. The lone star ticks are capable of transmitting *Ehrlichia chaffeensis* and *E. ewingii*, both of which cause the disease.

Symptoms of Ehrlichiosis

Non-specific symptoms similar to those of influenza are the predominant characteristics of the symptoms of ehrlichiosis. The complaints by patients requesting medical treatment and who are diagnosed with ehrlichiosis will often resemble symptoms of a number of other infectious and some non-infectious diseases. These clinical features generally include fever, general malaise, fatigue, leukopenia (low white blood cell count), thrombocytopenia (low platelet count), headache, and muscular aches and pains. Other signs and symptoms may include nausea, vomiting, diarrhea, cough, joint pains, confusion, and occasionally a rash. Symptoms typically appear after an incubation period of 5 to 10 days following the tick bite. It is possible that some individuals who are infected with an ehrlichial agent will not become ill enough to be aware of a disease state or they may develop only mild and innocuous symptoms that are spontaneously resolved.

Endemic Areas of the United States

Most cases of ehrlichiosis are reported within the geographic distribution of the three vector ticks, namely *Amblyomma americanum*, *Ixodes scapularis*, and *I. pacificus*. Occasional cases may occur from areas outside the normal distribution of the tick vector. But in most of these instances the cases have been traced to persons who have recently traveled to areas where the tick-borne diseases are endemic. Therefore, it is reasonable that these individuals were unknowingly bitten by an infected tick and did not develop symptoms until after returning to their home areas. Therefore, travel to an area that is considered endemic for ehrlichiosis within the past 2 to 3 weeks prior to developing symptoms should alert the physician that there is a possibility of a tick-borne illness, including that of ehrlichiosis.

Diagnosis and Treatment for Ehrlichiosis

Ehrlichiosis is a febrile illness with significant systemic symptoms including severe headaches, chills, muscle pain, and sometimes a rash along with other assorted subjective symptoms dependent upon the severity of the infection and the victim's general health. Laboratory findings may include anemia, a decreased white blood cell count where certain types of white cells are specifically affected and which include a lymphocyte count and a blood platelet count. Biochemistry levels with plasma electrolyte imbalances (sodium, potassium, and chloride) may reveal low sodium values perhaps related to nausea along with elevated liver enzymes that would indicate a degree of liver damage. Examinations of cerebral spinal fluid (CSF) may reveal an increased white blood cell level as well as an increased total protein level, values that are commonly found during infections. The antibiotic doxycycline is the most effective, whereas antibiotic susceptibility tests appear to show resistance of some strains of the organism to a powerful antibiotic called chloramphenicol.

Southern Tick–Associated Rash Illness (STARI)

A rash similar to that of Lyme disease has been described in humans following bites of the lone star tick, *Amblyomma americanum*. The rash may be accompanied by general malaise, fatigue, fever, headache, muscle, and joint pains. This condition has been descriptively named Southern Tick–associated Rash Illness (STARI) because of the characteristic "bull's eye" rash called **erythema chronicum migrans** that develops immediately around the bite of a tick. This manifestation of the infection mimics that of the circular rash typically observed in most cases of Lyme disease. *Borrelia lonestari*, a pathogen associated with STARI, also infects lone star ticks. Research suggests that up to 10 percent of the lone star ticks in an endemic area can be infected with any one of these pathogens. These ticks may also be infected with a spotted-fever group of rickettsia, *Rickettsia amblyommii*, but it is unknown at this time if this bacterium causes a similar or the same disease.

Symptoms of STARI

The symptoms accompanying this disease are somewhat vague and are the same as or similar to several other tick-borne diseases. Symptoms of STARI infections are mild and resemble respiratory illnesses similar to those found in cases of influenza, accompanied by symptoms of muscle pains, headache, and fatigue. These symptoms may also include a clinical finding of an elevated temperature, but this is by no means characteristic. The rash found in STARI usually appears within 7 days of a tick bite and may expand to an area of the skin around the bite site spanning up to 3 in. in diameter or even perhaps slightly larger. Quite frequently, the mechanical act of having been bitten will cause some redness and slight pain. But an accompanying rash found in cases of STARI is much more pronounced than any localized damage to the skin from an uncomplicated tick bite and the two should not be confused. But unlike Lyme disease, STARI has not been associated with any arthritic, neurological, or chronic symptoms.

Causative Organism of Lyme Disease

The causative organism for STARI is currently not clear and studies have shown that the disease is not caused by *Borrelia burgdorferi*, the organism that causes Lyme disease. Another spirochete, *Borrelia lonestari*, was detected in the skin of one patient and in the lone star tick that delivered the bite. Studies conducted on a number of patients exhibiting the signs and symptoms of STARI

have yielded no evidence of serological antibodies to the organism *B. lonestari*. In all the cases of this disease that have been studied to the current time, the rash and accompanying symptoms have resolved promptly following treatment with oral antibiotics.

It is a certainty that STARI may be specifically linked to bites from the tick *Amblyomma americanus,* which is commonly known as the lone star tick, even though the identity of the causative organism is unknown. The adult female is distinguished by an irregularly shaped white dot or lone star on her back but all three life stages including the nymph, larval, and adult forms of *A. americanum* tend to aggressively bite humans.

Preventing Infection Related to STARI

In general, tick-borne illness may be prevented by avoiding tick habitats such as the edges of dense wooded areas with tall grasses and brushy areas. The same precautions that are used for other tick and insect vectors include the use of repellents containing DEET or permethrin and wearing light-colored clothing that includes long trousers tucked into socks. Carefully conducted body searches to remove ticks before the vectors have the opportunity to explore the body and to eventually become embedded is paramount following outdoor activity, particularly in an endemic area.

Victims of tick bites should monitor their health closely for several days to a few weeks following the incident and should consult a physician if a rash appears of if headaches, elevated temperature, or unusual feelings of fatigue are experienced. If muscle pains and particularly if swollen lymph nodes occur within a month of receiving a tick bite, these symptoms and signs should prompt a visit to a physician. In most cases any treatment of persons who merely have a tick bite without prolonged exposure to an imbedded tick is not necessary. Epidemiologists at the CDC perform ongoing surveillance of STARI and are actively involved in seeking blood samples from patients who exhibit the signs and symptoms of STARI with the goal of eventually identifying the infectious organism that causes the disease called STARI.

Causes of STARI

The only certainty in the contraction of this disease is that the illness is a tick-borne disease undoubtedly transmitted by the lone star tick *Amblyomma americanum*. This tick was first postulated as a probable vector of the disease in 1984, which at the time was called a "Lyme-like disease." In the late 1990s it was recognized that the disease had some similarities to Lyme disease but there were separate and distinct differences also. One example of a difference lies in the fact that Lyme disease transitions through three distinct stages that have extremely serious ramifications if untreated. Several studies have failed to detect *Borrelia burgdorferi*, the causative agent of Lyme disease in patients from the southeastern region of the United States.

Some investigators have proposed that Southern Tick–associated Rash Illness may be caused by a related bacterium called *Borrelia lonestari*, a spirochete that was initially isolated in 2004 from a bacterial culture. But this conclusion was shown to be inconsistent with later cultures that showed that the spirochete has not been detected in all cases of the illness as would be expected. This has led some scientists to the conclusion that the disease is not based on a bacterial pathogen. Because viruses are more difficult to culture than bacterial ones, as they require live cells in which to grow, perhaps a breakthrough will occur in the near future and that will provide a definite identity for an organism that is without doubt the culprit.

TULAREMIA

Tularemia is a potentially deadly disease and occurs naturally in the United States, because a ready reservoir of aquatic animals is available for maintaining the causative organism in large numbers. This is a disease that has been widely known for many years and is also known variously as "rabbit fever," "Deer fly fever," and sometimes as "Ohara's fever." Tularemia is a contagious disease caused by a bacterial infection by an organism called *Francisella tularensis* (Figure 11-18). The organism is a Gram-negative coccobacillus with several subspecies that are associated with varying degrees of virulence.

The term *Gram-negative coccobacillus* means that the organisms stain a light pink color with Gram's stain and indicates that the shape is intermediate between that of a round or coccal shape and of a rod or bacillus (Figure 11-19). Little is known of the virulence of the organism but evidence leads to the conclusion that the

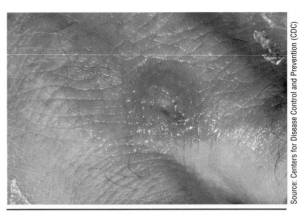

FIGURE 11-18 Tularemia lesion on the hand, caused by the bacterium *Francisella tularensis*

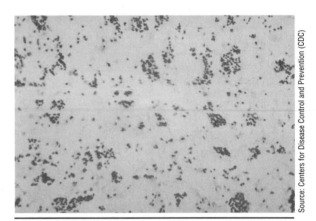

FIGURE 11-19 Photomicrograph of *Francisella tularensis* bacteria using a methylene blue stain

bacteria are intracellular pathogens that invade a type of large white cells called macrophages (large feeders). The course of the disease involves the spread of the organism to multiple organ systems, including the lungs, liver, spleen, and lymphatic system. The most clinically significant of the subspecies is that of Type A *F. tularensis tularensis*, which is found in rabbit herds in North America and is highly virulent for both humans and domestic rabbits. *F. tularensis* is an intracellular bacterium, which means that it is able to live in a similar manner of a parasite that inhabits host cells. Bioterrorism using this bacterium would be quite simple, when dispersed widely. *F. tularensis* is extremely infectious and can easily be disseminated by explosive military shells or bombs and possesses the capacity to cause widespread illness and death.

F. tularensis palaearctica, Type B, occurs mainly in water-dwelling rodents such as beavers, otters, and muskrats in North America. This serotype of *Francisella* is also found in hares and small rodents such as mice, voles, and ground squirrels in the northern regions of both Asia and Europe. The Type B organism is less virulent than Type A for humans and rabbits. Primary vectors for *Francisella* are ticks and deer flies, but in addition the disease can be spread somewhat easily by insects other than ticks and deer flies. In addition to the vectors, tularemia may be readily spread by the handling of infected animal carcasses, eating or drinking water and food contaminated by the organism, and by breathing the organism.

Tularemia has not been found to be spread from person to person and those infected with *F. tularensis* do not require isolation to prevent the spread of disease. Rapid treatment upon exposure and subsequent infection should be initiated quickly as the disease may be fatal if untreated. Again, as with other pathogens, those who are pregnant or who have weakened immune systems may be more susceptible to contracting the illness. Humans can become infected in many ways, particularly through exposure due to environmental activities. Methods of transmission are through bites by infected arthropods, by the handling of the carcasses of infectious animals or their body fluids, working with or eating and drinking water or food containing the organisms, or from exposure to bodies of water or soil contaminated by rodents and the inhalation of infectious aerosols (Figure 11-20).

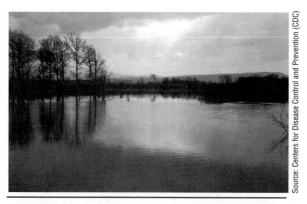

Source: Centers for Disease Control and Prevention (CDC)

FIGURE 11-20 Waters from which many muskrats were trapped, infecting a number of Vermont trappers with tularemia

History of Tularemia

In North America, *F. tularensis* was first discovered during an outburst of "rabbit fever" in 1911. The organism and subsequently the disease received its name from the area of Tulare Lake in California, after the local population of ground squirrels was decimated by infections with the organism. Scientists at the time determined that tularemia could be dangerous to humans and that contact with an infected animal may lead to contraction of the disease. Soon after this initial outbreak it became apparent that hunters, cooks, and agricultural workers were quite susceptible to the infective organism. As previously mentioned, there is a pneumonic form of the disease that could easily lend itself to bioterrorism with an air burst of a bomb that could disperse the disease to many individuals. This has led to the stockpiling of effective antibiotics in the event such an occurrence comes to fruition. In addition, there is a possibility that an unlicensed vaccine not controlled and tested by governmental agencies could be useful in preventing the infections from occurring as emergency procedures.

Epidemiology for Tularemia

Tularemia occurs throughout the more temperate regions of the Northern Hemisphere. Besides North America and continental Europe, the original areas of the former Soviet Union, and the Asian countries of China, Korea, and Japan are affected by this disease. All states within the North American continent (the exception is Hawaii) have reported cases of tularemia but some reported only an occasional rare case. The disease in humans is one required to be reported in the same way as for many venereal diseases and other infectious diseases. During the first 50 years of the 1900s, tularemia infections in the United States reached a peak with several thousand cases but since then the number of cases has declined greatly to only a little over a hundred per year in the entire country.

Clinical Symptoms and Microbiological Diagnosis of Tularemia

Depending on the site of infection, tularemia has six characteristic clinical syndromes. The most common type is that of the ulceroglandular variety that comprises

75 percent of the cases of tularemia. The other 25 percent of cases are spread over those called glandular, oropharyngeal, pneumonic, oculoglandular, and typhoidal. The incubation period is widely variable and ranges from only a few to 14 days, with most human cases appearing within 5 days of exposure. Humans characteristically experience skin lesions while infected wild and domestic animals do not. The victims may experience a moderately elevated temperature, but in some cases the body temperature rises to a high degree in severe illnesses. When fever is moderate to very high levels the tularemia bacillus can often be isolated from blood cultures during this stage of the disease (Figure 11-21). Face and eyes may redden and become inflamed and the inflammation spreads to the lymph nodes which enlarge and may suppurate (form pus that mimics bubonic plague).

Lymph node involvement usually occurs during a high fever and death occurs in less than 1 percent of cases if therapy is initiated quickly following diagnosis of an infection. The drug of choice is the antibiotic called streptomycin although tularemia may also be treated with gentamycin for 10 days or a tetracycline-type antibiotic such as doxycycline for 2 to 3 weeks. The more toxic chloramphenicol or fluoroquinolones may be prescribed and administered as well. The vaccine produced by attenuated (dead or damaged) live vaccine is available to vaccinate at-risk individuals but its use is restricted to these groups who may be occupationally exposed to *F. tularensis*.

TICK IDENTIFICATION

It may be important to determine the identity of a tick when assessing the potential for various infections. The following information and images may be useful when performing a body search and in finding foraging or embedded ticks in order to determine the potential risks.

Dermacentor variabilis: The American dog tick is found throughout the eastern United States and in Colorado and the Pacific Northwest (Figure 11-22). It occurs in some areas on a cyclical basis by becoming more abundant in certain habitats during alternate years. Adults are characterized by creamy-gray markings on the scutum and by short mouthparts. Larvae and nymphs feed on small mammals, especially meadow mice which inhabit vegetation where ticks are often found, and are seldom seen by people. Adults appear in April and reach peak numbers in June but are seldom seen after early July. They feed on a wide range of mammals that includes deer and other wild animals, livestock, pets, and humans. A female may deposit more than 6000 eggs before she dies.

The American dog tick is the most common tick found on humans and dogs in many areas of the country. Engorgement by adult females has been associated with tick paralysis. This species is the primary vector of spotted fever and also can be a vector of the diseases tularemia and anaplasmosis. Evidence to date does not support involvement in the transmission of Lyme disease by the dog tick but researchers continue to pursue this possibility.

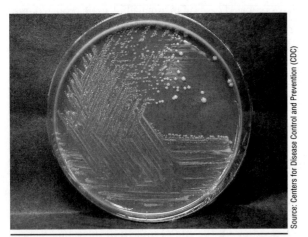

Source: Centers for Disease Control and Prevention (CDC)

FIGURE 11-21 *Francisella tularensis*, colonies grown on Chocolate Agar, 72 hours

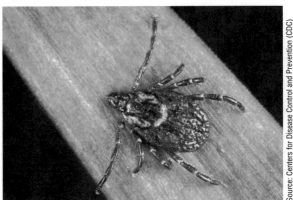

Source: Centers for Disease Control and Prevention (CDC)

FIGURE 11-22 Female *Dermacentor variabilis*, American dog tick

Amblyomma americanum: The lone star tick occurs across the southeastern and south-central United States. It is most common as one travels further south but is found in significant numbers in mostly moist woodlands. Adult females are characterized by a pearly white spot at the tip of the scutum and by long mouthparts. A wide range of animal hosts serve as a source of blood, including ground-dwelling birds, small mammals, and large mammals such as deer, livestock, and pets. All developmental stages of the lone star tick feed readily on humans. Larvae, which are sometimes referred to as either "seed ticks" or "turkey ticks," most often appear in the spring and again in the fall. The nymphs of this species over-winter and are active from April into July. Adults also over-winter and are active from late March into June. A female can produce up to 8000 eggs before she dies.

The lone star tick is the second most common tick found on humans especially in most of the southern states. The long and barbed hypostome of female adults inflicts a deep feeding wound and engorging females have been associated with tick paralysis. This species is a vector of spotted fever and the two recently recognized diseases of ehrlichiosis and Southern tick-associated rash illness (STARI).

Ixodes scapularis: The black-legged tick occurs throughout the eastern United States, and can be locally abundant in moist woodlands with thick leaf litter. Adults are significantly smaller than *Amblyomma* and *Dermacentor* ticks and have a characteristic uniform deep mahogany color. Female black-legged ticks are somewhat tear drop–shaped and have longer mouthparts than other species. Males are smaller than females and in comparison have shorter mouthparts. The areas in which these ticks range have tended to increase since the late 1980s but appears to be much more abundant in the more northern sections of the United States than is the lone star tick.

The black-legged tick has a very wide host range. Specimens have been collected from more than 100 species of birds, mammals, and lizards, with roughly half found on birds and about 10 percent found on lizards. Black-legged tick larvae feed primarily on white-footed mice and are most abundant from July into September. Nymphs feed primarily on a variety of small, ground-dwelling vertebrates, but are also found on humans and

their pets. Nymphs are most abundant from late spring into early summer. After the development of the nymphs into adults, they feed primarily on deer, as deer are very important to the reproductive success and spread of the black-legged tick. Adults are found in late summer into fall and again in early spring. A female lays about 3000 eggs before she dies.

Adult western black-legged ticks are rarely found on humans, but they do feed on dogs and cats (Figure 11-23). Nymphs appear to be the main vectors of Lyme disease to humans and pets. Nymphs are approximately the size of a poppy seed and are therefore almost never seen by a human. For this reason, people entering areas in which Lyme disease is transmitted are strongly encouraged to wear proper clothing and to use a repellent. In addition to Lyme disease, the black-legged tick is a vector of human anaplasmosis and babesiosis. More information on *Ixodes scapularis* is available from Purdue Extension publication E-244-W Lyme disease.

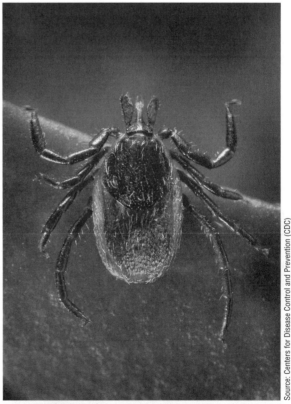

Source: Centers for Disease Control and Prevention (CDC)

FIGURE 11-23 Dorsal view of adult female western blacklegged tick, *Ixodes pacificus*

Rhipicephalus sanguineus: The brown dog tick is a species that is a worldwide pest of dogs and occurs in the southern United States. It is not native to the midwestern states and the northeastern and western states but has been repeatedly introduced into these states by infested dogs being brought there. Adults are small and almost uniformly brown with short mouthparts. Domestic dogs are the primary host for the developmental forms of larvae, nymphs, and adults, all of which conceal themselves in places near where dogs sleep, and will aggressively pursue their prey. This is a tick species known to inhabit homes and they are capable of reproducing indoors and tend to secrete themselves in homes and dog kennels that have source of heat including animal heat. A female can lay about 4000 eggs before she dies. Larvae, nymphs, and adults of the brown dog tick rarely bite humans, but infestations in kennels and homes occur all too frequently. These ticks may overwinter in houses and are sometimes seen crawling up walls, curtains, and on furniture (Figure 11-24). This species is a vector of a dog disease known as "canine ehrlichiosis."

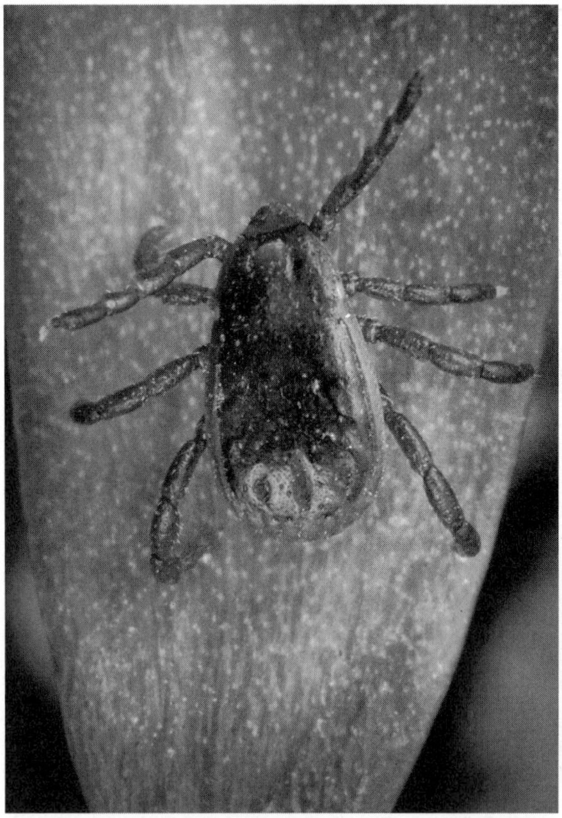

Can the Brown Dog Tick Transmit a Disease-Causing Agent of Humans in the United States?

The brown dog tick has not been known to transmit a disease-causing agent of humans in the United States. However, a recent outbreak of spotted fever in Arizona appears to have been associated with the brown dog tick, based on a research publication by Demma *et. al.,* in 2005, "Rocky Mountain Spotted Fever from an Unexpected Tick Vector in Arizona," an article that was published in the *New England Journal of Medicine.* The authors found that homes of several patients were infested with brown dog tick larvae, nymphs, and adults, many of which were infected with *Rickettsia rickettsii,* the bacterium that causes spotted fever. But remember that to date, no definite transmissions of tick-borne disease by the brown dog tick has occurred.

Source: Centers for Disease Control and Prevention (CDC)

FIGURE 11-24 Male brown dog tick, *Rhipicephalus sanguineus,* a hard tick, from dorsal view

MACROSCOPIC DIAGNOSTIC FEATURE (REQUIRES MAGNIFYING GLASS IN SOME CASES)

General Classification—Tick

Organism	*Ixodes scapularis*
Specimen Required	Organism (often found on host)
Stage	Adult
Color & Appearance	Dark brown to black
Size	3 mm in length
Shape	Elongated oval
Motility	Fall from vegetation onto host, or crawl over the body of the host after contact with vegetation

SUMMARY

Ticks operate as both parasites and as vectors of parasites. In this way the tick is able to gain nutrients from the host and to infect its benefactor with bacterial, rickettsia, and viral diseases. Some of the organisms transmitted must live inside blood cells in order to complete part of their life cycle. Some of these bacterial diseases are not between parasitic and basic bacterial infections.

Ticks are blood-feeding parasites that are often found predominantly at the edges of woods, in tall grass and shrubs, where they await the opportunity to attach themselves to a passing warm-blooded animal host. Ticks can be found in most wooded or forested regions throughout the world and are most common in areas where there are deer trails or human pathways. In these areas, a tick attaches itself to its host by inserting its sharp mandibles called chelicerae and a hollow feeding tube called a hypostome into the skin of its host. Ticks are also quite proficient at transmitting parasites and other organisms into the bodies of their hosts while they are feeding on the host's blood.

Because ticks do not have wings and are unable to jump, as they have somewhat short legs that are not adapted for jumping, physical contact, or close contact is the only method of infestation for ticks. Ticks often fall onto their hosts from vegetation but some actually stalk the host on foot. Ticks often take several days to complete a blood meal, and the attachment must last for roughly a day in order to pass infective organisms on to their hosts.

Ticks require hosts to support the maturation of the organisms. The significant species of ticks in the United States that transmit most of the tick-borne diseases are as follows. White-tailed deer in the eastern United States carry the *Ixodes scapularis* tick, which may be found as "seed ticks" on the deer, and the tick population is directly proportional to the white-tailed deer. The *Ixodes pacificus* ticks from the western portion of the United States are responsible for the majority of Rocky Mountain spotted fever cases in that area, as are the *Ixodes scapularis* for Lyme disease in the eastern parts of the country.

Immature stages of the *Ixodes scapularis* tick also feed on small mammals or birds until they are ready to infest a deer, and are capable of laying up to 2000 eggs following a blood meal of several days. Another hard tick,

as are *I. scapularis* and *I. pacificus*, is that of the lone star tick, *Amblyomma americanum*, also a member of the Ixodidae family. This species is blamed for the transmission of Southern Tick–associated Rash Illness (STARI), by a *Borrelia* organism, the same genus that causes Lyme disease.

Many diseases of the United States and the world are responsible for spreading diseases over wide areas of the world. Other than the lone star tick and the deer tick, there are two species of dog ticks of importance in North America: *Dermacentor variabilis*, commonly called the American dog tick or the eastern wood tick, and the *Rhipicephalus sanguineus*, or the brown dog tick.

A veritable multitude of diseases that are tick borne are covered in the chapter. Lyme disease is a disorder that involves multiple systems of the body, with chronic and serious permanent problems if not treated at the right time. Some other countries, particularly several that are located in Europe, also suffer Lyme-like diseases transmitted by species of ticks other than those found in the United States.

Rocky Mountain spotted fever (RMSF), a rickettsial disease, is another disorder that is named for a particular region of the country but is now found in many areas of the United States and even extends into Canada and Latin and South America. And despite effective treatment, the mortality rate stands at approximately 5 percent, even with the progress in treatment. RMSF is sometimes transmitted through breaks in the skin, because the organisms are spread throughout the infected tick's body.

Babesiosis is called the "malaria of the Northeast." Babesiosis is a parasitic disease caused by the genus *Babesia*, and like malaria, is also caused by a protozoan. However, a chief difference is that babeosis does not have an extracellular phase in its life cycle, as does the causative organism for malaria. Babesiosis is a somewhat rare infection of the blood caused by a parasite that lives in some species of ticks. Another similar disease is that it is intracellular caused by the genus *Trypanosomiasis* is also attributed to a blood parasite, also a protozoan, but is caused by a true bug rather than by ticks or mosquitoes, as are babesiosis and malaria, respectively. Other species of *Babesia* have been reported in other countries and the disease may be self-limiting without treatment, except in the immunocompromised and somewhat seriously ill victims. A number of animals also fall victim to babesiosis, at a greater rate than their human counterparts. The learner should note that babesiosis may be so mild as to be self-limiting with no long-term damage to the victim.

The term *ehrlichiosis* also applies to tick-borne illnesses, and is used to describe any of several bacterial diseases that affect both animals and humans. These diseases are caused by the organisms chiefly of the genus *Ehrlichia*, of which there are four species that cause human disease. All of these four *Ehrlichia* species are capable of infecting two types of white blood cells called monocytes and granulocytes.

Southern Tick–associated Rash Illness (STARI) is a Lyme-type disease transmitted by the lone star tick, *Amblyomma americanum,* and causes a rash with malaise, fatigue, fever, headache, and muscle and joint pains. Diagnosis is based on a circular and expanding "bulls eye" rash at the site of infection called erythema chronicum migrans and is similar to the rash in Lyme disease, and the causative is again the same as or similar to by *Borrelia burgdorferi*, the same organism that causes Lyme disease. Another spirochete, *Borrelia lonestari* has been isolated from one patient. But unlike Lyme disease, STARI is not been linked to arthritic, neurological, or chronic symptoms.

Tularemia, also called "rabbit fever," "deer fly fever," or "Ohara's fever," is a potentially deadly disease and occurs naturally in the United States, caused by a type of bacterial called Gram-negative coccobacillus. The disease is contracted variously by ticks, other blood-sucking insects, direct contact with infected animals, poorly cooked meat, or contaminated water. Water-dwelling rodents such as beavers and muskrats, as well as ground-dwelling animals may harbor the disease. Tularemia is a highly contagious disease caused by a bacterial infection by an organism called *Francisella tularensis* with several subspecies of varying levels of virulence.

Tick identification may be necessary to help in identifying the disease present. Images of the various ticks are helpful as well as knowing the likely tick inhabitants of a particular region of the country. The American dog tick, *Dermacentor variabilis*, is found throughout the eastern United States, in Colorado, and the Pacific Northwest. Adults are characterized by creamy-grey markings on the scutum and by short mouthparts. Larvae and nymphs feed on small mammals and are seldom seen by people. Adults appear in the spring and early summer, where they feed on mammals such as deer, other wild animals, livestock, pets, and humans. This species of female tick may deposit over 6000 eggs before she dies. Tick paralysis has also occurred from bites by these ticks.

The lone star tick, *Amblyomma americanum*, occurs across the southeastern and south-central United States, most commonly in moist woodlands. Adult females are characterized by a pearly white spot at the tip of the scutum and long mouthparts. A range of hosts are a source of blood, such as ground-dwelling birds, small mammals, and larger mammals such as deer, livestock, and pets. The long, barbed hypostome of female adults inflicts a deep feeding wound, and embedded females engorging themselves have been tied to tick paralysis. This species is also capable of transmitting spotted fever, ehrlichiosis, and Southern Tick–associated Rash Illness (STARI).

The black-legged tick, *Ixodes scapularis*, occurs throughout the eastern United States, and may be abundant in moist woodlands with thick ground cover. Adults, somewhat smaller than *Amblyomma* and *Dermacentor* ticks, are a deep mahogany color, with the female being tear drop–shaped and with long mouthparts. The larvae feed mostly on mice, and are abundant through the summer and into September. Adults feed readily on deer, important to the reproductive spread of the black-legged tick.

The brown dog tick has not yet been shown to pass disease-causing agents to humans in the United States. But a relatively recent outbreak of spotted fever in Arizona may be associated with the brown dog tick. The authors found that the homes of several patients were infested with brown dog tick larvae, nymphs, and adults, many of which were infected with *Rickettsia rickettsii*, the bacterium that causes spotted fever.

CASE STUDY

1. Roberto lives in a northeastern state bordering the Atlantic coast. He spends time in the woods during the summer, searching for small lakes where his goal is to catch a prize bass that he can mount over his mantel. A few weeks after returning from such a fishing trip that lasted several days, Roberto experienced a mild fever and a circular rash on the inside of his forearm. At first he ignored the rash, thinking it resulted from contact with a poisonous plant while working in his yard, but as the rash grew larger, Roberto continued to experience a low-grade fever and headaches. He visited his physician, who placed him on antibiotics for a possible tick-borne illness. What is the name of the probable disease, and what organism is implicated in this type of infection?

STUDY QUESTIONS

1. How long does a tick need to be imbedded in the skin of its victim before transmitting most illnesses?

2. What are some of the ways a tick becomes aware of and is attracted to a potential victim?

3. How do some insect repellents work in keeping insects away from their intended victims?

4. What is a serious consequence of Lyme disease that occurs when the condition is untreated and progresses to Stage Two?

5. What are the major clinical signs of Stage Three of Lyme disease, where permanent damage may occur?

6. Where was the disease now called Lyme disease first described?

7. What tick-borne disease results in up to 5 percent fatalities even with the effective treatment available today?

8. What is the major difference between babeosis and the *Plasmodium* parasites that cause malaria?

9. What clinical features, signs, and symptoms occur with the condition of ehrlichiosis?

Laboratory Procedures for Identifying Parasitic Organisms and Their Ova

LEARNING OBJECTIVES

Upon completion of this chapter, the learner will be expected to:

- Relate the important components of properly collecting specimens to include blood, feces, and sputum in order to enhance the recovery rate for parasites present
- Explain to a simulated patient by role-play the steps involved in collecting and safely transporting a specimen to the clinical laboratory
- Discuss the theory for making both thick and thin smears for blood pathogens
- List the four species of malaria that are common human pathogens
- Describe the symptoms of malaria and how the fever cycles vary among species
- Prepare and stain both thick and thin smears
- Discuss the necessity of safety precautions in using blood specimens for parasite studies
- Contrast the two hematological stains, Wright and Giemsa, and when each are used
- Use tables, images, and narrative to identify parasites in a variety of specimens

KEY TERMS

Axoneme	Gametocytes	Sigmoidoscope
Coplin jars	Gomori stain	Supernatant
Crustaceans	Indirect method	Thin smear
Direct smear	Malarial stippling	Trichrome
Duodenal aspirates	Meningoencephalitis	Wet mount
EDTA	Mortality	Zinc sulfate
Ethyl acetate	Ocular units	Zygote
Flotation	Schizont	
Formalin	Sedimentation	

INTRODUCTION

Skill must be exercised in determining the method for preparing specimens and identifying parasites that infect humans, which number into the hundreds. Professional knowledge and technical skills are both required to provide the optimum care and diligence necessary to produce a meaningful examination of a specimen for the presence of parasites.

INTRODUCTION TO DIRECT AND INDIRECT IDENTIFICATION OF PARASITES

The first 11 chapters of this book are devoted to the history of the development of parasitology as it relates to human civilization and the life cycles and identifying characteristics of most of the parasites that afflict humans. The medical impact of an infection by a parasite or parasites requires that the types of specimens necessary for optimizing the chances of recovery of the organisms receive sufficient attention. Proper collection, transport and storage of the specimen should precede the procedures for isolation and identification of the parasites, setting the stage for accurate identification leading to proper treatment for the victim of an infection with a parasite or parasites. The purpose of this summary of preliminary information is to provide a background to consider in beginning the quest for recovery and identification of a variety of parasites.

As the student has learned from the previous chapters, the most important step is the recovery of and identification of the organisms. Prevention is an important step, but in some areas of the world, it is virtually impossible to avoid or prevent parasitic infections. Only a small percentage of parasitosis cases are resolved without properly timed and handled specimens and careful examination of the samples by educated and trained professional personnel. Chapter 12 includes the most basic procedures in the files of parasitology, and when used in conjunction with the previous chapters, the student should be successful in recovering, preparing, and identifying the bulk of parasites that impact the health of humans.

Worldwide, parasite infections are an important component of human morbidity (illness) and mortality (death). The infestation or infection (those inside the body) of parasites is normally considered the domain of lesser developed countries and regions of the world. However, it has been estimated that in some rural areas of the United States, intestinal parasites may be found in large numbers. For instance, some rural medical clinics with patients who primarily drink well water have reported extremely high intestinal parasite infections in today's modern world with advanced medical practices available in even the most remote locations.

Increasing numbers of people are traveling on a routine basis to endemic areas of the country and to other countries with regularity. Primary health care practitioners must become increasingly aware that parasites not ordinarily found in a geographical area may be found during examination of patients and clinical specimens who are being treated for other medical conditions. Clinical laboratory technicians and technologists should communicate with clinicians when patients have nonspecific clinical symptoms that may be due to parasite infections, and particularly for those patients who have traveled to other countries. There will no doubt need to be more awareness among both clinical personnel with patient care responsibility and for those who provide diagnostic services such as radiography and labs. Education and training components relative to the broad spectrum of both vectors and parasites should be stressed as the world shrinks and more medical challenges arise.

IMMUNITY AND PREVENTION OF PARASITIC INFECTIONS

Many medical conditions that result in an impaired or altered immune status may result in an infection of a variety of parasites. In some cases, a human is an accidental host for a parasitic infection and may be entirely unsuitable for the conditions necessary for a parasite to maintain a population and to reproduce within a host. In these cases the human may be an accidental host but the parasites are unable to reproduce and be transmitted to others. But total lifetime immunity to parasitic infections, unlike those for viruses and for some bacteria, is almost never the case. In some countries or locales where large numbers of the population are infested with a particular parasite, the victims may be asymptomatic, but this is not the same as being immune. This situation occurs most frequently in areas with hosts suffering from poor nutrition and low socioeconomic conditions. The host's body has merely reached an equilibrium where the population of parasites is somewhat controlled and do not cause overt reactions to the organisms.

IMMUNITY TO PARASITIC INFECTIONS

In endemic areas of the world, some individuals show a tolerance or a resistance for becoming infected by parasites with which the individual invariably comes in contact. Some immunity may be hereditary for some individuals. In others, some become asymptomatic (show no signs of infection) and harbor at least a small number of parasites indigenous to the area. These persons may be carriers that are capable of transmitting the organisms to others. In some areas, those who work in food services are required to be screened periodically for a variety of organisms, both for parasites and for other microorganisms. It should be remembered from earlier chapters that in many cases, certain animals are natural hosts for specific parasites and may suffer no ill effects from the infection, but are nevertheless able to pass the organism to others, including humans.

Natural and Acquired Immunity

Antibodies may develop in the healthy individual against parasites, and cell-mediated reactions, vital components of an individual's immune system, develop. This may cause tissue damage in the infected regions of the body, but serves to hold the infective organisms at bay when a human or other animal host with good nutrition and health becomes chronically infected. This group is much less likely to develop the severe symptoms observed in those with poor health. Tests for identifying certain parasites such as *Giardia lamblia* and *Trichomonas vaginalysis* have been developed that use the immunological system where the patient's response to the infection can be utilized.

Most of the procedures for determining the presence and identification of parasites use a direct method, which means the parasites themselves are recovered and are concentrated and sometimes stained to make the identification easier. The treated samples are placed on microscope slides and studied microscopically. An indirect method of identification occurs when the patient's immune response is used for determining the presence and identification of the parasite(s) since infections with multiple organisms sometimes occurs. When a patient is infected, the level of antibodies against the particular parasitic organism will greatly increase due to the patient's body recognizing the organisms as foreign agents, and an immune response is elicited. Antibody production is specific for each organism and tests have been developed for a few parasites. These tests are called *indirect tests* because the procedure determines whether antibodies are present against a specific parasitic organism rather than determining the actual physical presence of the parasite. In addition to microscopic methods for direct identification, direct serological tests for some parasites (e.g., *Giardia lamblia*) have a test kit that provides antibodies that will react even against fragments of the *G. lamblia* present in a stool sample. This method is called a *direct test*, even though antibodies are a component of the test procedure, because the reaction is against the organism itself and not a measure of the patient's immune response.

Preventing Infection or Infestation by Parasites

Just as there is a cycle of infection, similar to the chain of infection for other infective organisms such as bacteria and viruses, a link in the chain must be broken to stop the spread of a parasitic organism. In order to do this, knowledge of the organism's life cycle is important. This includes both primary and intermediate hosts, method of reproduction, and the routes by which transmission of the infectious agent gains entry into the body, such as vectors, or lifestyles of the victims. Various species of parasites may be found in almost any body site or body fluid, from solid tissue such as muscle, feces, sputum, aspirations from atria of the body, blood, and urine. Methods for preventing the transmission of parasites include:

- Personal sanitation
- Safe food and water supply
- Health education
- Determining infective form and preventing its development

- Identifying infected persons and requiring treatment
- Effective vaccines as well as more effective parasiticides

CLASSIFICATION OF PARASITES FOR IDENTIFICATION

There are two broad groups of parasites that are easily determined. The first and most elementary step is to place the organism into one of the following broad groups. *Ectoparasites* live on the exterior of the body, on the skin and in the hair, and are said to cause infestations. They may also function as vectors, or organisms that transmit disease into the human body. The second group, called *endoparasites*, are defined as those that dwell in cavities, tissues, and organs of the body and this group of parasites is said to initiate an infection in the body. Each of these two groups is further defined as follows:

Ectoparasites   Lice, mites, and other arthropods (jointed legs)

Includes crustaceans, insects, and arachnids (spiders, ticks, scorpions)

Parasite

Endoparasites   Protozoa (amoebae, ciliates, flagellates, sporozoans)

Includes helminths (worms) such as flukes, tapeworms, and roundworms

1. Intestinal and atrial (body cavity) parasites
2. Blood and tissue parasites

SPECIMEN COLLECTION

The collection of specimens includes feces, sputum, blood, skin scrapings, tissue specimens, and even urine and other body fluids such as cerebrospinal fluid (CSF) and duodenal aspirates. Ectoparasites are often scraped from the skin with a scalpel blade or the edge of a microscope slide and examined using a solution that might provide for staining or differentiation of the organism by microscopic exam. CSF requires a needle aspiration of the fluid of the brain and spine meninges; aspiration of

duodenal fluid is collected in the same manner. Sputum is collected following a deep cough or as bronchial washings performed by a physician. Specimens to be examined for parasites of the blood, such as intracellular malaria, require a simple phlebotomy procedure. Occasionally *P. westermani* or *Schistosom hematobium* ova may be found in the urine, or when fecal contamination is the source of the parasite or its ova, as well as a chance ectoparasite such as scabies that falls into the urine. Nits may also be plucked from the hair with forceps for microscopic examination and identification. It is rare when any of the other body fluids would harbor a parasite, and if so would be a special procedure using some of the same techniques as used routinely in the parasitology department.

Endoparasites that require a fecal specimen are the simplest to collect. The chances of recovering a parasite from a clinical specimen are drastically increased when certain collection procedures are followed. It is sometimes necessary to perform identification procedures on more than one sample, and in a timed manner, in order to optimize the percentages of recovering and identifying the organism. In addition, it is necessary to know about the life cycle and epidemiology of the suspected organism and the criteria for specimen collection, handling, and transport of the sample. It is also wise for the laboratory professional to follow safe practices such as the use of hand hygiene before and after gloving and removal of the gloves, and thorough cleaning of work surfaces following the handling of clinical specimens. Many of these parasitic organisms are highly contagious, and are easily passed to the unwary person handling the sample.

Specimens should be obtained with the use of specially designed containers or in a clean but dry leak-proof receptacle with a lid to prevent leakage. Specimens should not be mixed with urine if collected in a bedpan, or with any other contaminants. In addition, they should be collected prior to the initial doses of any antiparasitic medications, or any dyes. Those patients taking medications for diarrhea or laxatives, as well as barium for X-rays of the intestine should stop taking these medications or following a barium X-ray for one week before attempting to collect a viable sample.

When specimens are collected at home, in a clinic, or in a physician's office and must be transported, they must be preserved to enhance recovery of any parasites present, but it should be remembered that trophozoites in fixed or preserved samples are destroyed in the process. New preservatives have been developed due to Occupational Safety and Health Administration (OSHA) regulations requiring safety in disposal of materials. Formerly PVA emitted toxic fumes from formalin and also contained mercury, so these have been largely replaced by environmentally safe zinc and copper-based PVA (polyvinyl alcohol). The new fixative kits to preserve specimens serve to provide for adequate studies of morphology. In addition, they, do not interfere with staining procedures or in the subsequent performance of other immunological tests (see Figure 12-1). These kits containing specimens should also be shipped in a leakproof container or bag which is placed into an approved shipping container for biological materials as required by the United States Postal Service and other commercial transporters (see Figure 12-2).

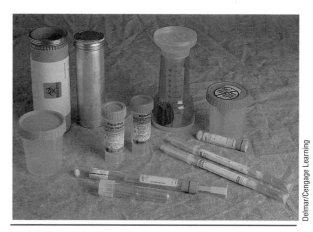

FIGURE 12-2 Suitable and approved containers for shipping biological samples

Collection and Preparation of Fecal Specimens

The eggs and various stages of the parasite itself, such as a trophozoite or cyst stage of a protozoan, may be present only at irregular times, and a single stool sample may not enable the correct isolation of an infective parasite. It is common practice to collect up to three stool samples over a 7- to 10-day period, a couple of days apart for each sample, in order to provide the best opportunity for "catching" the parasite in a form that can be easily seen and identified. Samples should be concentrated in order to optimize the effectiveness of the procedure. A number of commercial kits and some manual methods are available for concentrating fecal specimens and clearing the sample of fecal debris. However, visual observation of the sample and preliminary microscopic direct examinations of the sample may yield valuable clinical data prior to engaging in the more labor-intensive procedures, as discussed in this chapter.

Initial Step for Evaluating Stool Samples

The first step that is often included in the procedure manual for parasitology in a clinical laboratory is a direct smear called a wet mount. This method is practiced *only* on unformed and somewhat liquid stool samples, as the yield is extremely low for formed stools. This direct wet mount of unpreserved fecal matter is used to detect protozoan trophozoites (growth stage) which may be motile in a fresh liquid stool or a sample obtained through a sigmoidoscopy procedure which is performed by a physician. Wet mounts and stained smears are also made from the stool sample following a concentration procedure, which is valuable in detecting the cysts (inactive)

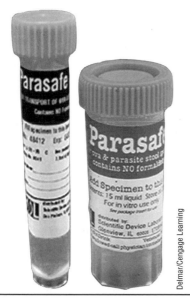

FIGURE 12-1 Vials containing fixative for preserving stool specimens

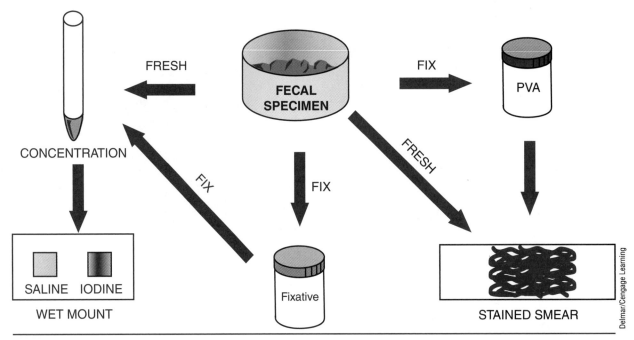

FIGURE 12-3 Initial preparation for the direct examination of fecal material

stage of protozoa and the eggs and larvae of helminthes (worms). When preparing stool specimens for basic staining and initial microscopic examination, the laboratory professional is exposed to potential biological hazards from exposure to both parasites and bacteria, as well as the chemicals used in preparing the sample (see Figure 12-3).

Wet mounts from fresh liquid stools and those obtained directly from the colon by a physician are entirely suitable for a direct and quick examination, which is sometimes fruitful. The entire wet mount, as described previously, should be scanned used the 10- or 20-power objective, and then the 40-power (high power) objective should be used to examine the slide for protozoa. It is helpful when trophozoite motility from fresh specimens can be observed, as preserved trophozoites are extremely small and are easily missed by the microbiologist or technologist. The wet mounts should not be extremely thick, as fecal detritus obscures some of the field and may cause the examiner to fail to see small protozoa. A good rule to follow is to make the mount thin enough that newspaper print can be read through

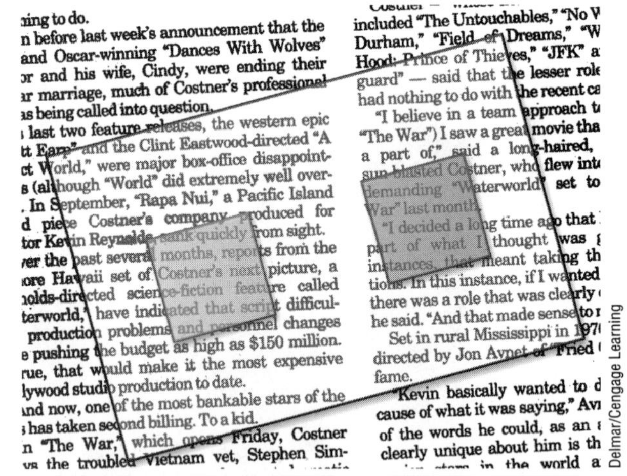

FIGURE 12-4 Concentration of properly prepared iodine and saline mounts may be easily checked by laying the slide over ordinary newsprint

both the saline and the iodine mounts (see Figure 12-4). It is vitally important to have a calibrated micrometer for measuring organisms seen, as a characteristic important in identifying the parasite.

PROCEDURE 12-1

INITIAL WET MOUNT

Clinical Rationale

There are three specific steps in performing the fecal samples for routine microscopic evaluation. The wet mount is a preliminary and direct procedure that will not only sometimes yield identification of certain parasites, but will enable visualization of WBCs or RBCs. The direct wet mount is the initial and perhaps the most important step and is used as a screening test in which trophozoite motility can be observed. The wet mount is followed by the second step, that of a concentration method procedure which affords the greatest opportunity for recovering parasite eggs or organisms. The third step involves preparation of and staining of permanent stains that are prepared from concentration methods. The process of staining shows important identification features such as intracellular components that include nuclei, organelles, and ingested materials, and a variety of stains are available for staining various features characteristic of the various organisms.

In diarrheal stools, trophozoites may be active and easily viewed with details that will provide an early diagnosis and therefore quicker treatment for the patient. Negative wet mounts should be followed by concentration procedures and the making of permanent stains of the feces for microscopic examination. Only fresh stools are used for the direct wet mount, while motile trophozoites will still be able to be viewed by the laboratory professional. The smear should be thin enough that a printed page such as a newspaper can be read through the mixture. Air bubbles should be avoided and the slide should be viewed systematically in order to cover the entire slide. The light source should be carefully adjusted, as some protozoa are colorless, by using the condenser and the iris diaphragm of the microscope to ensure that all details of the slide such as WBCs, RBCs, yeast, and the organisms are able to be seen. A systematic manner of viewing the slide should be employed to insure complete coverage of each slide (Figure 12-5).

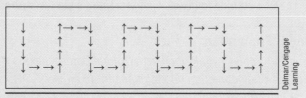

FIGURE 12-5 Systematic pattern for examining direct wet mount

Equipment and Supplies

1. Protective gloves and disposable gown
2. Standard microscope slides
3. Applicator sticks for obtaining and mixing saline and fecal material

(*continues*)

PROCEDURE 12-1
(continued)

4. 22-mm cover glasses
5. Lugol's iodine for demonstrating eggs and cyst structures more easily (iodine will kill trophozoites, so a preliminary examination for trophozoites should be conducted first)
6. Normal saline for suspension of fecal material
7. Binocular microscope with low- and high-power objectives
8. Ocular micrometer for determining sizes of organisms and ova

Procedural Steps

1. Obtain a standard 1 × 3 inch microscope slide and place one drop of normal saline on one end of the slide. A drop of iodine (1:5 dilution of Lugol's iodine) may be placed on the other end to be incorporated into the feces-saline mixture after an initial examination for motile trophozoites.
2. A small amount of stool (the amount clinging to the end of a wooden applicator stick may be sufficient) should be introduced to the drop of saline and another similar specimen into the diluted iodine.
3. Mix the stool samples and the two solutions with the applicator sticks.
4. Place a #1, 22-mm cover glass over each of the preparations by touching a long edge of the cover glass to the liquid and then allowing it to gently fall onto the mixture to avoid air bubbles.
5. The resultant preparation should be sufficiently transparent as to be able to read newsprint through it.
6. The edges of the cover slip may be sealed with clear nail polish or with equal mixtures of petroleum jelly (Vaseline) and melted paraffin.
7. Sealing the slides is desirable to avoid drying the specimen, which prevents clear visualization of the organisms if present. In addition, white and red blood cells, as well as yeasts, may be visible, all of which may be clinically significant. The cover glass can be removed from a well-made slide and after drying and fixing the slide, it can be stained to prepare a permanent slide for further identification and study.

Clinical Precaution:

Use of PVA (polyvinyl alcohol) as a fixative before making the wet mount will cause a cloudy condition due to exposure to air, so PVA-fixed samples should not be used for wet mounts.

---

8. If specimens submitted have been preserved with 10% formalin, saline drops may be avoided on the unstained sample on the slide.
9. Saline samples with unfixed samples enable more accurate examination of helminth (worm) eggs and larvae, as well as motile trophozoites and cysts, which are quite refractile.
10. The iodine solution enables the visualization of nuclear detail and darkly stains any glycogen masses that are diagnostic for some protozoa, but will kill trophozoites. Sometimes methylene blue is substituted for iodine for wet mounts.

11. Perform a thorough examination for both preparations at low power, starting at one corner of the cover slip and making sweeping moves either horizontally or vertically in order to cover the entire slide. High-power objectives are used for closer examinations of suspicious features.

12. Record the presence of white or red blood cells and any organisms observed on the appropriate form. Any parasites observed should be reported by both genus and species if possible and the stage of the parasite (ova, larvae, cyst, trophozoite). Cellular components such as RBCs, WBCs, yeast, etc., are reported in a semiquantitative form, as few, moderate, or many. Charcot-Leyden crystals are also reported semiquantitatively.

Microscopic Examination of Wet Mount

The prepared samples on microslides from the simple test tube **flotation** method, the simple flotation method, and the **sedimentation** method are examined under a microscope at the magnifications listed in Table 12-1.

TABLE 12-1 Magnification Table for Microscopic Examination of Wet Mounts

MAGNIFICATION	PARASITES
10 × 10	Nematode and cestode eggs
10 × 40	Protozoa
10 × 4	Trematode eggs

Clinical Precaution:

For oocysts of the Cryptosporidium *spp., special flotation procedures such as the Sheather sugar flotation method is the best procedure as it allows better visibility of the oocysts. The* Cryptosporidium *spp. oocysts are more refractive with this method against the background solution than they are with the zinc sulfate flotation method.*

Clinical Precaution:

Use of oil immersion lenses of the microscope for wet mount preparations should not be attempted unless the slides are well sealed!

Results and Report for Wet Mount Procedures

It is important to determine the genus and species if possible of any parasites observed, along with the stage of the parasite identified, such as that of eggs, larvae, cysts, or trophozoites. Ingested cellular components such as RBCs, WBCs, yeast, etc., are reported in a semiquantitative form, as few moderate or many. Charcot-Leyden crystals are also reported in the same manner. Any other identifiable elements such as artifacts or undigested materials may provide clues as to a medical condition requiring treatment.

PROCEDURE 12-2

CONCENTRATION TECHNIQUE—FORMALIN-ETHYL ACETATE

Clinical Rationale

Fecal concentrate procedures by the sedimentation method increase the probability of finding parasites and their ova when low numbers are present in the stool specimen. This is a routine technique and is often used in conjunction with a flotation method that is particularly valuable in detecting ova of parasites but the **ethyl acetate** method is most commonly used for concentrating eggs and cysts. A single concentrated sample from an infected patient is sometimes adequate for detecting helminths (worms). It is often necessary to utilize several specimens in order to detect protozoal organisms due to the difficulty in finding stages that are somewhat easily identified (Figure 12-6).

SEDIMENTATION

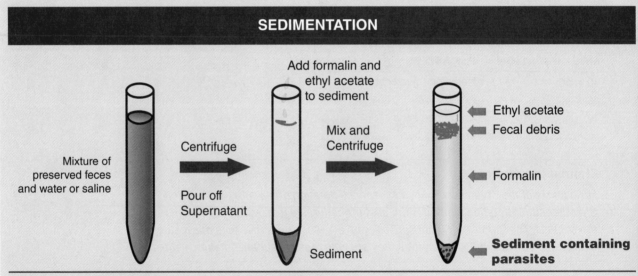

FIGURE 12-6 The sedimentation concentration method concentrates the parasites and their ova as a button in the tip of the centrifuge tube

Safety Alert:

Standard precautions must be employed when handling fecal samples and other tissues and body fluids being examined for parasites. Both biological hazards and chemical hazards may be present. Specimens may still be potentially infectious after the addition of fixative, because helminth eggs and cysts of protozoa are resistant to PVA.

Concentration methods are necessary in most examinations as the numbers of organisms present may be few. Several prepackaged kits are available for preparing the stool sample in the second process of a complete examination of a fecal specimen. However, these commercially prepared kits are more expensive than using bulk reagents and supplies. These kits are used most often for convenience, ease of cleaning of the environmental surfaces, and the substitution for some of the volatile formalin-ether mixture. It is possible to use both fresh and preserved stool specimens when performing a concentration procedure.

Because concentration processes enhance the chances of finding parasites, this is the second step following the initial wet mount to be performed in a complete analysis of a stool sample, and is preparatory to performing a sedimentation or flotation technique. Concentration procedures serve to increase the density of the parasites from a specimen into a small amount of liquid from which much of the fecal debris is also removed, leaving a clear view of the contents of the concentrating tube. It should be noted that trophozoites of protozoans are destroyed during this process, but cysts of protozoa and the larvae and eggs of helminthes are frequently found when using this technique.

It is often necessary to use both the sedimentation and flotation procedures for performing concentration techniques designed to increase the numbers of organisms or ova that may be present. The two methods accomplish basically the same goal but one may be more useful than the other depending upon the species of parasite or parasites present. Both of these methods are based on differences between the specific gravity, which is best described as the density of a solution based on dissolved materials, to consolidate the organisms or ova into a smaller area. In the sedimentation procedure, organisms and ova are compacted into the bottom of a conical-shaped centrifuge tube. Flotation methods serve to suspend the organisms and ova at the top of a solution of great density. The sedimentation method tends to give a greater diversity of organisms and their various stages as well as eggs and concentrates a large amount of feces into approximately 2 grams of sediment. The flotation method is primarily advantageous for concentrating the ova, but other stages and forms may also be found with this method.

Equipment and Supplies

1. Protective gloves and disposable gown
2. 15 mL conically shaped glass centrifuge tubes
3. Applicator sticks for obtaining and mixing saline and fecal material
4. 10% formalin
5. Saline for washing samples
6. Method for straining feces such as dampened surgical gauze that will allow ova and parasites to pass through but will retain large fecal debris (care should be exercised in mucoid sample, where oocysts and microsporidia may be trapped in the mucus).

(*continues*)

PROCEDURE 12-2
(*continued*)

7. Centrifuge with holders that will accommodate the large centrifuge tubes
8. Fresh fecal specimen collected in a suitable container free of contaminants including urine
9. Ethyl acetate
10. Cotton-tipped applicator sticks
11. Iodine stain
12. Standard microscope slides
13. 22-mm cover glasses
14. Parafilm or rubber caps sized to fit centrifuge tubes

Procedural Steps

1. Obtain a standard 1×3-in. microscope slide and place one drop of normal saline on one end of the slide and a drop of iodine (1:5 dilution of Lugol's iodine) on the other.
2. Add ½ to 1 teaspoon of fresh species to a container, such as a glass dish, and use applicator sticks to mix the stool sample with 10 to 15 mL of 10% formalin.
3. Strain the mixture through two layers of dampened gauze squares into the 15-mL glass centrifuge tube. The use of larger thicknesses of gauze may trap oocysts or microsporidia.

Clinical Precaution:

If the sample is extremely mucoid, the sample should not be strained but should be centrifuged for 10 minutes at 1500 rpm and then placed on a slide with a drop of iodine stain and a cover glass.

---

4. Centrifuge the suspension at 1500 rpm for 10 minutes and then carefully pour off the **supernatant** into a container containing disinfectant. If the sample still contains a large amount of fecal debris, resuspend the sample in 10 to 15 mL of saline or formalin and recentrifuge. This procedure may be repeated in the presence of excess fecal debris.
5. Resuspend the rinsed sample (step 4) in 7 to 8 mL of formalin and 4- to 5-mL ethyl acetate (this step is not necessary if only a small amount of fecal debris is present following the previous step).
6. Cover the tube with Parafilm or a rubber cap and shake the mixture vigorously for at least 30 seconds.
7. Remove the Parafilm or cap carefully to avoid splashing into the face or eyes.
8. Recentrifuge the suspension at 1500 rpm for 10 minutes.

9. Carefully "rim" the top layer to remove the debris on the edges of the upper layer. Quickly and smoothly empty the supernatant into a container of disinfectant only one time, taking care not to shake and disturb the "button" in the tip of the centrifuge tube. If necessary, while holding the tube in an inverted position for emptying, excess ethyl acetate that appears as bubbles can also be carefully removed with a cotton-tipped applicator stick.

10. Place a small amount of fecal sediment on a microscope slide and place a #1, 22-mm cover slide over each of the preparations.

11. The resultant preparations should be sufficiently transparent as to be able to read newsprint through them.

12. An unstained and an iodine-stained specimen should be examined. The unstained sample is necessary because cyst forms are refractile and can be more easily observed if unstained with the iodine. The iodine solution enables the visualization of nuclear detail and darkly stains any glycogen masses, which are diagnostic for some protozoa.

13. Perform a thorough examination for both stained and unstained specimens at low power, starting at one corner of the cover slip and making sweeping moves both horizontally and vertically to cover the entire slide. The use of a high-power objective with immersion oil may be used for closer examinations of suspicious features but the slide should be sealed to avoid oil entering the specimen underneath the cover glass.

14. Any parasites observed should be reported by both genus and species if possible and the stage of the parasite (ova, larvae, cyst, trophozoite). Cellular components such as RBCs, WBCs, yeast, etc., are reported in a semiquantitative form, as few moderate or many. Charcot-Leyden crystals are also reported semiquantitatively.

Summary for Concentration of Fecal Specimens

To summarize the sedimentation method for concentrating fecal parasites and their ova, this method is most effective for helminth ova, larvae, and protozoan oocysts (Figure 12-5). The method requires the use of both ethyl acetate and formalin, both of which may prove toxic to humans if not handled carefully.

Results and Report for Sedimentation Methods

Any parasites observed should be reported by both genus and species if possible and the stage of the parasite (ova, larvae, cyst, trophozoite). Cellular components such as RBCs, WBCs, yeast, etc., are reported in a semiquantitative form, as few, moderate, or many. Charcot-Leyden crystals are also reported semiquantitatively. Any other identifiable elements such as artifacts or undigested materials may provide clues as to a medical condition requiring treatment.

ZINC SULFATE CENTRIFUGAL FLOTATION PROCEDURE

Clinical Rationale

When properly performed, the flotation procedure will concentrate the organisms from a small amount of fecal material that is then cleansed of debris with water. The density of the **zinc sulfate** enables the lighter elements such as larvae, protozoa, and ova to be found at the top of the centrifuge tube. The flotation method is the most effective way for concentrating protozoa and their cysts, along with *Cryptosporidium* oocysts. Several commercial methods exist for concentrating fecal parasites and their ova. These kits are disposable and contain all the necessary materials in a closed system for performing the flotation procedure. The manual method is also quite effective but requires the making of the main reagent, that of zinc sulfate. The manual procedure perhaps exposes the laboratory worker to the specimen and the chemicals used to a greater extent than one of the commercial kits (see Figure 12-7).

FLOTATION

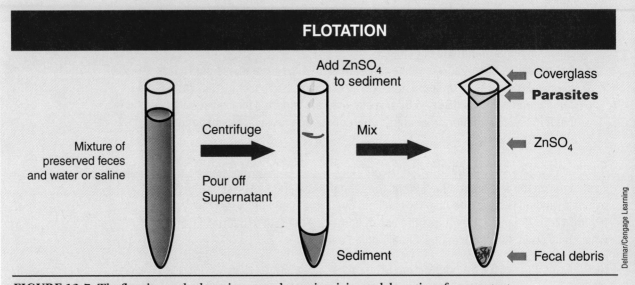

Mixture of preserved feces and water or saline

Centrifuge

Pour off Supernatant

Add ZnSO$_4$ to sediment

Mix

Sediment

Coverglass

Parasites

ZnSO$_4$

Fecal debris

Delmar/Cengage Learning

FIGURE 12-7 The flotation method requires several steps in mixing and decanting of supernatant

The method called *flotation* uses liquids with a relatively high specific gravity, greater than that of parasite cysts or eggs, so that they will float to the surface. This concentrate found at the top of the tube will contain the organisms and their eggs that can be skimmed from the top and used to prepare slides for microscopic examination. The concentrating solution has a final specific gravity of 1.18 (compared with water which has a specific gravity of 1.000). Most often zinc sulfate is used in the flotation procedure but it should be noted that the flotation method is not particularly effective in the recovery of operculated eggs and unfertilized *Ascaris lumbricoides* ova. And with iodine, the zinc sulfate kills trophozoites and alters the morphology of some fragile eggs such as those of *Hymenolepsis nana.* If these organisms are suggested from history and from the wet mount, the formalin-ethyl acetate sedimentation method should be utilized.

Equipment and Supplies

1. Protective gloves and disposable gown
2. Clean water (deionized or distilled water may be preferable to avoid contaminants)
3. 13 × 100 round-bottom test tubes
4. Fixed and washed fecal sample obtained by the following steps.
5. Centrifuge with head adaptable for the 13 × 100 test tubes
6. 22 × 22 mm cover glasses
7. Test tube rack configured to hold tubes in vertical position
8. Pasteur pipettes
9. Microbiological wire loop
10. Standard microscope slides
11. Zinc sulfate of 1.20 specific gravity
12. Saline for washing samples

Clinical Precaution:

Specific gravity of zinc sulfate should be verified by use of a hydrometer.
A specific of 1.20 is preferable for formalin-preserved specimens.

Procedural Steps

33% Zinc Sulfate Solution Preparation

330 g zinc sulfate
Water added to reach (QS) a volume of 1000 mL

Additional water or zinc sulfate to produce a specific gravity (SpG) of 1.18. Specific gravity can be determined with a hydrometer and adjusted to 1.20 by adding small amounts of zinc sulfate. Zinc sulfate centrifugal flotation has the unique ability to float *Giardia* cysts as well as other parasite structures. It is a simple, accurate, and inexpensive procedure that can be performed in almost any basic clinical laboratory.

1. Prepare washed and fixed fecal sample in a 13 × 100 mm test tube. The sample is prepared by centrifuging the suspension at 1500 rpm for 10 minutes and then carefully pouring off the supernatant into a container containing disinfectant. If the sample still contains a large amount of fecal debris, resuspend the sample in 10 to 15 mL of saline or formalin and recentrifuge. This procedure may be repeated in the presence of excess fecal debris.

(continues)

PROCEDURE 12-3
(continued)

2. Wash the sample one or two times with saline, centrifuging for 10 minutes at 1500 rpm to obtain 1 mL or less of the sample.
3. Resuspend the sample, mixing it well, into 12 mL of zinc sulfate (see note on preparing the zinc sulfate solution).
4. Centrifuge at 1500 rpm for two minutes, allowing the centrifuge to stop of its own volition in order to avoid vibration and disturbance of the sediment.
5. Carefully place the tube in a vertical position in the rack and slowly add drops of zinc sulfate with the Pasteur pipette until a meniscus that rises above the top of the tube is achieved.
6. Without disturbing the tube, place a cover glass over the top of the tube and in contact with the meniscus, which should not be so high as to cause liquid to run down the side of the tube.
   a. An alternate method involves the use of a sterile Pasteur pipette or a clean microbiological wire loop to the surface of the fluid in the tube.
   b. Several loopsful of the fluid are transferred onto a microscope slide.
7. The cover glass from the tube is placed on a microscope slide, and in the alternate method, a few loopsful of fluid are placed on a microscope slide and are covered with a 22 × 22 or a 22 × 40 mm cover glass, and the initial examination using the 10 × objective is conducted.
8. A drop of iodine may be added, following an examination for refractile and colorless organisms.

Characteristics of Organisms for Microscopic Examination

Giardia lamblia

1. Floats in 33 percent zinc sulfate solution under centrifugal flotation, but not as readily in other flotation solutions.
2. The size of G. lamblia is 11 to 15 μm in length and somewhat consistent in size, being most often oval-shaped, and refractile green in color.
3. Contains **axoneme**/nuclei/median bodies; however, these structures are not always visible. The use of oil immersion (100 x) objective is helpful in seeing these structures when one is having difficulty at a lower magnification. Usually the median bodies are the most visible of the three structures.
4. Some cysts have a crescent-shaped indentation caused by high salt concentration.
5. Cysts appear to reach their own focal plane by floating just below the cover glass.
6. When scanning the slide, use 10 x objective magnification with a moderate amount of light and a reduced diaphragm aperture for optimum light contrast.

Yeast Bodies

1. Float in almost all commonly used flotation solutions.
2. Similar to *Giardia* in size, shape, and color but may be mistaken for red blood cells, except for greenish-gray cast. Yeast bodies are often more common than *Giardia*.
3. Contains circular vacuoles, but no body structures such as axonemes, nuclei, or median bodies are visible.
4. If yeasts are actively growing, buds can form on the yeast bodies.

Sarcocystis spp. and *Cryptosporidium* sp.

1. ***Sarcocystis*** spp. sporocysts are about the same size as *Giardia* cysts. They float in all commonly used flotation solutions. Their internal structure consists of four banana-shaped sporozoites and a clump of material called a *residium*. Because of its relatively thicker cyst wall, *Sarcocystis* is more easily seen than *Giardia*.
2. ***Cryptosporidium*** sp. is spherical and measures 3 to 5 μm in diameter. They are so small that they are often missed during the fecal examination.

Other Considerations

1. Oocysts of *Isospora belli* are lightweight and may float near the top of the meniscus.
2. A phase-contrast microscope may be used to determine the presence of *Cryptosporidium, Cyclospora,* and *Isospora*.
3. Centrifugation may distort the helminths eggs that are thin-shelled and some protozoan cysts.
4. It may be important to examine the sediment following the flotation method, because the heavier operculated eggs and the unfertilized *A. lumbricoides* eggs do not float.

Results and Report for Flotation Procedures

Any parasites observed should be reported by both genus and species if possible, using the characteristics in the descriptions listed previously. The stages exhibited by the parasite (ova, larvae, cyst, trophozoite) are important clinical items leading to appropriate treatment for the victim of the infection. Cellular components such as RBCs, WBCs, yeast, etc., are reported in a semiquantitative form, as few, moderate, or many. Charcot-Leyden crystals are also reported semiquantitatively. Any other identifiable elements such as artifacts or undigested materials may provide clues as to a medical condition requiring treatment.

PROCEDURE 12-4

TRICHROME STAINING PROCEDURE

Clinical Rationale

Some of the trichrome stains are modified, in that they include iron hematoxylin and trichrome stains, called the Wheatley modification of the **Gomori stain**. The technique for a trichrome procedure requires less detail and is less time consuming than the others. The stain may be made on a fresh sample or a PVA-preserved specimen. SAF-preserved specimens do not stain as well with trichrome as with iron hematoxylin. The following procedure is a standard method, but with various brands of stain, the procedure may vary.

Stained fecal smears should be prepared from all stool specimens for positive identification of protozoan parasites in their various life stages. The Wheatley trichrome technique is a rapid procedure that is convenient for identification of intestinal protozoa in fresh fecal specimens. Nuclear material is easily visualized as important tools in diagnosing particular organisms due to colors imparted to the components of the organism. Fecal smears must be fixed using polyvinyl alcohol (PVA) or Schaudinn solution. Modifications of the procedure and the use of other stains are used by some to aid in observing microsporidia and acid-fast stains are often used for *Cryptosporidium, Cyclospora,* and *Isospora*. Several different stains may be used for parasite differentiation. Three basic varieties of the stain are used depending upon the species of the parasite being examined (see Table 12-2).

TABLE 12-2 Stains, Characteristics Associated with Various Species

STAIN	ORGANISM	APPEARANCE OF STAINED ELEMENTS
Trichrome	Protozoan Cysts and Trophozoites	Blue Green
	Exception is *Entamoeba coli*	Often stains purple
	Red Blood Cells	Dark red-purple
	Eggs and Larvae	Red
	Yeasts	Green
Iron hematoxylin	Organisms	Gray-black
	Nuclear material	Black
	Background material and debris	Light blue-gray
Modified Acid-Fast	Oocysts of *Cryptosporidium spp.,* *Isospora belli, Cyclospora cayetanensis*	Magenta-stained organisms against a blue background

Equipment and Supplies

1. Protective gloves and disposable gown
2. Applicator sticks
3. Standard microscope slides
4. Fresh fecal sample
5. Schaudinn fixative solution (without acetic acid)
6. 70% and 90% ethyl alcohol (ethanol)
7. Acidified 90% ehtanol
8. Absolute ethanol
9. Trichrome stain
10. PVA fixative for diarrheic stools
11. Xylene or xylene substitute
12. Permount
13. #1 cover glasses
14. Slide warmer or 37°C incubator
15. Immersion oil
16. Microscope

Procedural Steps

1. For a fresh stool sample, applicator sticks or similar implements may be used to smear the specimen as a **thin smear** of fresh feces on a 1 × 3-in. microscopic slide. Do not allow the smear to dry before initiating the staining procedure.
2. Place the moist smear in Schaudinn fixative solution for 5 minutes at 50°C or for 1 hour at ambient (room) temperature.
3. Rinse the slide in 70 percent alcohol for 5 minutes but avoid fixation of the smear for PVA-fixed material.
4. For PVA-preserved specimens, a few drops of the sample should be placed on absorbent filter paper for approximately 3 minutes and allowed to drain before collecting the material from the paper. Do not allow the specimen to dry before making a smear!
5. Using an applicator stick, prepare a smear as in Step 1 on a 1 × 3-in. microscopic slide.
4. Allow the smear to air dry overnight at room temperature or for 2 to 3 hours on a 37°C on a slide warmer or a 37°C incubator. If slides are dried too quickly, distortion of the morphology of the organism(s) may occur. But thorough drying is essential to prevent sloughing off of the material during the staining process.
5. Place the smear in 70 percent ethanol with enough iodine to make the solution the color of strong tea, for 2 to 3 minutes. A 10-minute period is required if the smear is PBA-fixed.
6. Place slide in two changes of 70 percent alcohol solutions for 5 minutes in each solution.

(continues)

PROCEDURE 12-4
(continued)

7. Place the slide(s) in a trichrome stain for at least 10 minutes.
8. Rinse in acid-alcohol (90 percent solution) for no more than 10 seconds. One to three seconds may be sufficient.
9. Again, briefly rinse the slides by dripping them several times in two changes of absolute methanol. This step should be used as a rinse for no more than 10 seconds. Prolonged de-staining in this step causes poor differentiation in some organisms.
10. Place in xylene or xylene substitute for 5 minutes.
11. Mount with a 22 × 40 mm cover slip (no. 1 thickness). A mounting medium such as Permount may be used to protect the slides but this step is optional.
12. Examine the smears using the oil immersion objective (1000 x). Read at least 100 fields of the slide. The reading time should be at least 10 minutes per slide.

Results and Report for Trichrome Staining Procedures

Any parasites observed should be reported by both genus and species if possible, using the characteristics listed above as well as images provided throughout the chapters of this book. The stages exhibited by the parasite (ova, larvae, cyst, trophozoite) are important clinical items leading to appropriate treatment for the victim of the infection. Cellular components such as RBCs, WBCs, yeast, etc., are reported in a semiquantitative form, as few, moderate, or many. Charcot-Leyden crystals are also reported semiquantitatively if they are identifiable. Any other identifiable elements such as artifacts or undigested materials may provide clues as to a medical condition requiring treatment.

When trichrome staining methods are used, trophozoites, cysts, human tissue cells and blood cells, and yeast or pseudohyphae are easily identifiable. Helminth ova and some larvae often are excessively stained and the features of them are difficult to visualize. Reportable artifacts are usually quantified as follows:

Average artifacts/ 10 oil immersion fields	Unit of report
Fewer than 2	Few
3–9	Moderate
Greater than 10	Many

PROCEDURE 12-5

THICK AND THIN SLIDES FOR IDENTIFYING BLOOD PARASITES
Clinical Rationale
Blood and Tissue Parasites

Blood, which is also considered a tissue, is an excellent medium for a number of blood parasites. The major so-called blood parasites are from the genera *Plasmodium* (malaria), *Babesia* (babesiosis), *Trypanosoma* (trypanosomiasis), and microfilaria from a variety of organisms. Malaria outnumbers all of the others listed here combined and it is estimated that up to one-half billion people in the world may be afflicted by a strain of malaria, and several million people die each year from the infection. Tissue parasites are obtained by surgical biopsy and include *Trichinella spiralis*, *Leishmania* spp., and *Toxoplasma gondii*. Biopsy specimens are needed to test for *Trichinella spiralis* encysted in muscle tissue, and amastigote stage of *Leishmania* spp. because these organisms are intracellular. *Toxoplasma gondii* is also identified from a pre-pared slide from a tissue biopsy. Depending on the species of certain organisms, amoebic **meningoencephalitis** may be caused by *Naegleria fowleri*, and the spinal fluid must be cultured to identify the pathogen.

Some bacteria are not classified as parasites but infect either/or red and white blood cells, which they require in order to survive and to reproduce. But the most common of these tissue parasites are those that infect the blood. Blood is stained by either Giemsa or Wright stain but the combination Wright/Giemsa stain is the most effective for observing both blood cell morphology and inclusions in the red blood cells. With a properly prepared blood film, and staining by a Wrights-Giemsa stain, most if not all parasites typically found in the blood may be detected by microscopic examination. The most common blood parasite occurring on a worldwide basis is that of four species of malaria, including *Plasmodium falciparum*, *P. ovale, P. vivax,* and *P. malariae*. But the laboratory professional must be alert for other possibilities, as travel throughout the world and to endemic areas for a large variety of parasitic infections is not uncommon.

Blood smears are necessary to determine the presence of malaria (*Plasmodium*), *Babesia, Trypanosoma*, and some species of microfilaria of *Wuchereria bancrofti* that circulate in the blood during the night. There they are ingested by mosquitoes, where they continue their development, becoming infective larvae in two weeks, and then are reinjected into other humans. Motile organisms such as *Trypanosoma* and microfilariae can be seen on direct wet mounts of fresh blood specimens under both low- and high-power magnification. But definitive identification is made from a permanently prepared and stained slide where morphological characteristics can be readily observed for specific identification.

(*continues*)

PROCEDURE 12-5
(continued)

Identification Procedure for Blood Parasites

Fresh anticoagulated blood is necessary for preserving the morphology of the erythrocytes and to stain the parasites themselves. For microfilaria, stains other than Wrights-Giemsa are used but it is possible to detect the presence of microfilaria from a slide stained by this stain. This stain gives better morphology with details of parasites that also exhibit more color intensity than slides stained with only Wrights stain. For suspected cases of malaria and other blood parasites, based on travel, clinical signs and symptoms, both a thick and thin blood film should be made. Methanol is used to fix the RBCs on the thin film. RBCs are lysed on the thick smear with water before staining. The thick smear is made to afford a higher concentration of malaria parasites and the thin film provides better morphology for identifying parasites by species.

Identification Procedure for Malaria

Malaria is identified by the fever cycle for the various species and history of travel, although infection with more than one *Plasmodium* species may cause some confusion. The morphology of the trophozoites and gametes as well as the presence of a few well-known phenomena is helpful. The four species of malaria that infect humans have varying geographic distribution but some zones overlap. A number of other species other than these four exist but only certain animals and birds are affected. Of the four species that infect humans, the "malignant" strain is *P. falciparum* (see Figure 12-8). The characteristic morphology of these four species may be used from microscopic examination to identify the species. Fresh blood from a fingerstick is the best specimen but a tube with the anticoagulant **EDTA** is adequate if stained within 1 hour of collection. With Giemsa stain, the parasite's cytoplasm is stained bluish, with red to purple-red chromatin. **Malarial stippling**, if present, will stain as faint, discreet pink-red dots in the cytoplasm.

For malarial determinations, the best time to make blood smears for identification of the parasite is halfway between paroxysms (see Table 12-3). In malaria, samples are examined every 6 to 8 hours for up to 3 days to allow for the differences the reproduction of the four species of malaria that affect humans. Usually during a paroxysm (a severe attack or increase in violence of a disease that

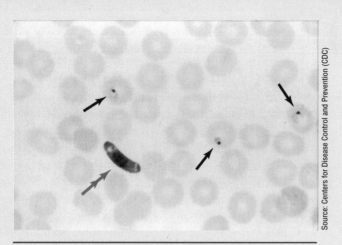

Source: Centers for Disease Control and Prevention (CDC)

FIGURE 12-8 Malarial parasites in blood smears. Micrograph of Giemsa-stained thin smear showing a *Plasmodium falciparum* gametocyte (bottom, double arrow) and several ring forms within erythrocytes (arrows).

TABLE 12-3 Fever cycles characteristic of malaria species that infect humans

SPECIES	DISEASE CAUSED	PAROXYSMS
P. vivax	Benign tertian malaria	Every 48 hours
P. ovale	Ovale malaria	Every 48 hours
P. malariae	Quartan malaria	Every 72 hours
P. falciparum	Malignant malaria	Every 36 to 38 hours

recurs periodically), each of the merozoite-filled red blood cells (RBCs) rupture releasing 12 to 24 free merozoites and malarial pigment into the bloodstream. Merozoites are formed by asexual reproduction through the breaking up of a **schizont** (another stage in asexual reproduction of some protozoans) and invade other red blood cells. These stages are ingested into the *Anopheles* mosquito in cases of malaria, where they mature into **gametocytes** that reproduce in the mosquito's blood.

(*continues*)

PROCEDURE 12-5
(continued)

Identification Procedures for Other Blood Parasites

Four species of *Trypanosoma* may be found in human blood (Table 12-4).

As with malaria, travel to endemic areas for non-malarial infections aids in identification of the parasite. *Trypanosoma brucei* is the hemoflagellate that causes sleeping sickness. It is spread by the bite of the tsetse fly requiring travel to the "tsetse belt" of sub-Saharan Africa where the organism is transferred from a host such as a cow or other grazing animal. The disease is endemic to Africa and two geographically isolated strains are known. It is also possible to find other parasites, including trypanosomes, microfilaria, *Babesia* spp., and *Leishmania* on the blood smears stained by the procedures outlined here. If parasites are not found in the initial blood specimen/smears, it is advisable to take additional thick and thin smears every 6 to 8 hours, for as long as 48 hours if necessary, regardless of the parasite suspected.

Filariasis Detection

For cases of blood parasites where microfilariae would be in the blood, initial scanning of a stained smear at 10-power should reveal the presence of this form of parasite. Patient history including travel is also helpful. If filariasis is probable based on the clinical history, both diurnal (day) and nocturnal (night) collections of blood are necessary to allow for differences in the activity of the various species.

TABLE 12-4 Species of blood parasites, how they are transmitted and the diseases caused

ORGANISM	TRANSMISSION	DISEASE CAUSED
Plasmodium spp.	Mosquito bite	Malaria
Babesia	Tick bite	Babesiosis
Trypanosoma brucei	Tsetse fly bite	African sleeping sickness, trypanosomiasis
Trypanosoma cruzi	Reduviid bug bite contaminated with bug's infected feces	Chagas disease, American trypanosomiasis
Wuchereria bancrofti	Mosquito bite	Filariasis, elephantiasis
Brugia spp.	Mosquito bite	Filariasis, elephantiasis
Leishmania donovani	Sand fly bite	Visceral leishmaniasis, Kala azar, dumdum fever
Toxoplasma gondii	Ingestion of oocysts, eating undercooked infected meat, congenital	Toxoplasmosis

Equipment and Supplies

1. Protective gloves and disposable gown
2. Wright-Giemsa Stain (Quick-Stain)
3. Absolute Methanol (methyl alcohol)
4. Distilled water
5. 3 **Coplin jars** or equivalent containers
6. 1 mL disposable pipet
7. Known positive controls slides are optional but important
8. Microscope slides

Procedural Steps

Most likely malarial parasite stages will be observed on the thick smears, and identification will be definitive from the stained thin smears.

Preparing the Slides (Thick and Thin)

1. Prepare both thin and thick smears (see Figures 12-9–12-11). Thick films must not be extremely thick as they will peel from the slide. The ability to barely discern newsprint with the initial wet drop for the thick film is optimum.
2. Use clean microscopic slides only. For thick smears, place six drops of blood on the slide, two each in the three points of triangular shape (see Figure 12-10). Use the corner of another slide to mix the drops in a circular motion and spread them out to the approximate size of a dime. Allow the slide to air dry for 6 to 8 hours, preferably overnight. Thin smears are made in the same manner as those for a routine blood smear performed during a complete blood count.

> **Clinical Precaution:**
>
> *Only air-dry the thick smears. Do not heat the thick smears with a flame or slide warmer; this tends to fix the RBCs. Recall that methanol as a fixative will prevent the RBCs from lysing when water is added to the thick drops.*

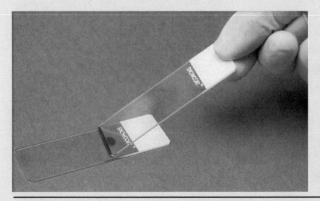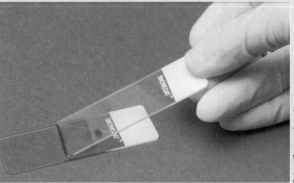

FIGURE 12-9 Preparing a thin blood smear for examination for parasites

(continues)

PROCEDURE 12-5
(continued)

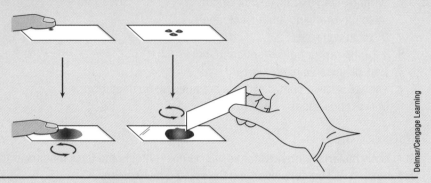

FIGURE 12-10 Demonstration of two methods of preparing thick blood smears, directly from finger puncture and triangular pattern of blood on slide

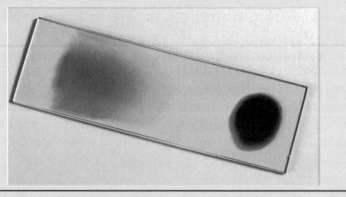

FIGURE 12-11 Image of both thin- and thick-stained blood smears on same slide

Staining the Thin Smears
1. For thin smears, place a drop of blood on a slide, and, using another slide, streak out the blood as in making a differential smear. It is important to use a technique that will result in a good feathered edge. Allow to air-dry.
2. When staining the thin smear, it is advantageous to have a positive control slide that is stained with all malaria specimens when available.
3. Dip the thin slide in a Coplin jar of Absolute Methanol five times, 1 second per dip.
4. Place the slide in a Coplin jar of Wright-Giemsa Stain (Quick-Stain) for 10 seconds.
5. Place slide in a Coplin jar of distilled water for 20 seconds or more to effect a more desired color balance. This may take practice and experience to perfect this step.
6. Drain the slide and allow to air-dry in an upright position, by standing the slide on its end. There are special racks available for this step.

Staining the Thick Smears
1. Place slide on a flat surface, such as a rack over a sink.
2. Carefully overlay the entire slide with distilled water.

3. Allow the water to lyse the RBCs, which usually takes approximately 3 minutes, and remove excess water from slide. Allow slide to air-dry completely before staining. If available, a positive control slide should be stained with all malaria specimens.
4. Place the slide in a Coplin jar containing Wright-Giemsa stain (Quick-Stain) for 10 seconds.
5. Place slide in a Coplin jar of distilled water for 20 seconds or more to achieve a desired color balance.
6. Drain the slide and allow to air-dry in an upright position, by allowing it to stand on its end.

Examining the Stained Slides
1. Examine the stained slide under a microscope using the oil immersion objective (1000 ×).
2. The various stages of blood and tissue parasites are often similar for different species. Determining the various stages (Table 12-5) of the life cycle for these organisms is invaluable in providing a diagnosis.
3. Examine thick smears thoroughly for the presence of malarial parasites. Remember that the cytoplasm of the *Plasmodium* species stains robin egg blue and the nuclear chromatin stains crimson or violet. Examine at least 100 oil immersion fields on each thick film.
4. The thin films are used primarily for speciating the *Plasmodium* organism. However, even if no parasites are discovered on the thick films, the thin films must still be examined. View at least 200 fields on each thin smear before reporting a negative result.
5. When malarial parasites are observed, identify the organism using the diagram (see Figure 12-12).
6. The results obtained from all positive malarial slide preparations should be phoned to the attending physician or his or her designate as soon as possible.

TABLE 12-5 Terms Related to Identification of Blood and Tissue Parasites

TERM	IDENTIFYING DEVELOPMENTAL CHARACTERISTICS
Gamete	Sex cell resulting from the maturation of a gametocyte; process occurs in mosquito
Gametocyte	Sexually differentiated cell capable of producing gametes that is passed from human to mosquito
Merozoite	Sexually differentiated cell capable of producing gametes that is passed from human to mosquito
Oocyst	Unencysted form of an ookinete in the mosquito
Schizogony	Asexual reproduction by the development of spores in the mosquito
Sporozoite	A form resulting from the division of the oocyst and is passed from mosquito to a human
Trophozoite	The vegetative or feeding stage of the parasite that occurs in the human
Zygote	The cell that results from the union of two gametes in the mosquito

(*continues*)

Malaria
(*Plasmodium spp.*)

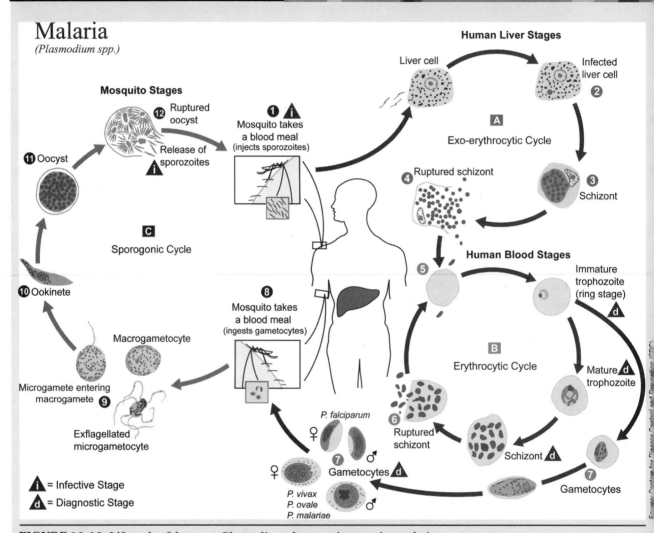

FIGURE 12-12 Life cycle of the genus *Plasmodium*, the organism causing malaria

Results and Reporting of Geimsa Staining Procedure
1. Stippling (dotted pattern) of the RBCs is best observed within 1 hour of collection for EDTA specimens.
2. The cytoplasm of *Malaria*, *Babesia*, trypanosomes, and leishmania stain blue, whereas nuclear material stains red.
3. The sheath of microfilaria may not be visible with the stain but the nuclei will stain blue or purple.
4. WBCs stain purple and RBCs stain pale red. Eosinophil granules will stain bright red and the granules of segmented neutrophils will be dark pink to lavender.
5. Organisms should be reported by genus and species if possible.

QUALITY CONTROL

As in all clinical laboratory procedures, quality control is paramount in order to provide accurate results. Commercial slides may be purchased and used to familiarize the learner or to enhance and challenge the skills of experienced parasitologists, or permanent slides from actual patient samples can be retained for review. Control samples may be preserved for examination on a periodic basis to ensure stains are still viable, or when new stains are prepared. WBCs from a centrifuged, anticoagulated blood sample may be incorporated into the control slides for comparison. Control samples should be reviewed at least on a quarterly basis and each time new stains are prepared. The ocular micrometer is initially calibrated for a particular microscope and should not be transferred to another microscope due to individual differences between instruments. Recalibration should be performed on an annual basis and anytime when doubt arises regarding the accuracy of the calibration.

It is wise for those performing parasitology procedures to maintain a familiarity with artifacts that may be encountered when examining a wet mount. Many artifacts may be mistaken for parasites by the inexperienced or unwary laboratory technician. Artifacts include pollen or plant cells, WBCs and RBCs, yeasts, hair, starch granules, macrophages (large white cells), and mucosal epithelium. Other areas of note are the presence of eosinophils and Charcot-Leyden crystals associated with the breakdown of eosinophils, which are often found in heavy parasitic infections. Quality control results should be recorded each time a procedure is performed and out-of-control results should be accompanied by an action plan that outlines the steps taken to determine the cause for aberrations from the expected results.

MISCELLANEOUS METHODOLOGY FOR RECOVERING SPECIFIC PARASITES

Several manual and commercial preparations are available for convenient recovery of specific parasites from body sites of the human. Recovery of these organisms by the methods described here are specific for a limited number of parasites. Some parasites do not lend themselves to being easily isolated from fecal specimens, one of which is the common pinworm that infects many children. Others that are not always found in the stool are recovered from certain body sites as is discussed in this section. Many of the following collection techniques do not require the care or elaborate preparations as the previous procedures do, so a step-by-step procedure is not necessary for each of these. Specimens gathered from the following sources are directly examined by microscope and reported if found.

Scotch Tape Prep for Pinworms

Because pinworms and their ova are rarely recovered from stool specimens, a low-tech method that has been in existence for decades is described here. The life cycle of the pinworm called *Enterobius vermicularis* entails movement from the colon to the anus, where the adult female lays eggs in the perianal area. Cellophane tape is used by stretching a several inch strip over a tongue blade with the adhesive side to the outside of the tongue blade (see Figure 12-13).

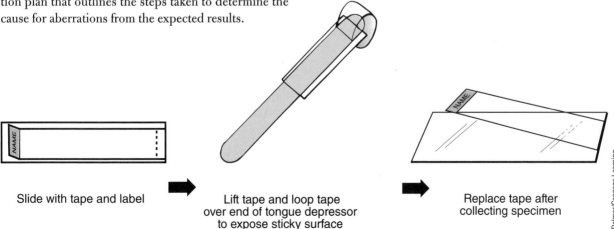

Slide with tape and label   Lift tape and loop tape over end of tongue depressor to expose sticky surface   Replace tape after collecting specimen

FIGURE 12-13 Cellophane tape/tongue blade device for recovering pinworm ova

Delmar/Cengage Learning

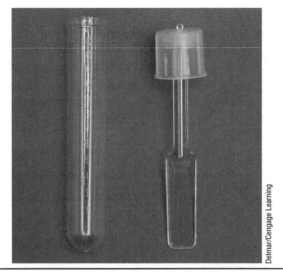

FIGURE 12-14 A commercially provided paddle swab is placed between the anal folds of the child, where pinworm ova adhere to the device

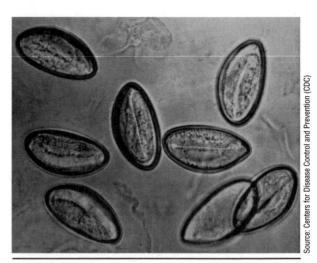

FIGURE 12-15 Microscopic appearance of *E. vermicularis* ova, oblong, opposite side flattened

Early in the morning, before the child rises from the bed, the tongue blade-cellophane device is placed between the folds of the hip cheeks, at the rectum. The tape is then removed and placed sticky side down against a 1 × 3-in. microscope slide. The slide is scanned on low power for eggs of the *E. vermicularis* parasite. A commercially provided flat swab called a *paddle swab* is also available and can be used in lieu of the cellophane tape and tongue blade apparatus (see Figure 12-14).

Pinworm ova are infectious for up to several weeks following the laying of them, as well as are ova of other helminths. Infection occurs by either airborne ova or accidental infection from contaminated surfaces and hands. Gloves should be worn for the collection, and the supplies should all be discarded as biohazardous wastes. Even the microscope should be disinfected following the examination of a pinworm prep. Microscope slides are placed in a "sharps" container due to the sharp corners of the glass. The ova appear as an oblong egg with one edge flattened or less rounded than the opposite side of an egg (see Figure 12-15).

Sputum

In some cases, parasites are found in sputum and may be swallowed, where they enter the gastrointestinal tract before continuing the infective cycle. *Entamoeba*, round-worm, hookworm, *Strongyloides*, and *Pneumocystis*

carinii are all found in the sputum on occasion. Both ova and larvae may be present in a wet mount of the sputum of an infected individual.

Duodenal Aspirates

This procedure is performed when a routine stool examination for parasites returned negative results, but where clinical findings indicate a possible infection with *Giardia lamblia* or *Strongyloides stercoralis*. A test is available where a gelatin capsule attached to a weighted string is swallowed into the upper small intestine, and the string end is taped to the patient's cheek. After 4 hours in the intestine, the gelatin capsule is carefully extracted by gently pulling the string from the patient's mouth while the gelatin remains attached to the distal portion of the string. Mucus that is covering the gelatin capsule is scraped off and placed on a slide, where a wet mount is performed. Motile trophozoites should be present in cases of active infection. A portion of the sample is also placed in a fixative and is used in a permanent stained smear. Ova of *Fasciola hepatica* (liver fluke) or *Opisthorchis sinensis* may be identified along with oocysts of *Cryptosporidium* or *Isospora belli* are occasionally identified from the stained specimen.

Specimens Collected by Sigmoidoscopic Procedure

Sigmoidoscopic examinations are performed for a variety of reasons. A **sigmoidoscope**, a tubular lighted speculum used for examining the sigmoid colon and the rectum, is passed through the anus and into the lower intestine to examine the sigmoid colon and the rectum. Aspirates and scrapings from the device are used for diagnosing amebiasis or cryptosporidiosis. Immediate examination by wet mount may yield trophozoites, and a part of the specimen is also placed in PVA fixative and fixed permanent slides are prepared by staining the specimen with trichrome or other stains designed for this purpose.

Urine, Vaginal, and Urethral Specimens

Urine sediment may reveal the trophozoites of *Trichomonas vaginalis* in women and occasionally in men, and is a sexually transmitted infection. These trophozoites are often extremely motile and are easily identified in urine sediment during a routine urinalysis examination in most cases. Ova of *Enterobius vermicularis* (pinworm eggs) may be recognized, along with *Schistosoma hematobium*, a fluke. *T. vaginalis* is also often identified by a wet mount of vaginal or urethral discharge, and can also be cultured, unlike many other parasites, in a medium that promotes growth and reproduction when incubated at 37°C, a normal human body temperature.

Immunological Tests for Diagnosing Infections of Parasites

Additional tests are currently being researched for the development of serological tests for antibodies to parasites. Several disadvantages exist to the use of these techniques that would prevent the use of the tests for routine diagnosis, because they cast much doubt as to a current infection. These tests are not suitable for determining if antibodies that may yield a positive result were there prior to the most recent illness, as would be the case in a past exposure to the parasite in question. Antibodies persist for years, and would be positive even with no current infection. Also, there are a number of cross reactions where similar antigens may give a positive result, limiting any usefulness in diagnosing an infection of parasites. The cost for some of these tests may also be prohibitive, and the number of types of tests available commercially is quite low. Some tests that are commercially available and that are quite useful are immunoassay or fluorescent antibody tests for *Toxoplasma gondii* and *Entamoeba histolytica*. Tests for soluble *antigens* (components of the parasites themselves) rather than *antibodies* to the parasitic antigens in clinical specimens do provide clinical information regarding current infection. But tests are only available currently for some of these organisms.

Serological tests may not be useful unless the parasite is of a type that invades the tissue, which provides the greatest stimulation of antibody production. But these tests may be useful where invasive procedures can be avoided if the parasites are identified by immunologic means. Kits are not always available from commercial vendors but the Centers for Disease Control and Prevention (CDCP) may be of assistance by providing diagnostic methods to clinical laboratories. A direct fluorescent procedure is available where an antibody against *Giardia lamblia* and *Cryptosporidium* antigens may be obtained.

Quality Assurance for Parasitology Procedures

Reference samples are necessary for comparison when performing parasitological procedures. In addition, written reference materials and pictures are necessary for those who seldom perform procedures for recovering and identifying parasites. Most laboratories do not have a dedicated laboratory professional to perform or oversee the supplying and maintenance of the section, and rotate various personnel through the department when specimens arrive. The recovery rate suffers in these cases, at an estimate of the finding of twice as many positive specimens when one person is in charge of the department. The parasitology department should also be enrolled in a proficiency program acceptable to the facility's accreditation requirements to ensure accuracy. And because size is important for stages such as the trophozoites, cysts, or ova of various species of parasites, a properly calibrated ocular micrometer should be available for each objective on the microscope used for parasitology.

CALIBRATION OF MICROSCOPES USING AN OCULAR MICROMETER

The purpose of calibrating the ocular micrometer is to correctly correlate ocular units of an entity being measured to the number of microns represented by these units. This process is necessary for each objective (10 ×, 40 ×, and oil immersion objectives). To determine how the ocular units correspond to actual millimeters in size, a stage micrometer must be used to calibrate the ocular micrometer. If a different microscope is being used other than the one that is properly calibrated, a calibration for that microscope must be performed, and there are subtle differences between microscopes. A correctly calibrated microscope is crucial because size is an important characteristic for identification of parasites. This section assumes that an ocular micrometer disk has been installed in one of the oculars and that a stage micrometer is available for calibrating the ocular micrometer. This calibration should be done for each of the microscope's objectives.

1. Place the stage micrometer on the microscope stage and focus on the micrometer scale, until you can distinguish between the large (0.1 mm) and the small (0.01 mm) divisions of the scale. Install an ocular micrometer disk in the eyepiece of the microscope by placing it underneath the eyepiece lens.

2. Using the low power objective, adjust the stage micrometer so that the "0" line on the ocular micrometer is superimposed with the "0" line on the stage micrometer.

3. Without changing the stage adjustment, find a point as distant as possible from the two superimposed "0" lines where *two other lines are also exactly superimposed.*

4. Determine the number of ocular micrometer spaces *and* the number of millimeters on the stage micrometer where the ocular micrometer directly aligns with a division line of the stage micrometer (Figure 12-16). Divide the number of stage units by the number of ocular units and then multiply the results by 1000. This calculation provides the micrometers for one ocular unit on low power.

5. Follow the above steps for each objective. Calibration readings should be posted on each microscope and the microscope should be recalibrated after every cleaning or changing of objectives or oculars. Before preparing a wet mount slide, the microscope should be calibrated. The objectives and oculars used for the calibration procedure should be used for all measurements on the microscope. The calibration factors should always

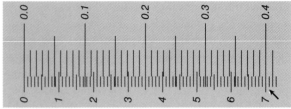

FIGURE 12-16 Stage micrometer and ocular micrometer superimposed

be posted on the side of the microscope for quick reference.

a. Look as far as possible along both sides until you see two lines exactly over one another. On this scale, the numbers that coincide are 70 and 0.4. At higher magnifications it may be necessary due to the thickness of the lines.

b. Divide 0.4 by 70 and multiply the result by 1000. The figure, 5.7 (rounded down), provides the number of microns per ocular unit.

In this example, 1 ocular unit = 0.40/70 × 1000 = 5.7 microns

Procedure for Calculating Size of Organism

1. Place the ocular lens containing a micrometer disc on the microscope.

2. Focus on the object to be measured and determine the size in ocular units.

3. Multiply the ocular units by the calibration factor for that specific microscope, objective, and ocular micrometer (i.e., 1 ocular unit = 5.7 microns for the microscope being used and that has been calibrated).

Example

A parasite cyst was measured using an ocular micrometer in the eye piece of a phase contrast scope and its 40 × darkfield objective. The organism was three ocular micrometer units wide. The calibration factor for that specific micrometer used on the phase scope with the 40 × darkfield objective is 5.7 um. three ocular micrometer units × 5.7 um = 17.5 um wide.

SUMMARY

A number of parasites from human blood must be stained with certain stains in order to identify the causative organisms for the blood-borne parasites. Human blood parasites, such as *Plasmodium,* which causes malaria; trypanosomes that cause African sleeping sickness; and American trypanosomiasis (Chagas's disease), as well as babesiosis, comprise most of these. Safety practices for those performing the tests, and scrupulous attention to detail are required to correctly identify these pathogens. Smear findings should only be released by competent technical personnel able to review, interpret, and evaluate sometimes nebulous results. The timing of blood and tissue collection, the manner in which the specimens are prepared and stained, must be followed carefully in order to enhance the chances of successfully finding and correctly identifying the causative organisms for the blood and tissue parasites.

No current technology comes close to recovering and identifying the numbers of parasitic infections that are actually in existence. A dedicated staff that insists on scrupulously performing the tasks for identifying definitively the causative organisms for parasitic infections is the best tool for accuracy and efficiency. Antibody studies that are available do not distinguish between current infections or past infections, and the manner of collection of samples, with the cooperation of the patient, is still not completely satisfactory, and many cases of infection are missed. No doubt newer detection methods, rather than those labor-intensive procedures currently used, will replace these methods, and more accurate determinations of infection may come to reality.

STUDY QUESTIONS

1. What are some methods used for diagnosing parasitic infections?

2. Name three major groups of human parasites.

3. In what ways does climate and region affect the types of parasites there?

4. Name three body sites where parasites may be found.

5. What are three ways parasites may be transmitted?

6. What are the procedures for diagnosing blood and tissue parasites?

7. What are the four species of *Plasmodium* that humans may contract?

8. Name the families for tapeworms and roundworms.

9. List the three helminthes.

10. Compare cysts and trophozoites of intestinal protozoa.

11. What dilutant is most often used for wet mounts?

12. Relate the two concentration methods for fecal specimens.

13. Why is it necessary to employ Standard Precautions when handling parasite specimens?

14. Why is it necessary to calibrate the ocular of the microscope with a stage micrometer?

15. Why are thick and thin preparations required for blood parasites?

REFERENCES

Acuna-Soto, R., J. Samuelson, P. De-Girolami, et al. 1994. Application of the polymerase chain reaction to the epidemiology of pathogenic and nonpathogenic *Entamoeba histolytica*. Am. J. Trop. Med. Hyg. **48**:58–70.

Ali, I. K. M., M. B. Hossain, S. Roy, P. F. Ayeh-Kumi, W. A. Petri, Jr., R. Haque, and C. G. Clark. 2003. *Entamoeba moshkovskii* infections in children, Bangladesh. Emerg. Infect. Dis. **9**:580–584. [PubMed].

Amaya, K. 2003. "Brugia malayi" (On-line), Animal Diversity Web. Accessed January 20, 2009 at http://animaldiversity.ummz.umich.edu/site/accounts/information/Brugia_malayi.html.

Avicenna (Ibn Sina). C1000. Al Canon fi al Tib. See Libri in re medica omnes qui hactenus ad nos pervenere, p. 1–966, Venetiis.

http://search.yahoo.com/search;_ylt=A0geu6VSSR1K6zsB6r
FXNyoA?p=Naunyn&y=Search&fr=yfp-t-501&fr2=sb-
top&sao=2 Bernhard Naunyn; Accessed 27 May, 2009.

Brumpt E. (1912). "Blastocystis Hominis N. sp et formes
voisines." Bull. Soc. Pathol.

Bryan, C. P. 1930. The Papyrus Ebers (translated from the
German). Geoffrey Bles, London, United Kingdom.

Clark, C. G., and L. S. Diamond. 1991. The Laredo strain
and other *Entamoeba histolytica*-like amoebae are
Entamoeba moshkovskii. Mol. Biochem. Parasitol.
46:11–18. [PubMed].

Clin Microgiol Rev. 2002 October; 15(4):595–612.

Cox, F., (2002). History of Human Parasitology. Retrieved
January 5, 2009, from http://pubmedcentral.nih.gov/

Cysticercosis, accessed 27 May, 2009; http://spinwarp
.ucsd.edu/NeuroWeb/Text/br-270cyst.htm doi:
10.1128/CMR.15.4.595-612.2002.

Estridge, B. H. and Reynolds, A. P. (2008). *Basic clinical laboratory techniques* (5th ed.). Clifton Exot. 5:
725–730.

Farr, G., 2002. Parasites. www.becomehealthynow.com/
ebookpring.php?id=674. From Wikipedia, the free
encyclopedia.

Gonzalez-Ruiz, A., R. Haque, A. Aguirre, et al. 1994. Value
of microscopy in the diagnosis of dysentery associated
with invasive *Entamoeba histolytica*. J. Clin. Pathol.
47:236–239. [PubMed].

Haque, R., I. K. M. Ali, C. G. Clark, and W. A. Petri, Jr.
1998. A case report of *Entamoeba moshkovskii* infection in a Bangladeshi child. Parasitol. Int. **47**:201–202.

Haque, R., I. K. M. Ali, S. Akther, and W. A. Petri, Jr. 1998.
Comparison of PCR, isoenzyme analysis, and antigen
detection for diagnosis of *Entamoeba histolytica* infection. J. Clin. Microbiol. **36**:449–452. [PubMed].

Haydon D.T., Cleaveland S., Taylor L.H., Laurenson M.K.
Identifying reservoirs of infection: a conceptual and
practical challenge. Emerg Infect Dis [serial online]
2002 Dec [date cited]; 8. Available from: URL: http://
www.cdc.gov/ncidod/EID/vol8no12/01-0317.htm

Hoeppli, R. 1956. The knowledge of parasites and
parasitic infections from ancient times to the
17th century. Exp. Parasitol. 5:398–419. [PubMed].

Hoeppli, R. 1959. Parasites and parasitic infections in early
science and medicine. University of Malaya Press,
Singapore, Singapore.

http://search.yahoo.com/search?p=sedimentation+
method+for+parasites&fr=yfp-t-501&toggle=
1&cop=mss&ei=UTF-8 (Accessed 21 May, 2009)

http://www.babylon.com/definition/Opisthorchiasis/

http://www.cvm.umn.edu/academics/course_web/current/
CVM6202/labs/giardia_pg2.pdf (Accessed 22 May, 2009)

http://www.dpd.cdc.gov/dpdx/HTML/Diphyllobothriasis
.htm (Accessed 8 June, 2009)

http://www.dpd.cdc.gov/dpdx/HTML/Schistosomiasis
.htm (Accessed 9 June, 2009)

http://www.tulane.edu/~wiser/protozoology/notes/intes.html

James H. Cassedy, "The 'Germ of Laziness' in the South,
1900–1915: Charles Wardell Stiles and the Progressive Paradox," *Bulletin of the History of Medicine,*
45 (1971): 159–169.

Jones J.L., Kruszon-Moran D., Sanders-Lewis K., Wilson M.
(2007). "Toxoplasma gondii infection in the United
States, 1999–2004, decline from the prior decade."
Am J Trop Med Hyg 77 (3): 405–10. PMID 17827351.

Jones, W. H., and E. T. Whithington. 1948–1953. Works
of Hippocrates. Loeb Classical Library, Heinemann,
London, United Kingdom.

M. Tanyuksel and W. A. Petri, Jr. (2003). Laboratory
diagnosis of amebiasis. *Clinical Microbiology Reviews,
Vol. 16, 4,* pp. 713–729.

Mary Boccaccio, "Ground Itch and Dew Poison: The
Rockefeller Sanitary Commission 1909-14," *Journal
of the History of Medicine and Allied Science,*
27 (January 1972): 30–53.

McMillan, A., H. M. Gilmour, G. McNeillage, and G. R.
Scott. 1984. Amoebiasis in homosexual men. Gut
25:356–360. [Abstract/Free Full Text].

Moe K.T., Singh M., Howe J., et al. (1996). "Observations
on the ultrastructure and viability of the cystic stage
of Blastocystis hominis from human feces." Parasitol. Res. 82 (5): 439–44. PMID 8738284. Park, NY:
Thomson Delmar Learning.

Niash, Darren, 2009. Evolution of avian locomotion:
scienceblogs.com/tetrapodzoology/2009/06/birds_
come_first_no_they_dont.php

Rhazes (abu Bakr Muhammad ibn-Zakariya-al-Razi).
C900. Al-Hawi (a summary of medical knowledge).

Taber's Cyclopedic Medical Dictionary, 20th Edition.
(2005). Philadelphia: F. A. Davis Company. www.new
worldencyclopedia.org/entry/Ebers_Papyrus

The Dreadnought Seamen's Hospital (2008). www
.greenwich-guide.org.uk/dreadnought.htm (Accessed
21 Nov. 2009)

Zaman V., Howe J., Ng M. (1995). "Ultrastructure of
Blastocystis hominis cysts." Parasitol. Res. 81 (6):
465–9. PMID 7567903.

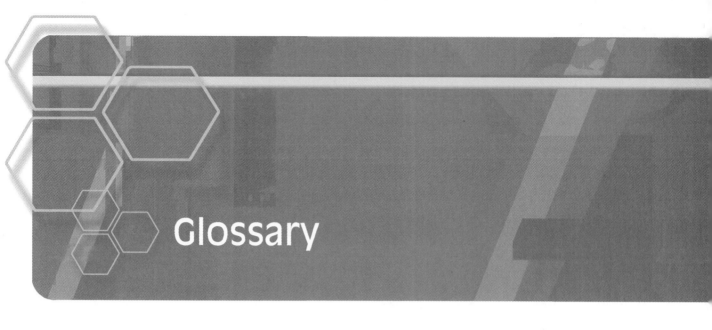

Glossary

A

Acaridae Family of mites that cause irritation to the skin.

Acarina Ectoparasites of the order Acarina includes many vectors such as ticks and mites.

Acellular Acellular organisms are not organisms at all, but rather viruses that are not considered living organisms.

Acetabula Structure of *Schistosomal cercaria* producing secretions glands used in the invasive process of the parasite.

Acetone Colorless and flammable liquid; used as a solvent for decolorizing and cleaning of the laboratory.

Aedes Genus of mosquito originally found primarily in tropical, subtropical zones but has spread by human activity to all continents; several species important in transmitting human diseases.

Accidental host One that may harbor an organism that does not actually infect it.

Agar plate A Petri dish that contains nutritive media (agar) to promote bacterial growth.

AIDS Acquired Immunodeficiency Syndrome.

Algae Source of food for some organisms; grows in both fresh and salt water as a photosynthetic organism.

Amastigote An amastigote is a cell that does not have any flagella and is used mainly to describe a certain phase in the life cycle of trypanosome protozoans.

American dog tick The American dog tick, *Dermacentor variabilis*, is found in the eastern United States and less frequently in the Pacific west. These ticks are encountered in grassy meadows, young growing forests along weedy trails, and roadsides.

Amicrofilaremic Inability to find microfilaria in the blood; refers to *W. bancrofti* and *Loa loa* microfilaria.

Amoebae Plural form of a type of a protozoan.

Amoebiasis Condition of being infected with amoebic parasites.

Amoebic colitis Refers to infection with the pathogenic protozoan, *Entamoeba histolytica*.

Amoebicides Chemotherapeutics for ridding the gastrointestinal system of amoebae.

Amoeboid pseudopodia Cytoplasmic extrusions used for motility as well as to engulf blood cells and bacteria.

Amputation Either traumatic or surgical removal of an entire limb or fingers and toes.

Anaerobic Condition of decrease or absence of oxygen; some bacterial require this condition in order to grow.

Anaphylactic A severe allergic condition of hypersensitivity may affect only certain organs and systems of the body or may include the entire body; previous exposure and sensitization necessary due to previous exposure to antigen (causative agent); anaphylaxis has a rapid onset and may lead to death if not quickly treated.

Anaplasma Prevalent tick-borne pathogen that causes considerable damage to the health of livestock throughout the world.

Annelids Large phylum of worms that appear to be ringed and segmented; includes leeches and earthworms.

Anemia A condition literally meaning "without blood"; caused by a red blood celldeficiency; may exhibit weakness and shortness of breath.

Anoperineal region Refers chiefly to the anus and perineum, the region between the thighs.

Anopheles Species of mosquito that transmits human malaria.

Anorexia An eating disorder mainly based on an emotional or psychological condition, resulting in willful self-induced starvation; may be called anorexia nervosa; persistent loss of appetite.

Antibodies Proteins produced by B lymphocytes in response to the presence of a foreign antigen.

Antigens Any substance capable of stimulating an immune response.

Antihistamines Drug used to reverse the production of histamines during allergic reactions.

Antiprotozoal drugs Designed to treat diseases caused by protozoa, animal-like, one-celled animals including amoebae.

Appendicitis Inflammation of the vermiform appendix, an appendage of the large intestine.

Apterygotes   Insects without flying wings; may have vestiges such as wing pads.

Arachnida   Class that includes spiders, scorpions, ticks, and mites.

Arboviruses   Examples of these organisms are those that cause yellow fever and viral encephalitis; may reproduce in both mammals and ticks.

Argasidae   Tick family called *soft-bodied ticks*; appear shriveled before becoming engorged by blood.

Arteriolitis   Inflammation of the arteries and arterioles.

Arthralgia   Joint pain; may include all synovial joints and vertebra.

Arthropods   Refers to insects with jointed legs, as well as other members of families of animals with jointed legs and hard segmented bodies (includes crustaceans, spiders, and insects).

Ascariasis   A condition of being infected with a parasite of the genus *Ascaris*.

Ascites   A medical condition in which fluids build up chiefly in the abdominal cavity.

Asexual   Non-sexual; often refers to process of reproduction.

Aspergillosis   Diseases of humans and animals caused by mold fungus from the Aspergillus family.

Asplenic   Condition of lacking a spleen; spleen removed by surgery (splenectomy).

Asthma   Chronic and sometimes allergic inflammation of the lungs where airways (bronchi and bronchioles) are narrowed.

Asymptomatic carrier   Organism infected with a pathogen that shows no symptoms itself of being infected but is capable of infecting other animals or humans.

Australian paralysis ticks   Of the genus Ixodes, the tick secretes a poisonous saliva that may cause severe paralysis and death.

Avian malaria   Most caused by *Plasmodium relictum*, and infects tropical birds.

Axoneme   An inner, central core, usually bisecting the organism that provides skeletal structure and carries a whip-like appendage (cilia or flagella).

Axostyle   Simple supporting structure that runs through the body of a trichomonad and protrudes at the posterior end.

B

Babesiosis   A category of tick-borne disease including humans and cattle, dogs, horses, sheep, and swine, and is caused by a babesia protozoan.

Bacillus   Bacterial strain with a rod-shaped morphology.

Balkh sore   Skin break caused by cutaneous leishmaniasis; traced to the ninth century.

Bedbug   A wingless bloodsucking hemipterous insect, *Cimex lectularius*, with flattened body morphology, that infests houses, furniture, and beds.

Benzene hexachloride   Insecticide used in agriculture and as treatment for lice and scabies.

Bile   Composed mostly of cholesterol and formed in the liver, bile is a bitter, alkaline, greenish to yellow fluid that facilitates breakdown of fats; in Asia, chronic infection of the biliary system occurs when parasitic infections are found in the bile ducts, causing increased bilirubin in the blood of these victims.

Bilharziasis   Also known as schistosomiasis, is a disease of nematodes contracted in fresh water in the Eastern countries.

Binucleate   Having two nuclei as occurs in some protozoa.

Biological life cycle   A life cycle includes one generation of an organism; refers to reproduction of both sexual and asexual means; includes hosts, reservoirs.

Bioterrorism   Use of microorganisms to kill or incapacitate large segments of a population.

Biting midge   Certain species of the midge are serious biting pests, and can spread diseases to livestock.

Blackflies   Small, dark flies that can give a painful bite, but unlike a mosquito which sucks up blood, blackflies break the skin and lap up the pooled blood; carry a variety of filarial diseases, particularly onchocerciasis.

Bladder worms   Larval forms of tapeworms (Cestodes) that inhabit a cyst formed in tissue; bladder worms include pork tapeworms, broad fish, and dog tapeworms.

Blastomeres   Cells resulting from fertilized ovum that has split (cleaved).

Blood flukes   Schistosomal infections referred to as blood flukes or bilharzia.

Boophilus   Genus of ticks transported to the New World by Spanish colonialists; transmit bovine babesiosis.

Borreliosis   Any of a number of diseases spread by the genus *Borrelia*; chiefly spread by insect vectors.

Bothria   Cestodes that attach to the intestines have muscular grooves that provide attachment by grasping host tissue between them.

Brightfield microscopy   General use microscopes that are not electron, phase contrast, dark field, or polarized light instruments.

Bronchioles   Smaller division of the bronchi that have no cartilage in the walls.

Bronchoconstriction   Reduction in air flow of small airways of the respiratory system.

Brown dog tick   Can complete its entire life cycle indoors but is not known to be a major transmitter or disease organisms.

Brucellosis   Refers to an infectious disease caused by a bacterium of the genus Brucella.

Bubo   Swelling of the lymph nodes found primarily in diseases such as bubonic plague, gonorrhea, TB, or syphilis; may appear as a large blister often occurring in the armpit, groin, or neck.

Bubonic plague   Bacterial disease caused by the bacterium *Yersinia pestis* (previously *Pasturella pestis*).

Bull's eye rash   A rash from infected ticks; chiefly refers to Lyme disease, although the phenomenon may be present in other tick-borne diseases.

C

Calcifies   Calcium salts build up in various soft tissues, resulting in hardening.

Canid species   Includes dogs, foxes, wolves, and coyotes.

Carcinomata   Plural term for cancers or malignancies.

Cardiac failure   Failure based on the heart's inability to effectively pump blood to organs of the body; trichinosis is the most common cause of cardiac involvement; trichinosis and hookworm anemia are common causes of cardiac failure in the tropics.

Carnivores   Animals whose diets are chiefly meat; scavengers and hunters.

Carriers   Human or animal that harbors a pathogen which may be parasitic and does not exhibit symptoms of an illness from the organism.

Cartilaginous   Structural support from cartilage within chiefly a lumen (tube).

Caudal   Tail-like structure or position near the end of an organ or at the hindmost area of an organism.

Cellulose   Structural component of the primary cell wall of green plants and many forms of algae; undigestible by humans.

CDCP   Centers for Disease Control and Prevention.

Cephalic ganglion   Solid nervous tissue as a cluster that contains many cell bodies and nerve synapses and frequently enclosed in a tissue sheath; may function as "brain" of small organisms; found in invertebrates and vertebrates.

Cercaria   Free-swimming stage of life cycle for some flatworms and roundworms; often parasitize snails and mollusks as intermediate hosts before entering final host.

Cerebral cysticercosis   Infection primarily of the brain or spinal cord with the larval forms of the genus Taenia, which is primarily *Taenia solium* in humans.

Cestode   Group of parasitic flatworms commonly called tapeworms.

Cestodiasis   Infection with tapeworms.

Chagas's disease   May be called American trypanosomiasis, and includes North and South America; caused by infection with a protozoan parasite *Trypanosoma cruzi*.

Charcot-Leyden   Crystallized structures of varying sizes that are found in feces, sputum, crystals and body tissues of those with helminth infestations; originate from white blood cells called eosiniphils and that are found as an immune response in allergic infections and parasitic infections.

Chelicerae   Mouth parts of certain spiders (arachnids), horseshoe crabs; chelicerae of spiders are pointed appendages for grasping food or prey serve as chewing mandibles found in other arthropods.

Chiggers   Larvae of a type of mite found in tall grass and weeds, and whose bites cause severe itching; scratching may result in secondary bacterial infections.

Chigoes   The chigoe flea, the smallest known flea, is also called a "jigger" and is a parasitic arthropod found in tropical climates, especially South America and the West Indies.

Chloramphenicol   Belongs to group of medicines called antibiotics; used for infections that are nonresponsive to other antibiotics; may be carcinogenic (cancer-causing).

Chlorosis   Type of chronic anemia, primarily of young women, accompanied by a greenish-yellow skin discoloration; may be associated with deficiency in iron and protein in part caused by parasitic infections.

Chromatin   Nuclear components that stain when appropriate staining materials and techniques are employed.

Chromatoid bodies   Bar-shaped inclusions in the cytoplasm that are stained but are not a part of the nuclear material, such as chromatin.

Ciliates   Former class of protozoa that move by use of cilia (hairlike projections).

Clade   Group of related organisms that share certain genes; also refers to a genetically distinct strain of a microorganism.

Clay   Natural earthy material that is formable when wet; consist of fine earth particles and includes hydrated silicates of aluminum.

Clindomycin   Antibiotic used in the treatment of anaerobic bacteria infections but may be used to treat malaria as well as some other protozoal diseases.

Clononorchiasis   Disease resulting from infestation with a liver fluke (*Clonorchis sinensis*) from eating raw fish; invades bile ducts of the liver and may cause edema (swelling), liver enlargement (splenomegaly), and often diarrhea.

Coccidia   A sporozoan of the order Coccidia; may be parasitic in the digestive tracts of certain animals and a cause of coccidiosis.

Coccidiomycosis   Coccidiodomycosis is a disease caused by the spores of the fungus, *Coccidioides immitis*, which grows on desert mouse droppings; also called coccidiosis or San Joaquin (pronounced Wah keen) Valley fever.

Coenurus larva   *Taenia* sp. larval form that normally infect rodents; but the coenurus larvae has also been reported in Africa as infecting humans; one case reported in Texas from Mexican visitor.

Colonoscopy   Endoscopic examination of the colon and the distal part of the small bowel with a fiber optic camera.

Commensal   A term literally meaning "eating at the same table," which refers to parasitic relationships with the host; neither harms the other and one organism gains a benefit such as nutrition.

Common name   Term used to identify an organism or object that does not include the scientific name of genus and species.

Congenital   Disease existing at birth is a congenital disease; may be genetic in origin.

Conjunctivitis   Inflammation of the conjunctival membrane, or conjunctiva (mucus membrane) of the eye or eyes.

Constipation   Condition of the digestive system where a person has difficulty expelling hard feces.

Contractile vacuoles   Organelles (little organs) that pump accumulated fluids from protozoa (unicellular organisms) to regulate internal pressure.

Copecod   Small crustaceans found in the sea and most freshwater habitats; drinking water containing a copecod that is infected with a certain parasite, such as *D. meninensis*. The infective larvae from the intestine of the copecod are liberated into the body of the host, and make their way to the deep tissues.

Coplin jar   Wide-mouthed glass jars with interior walls that are grooved and are used primarily for staining slides containing blood smears or tissue sections.

Coprolites   Also known as a coprolith; is fossilized solid animal wastes that give evidence of intestinal infections, diet, etc.

Coracidium   Eggs of the tapeworm are passed generally through feces and hatch in the water; the first larval stage, the coracidium, is produced from this hatching.

...teroids Involved in a wide range of physiologic ...ns such as a response to stress, regulation of inflammation, and the immune response to infection.

Crabs Crustaceans that live in marine environments and are capable of transmitted diseases contracted from water.

Crayfish Poorly cooked crabs or crayfish provide the basic way of contracting the lung fluke *P. westermani*, primarily in parts of Asia.

Crohn's disease Inflammation of the intestine, especially the small intestine, with swelling, redness, and loss of normal bowel functions. Inflammation may be caused by the immune system attacking the body itself instead of foreign cells.

Crustaceans A small crustacean, the copecod, is a diet of fish and in this way may infect the fish with parasites which are in turn eaten by humans.

Cryotherapy Destruction of tissue by use of extremely cold temperatures.

Cryptosporidium Protozoans comprised of at least four species; waterborne parasites found in dirty ponds with run-off from areas that cattle frequent; also found frequently in immunosuppressed individuals, such as people with AIDS; chlorination does not alleviate the contamination; large outbreaks sometimes occur where public water system is contaminated with sewage.

CT-scans Computerized tomography (CT) combines a series of X-ray views from various angles to produce cross-sections of the bones and soft tissues inside the body.

Culex Genus of mosquito important as a vector for important disease organisms that include the West Nile virus, various microfilaria, Japanese and St. Louis encephalitis, as well as avian malaria.

Cutaneous larva Skin disease in humans that is caused by larvae of some nematode parasites; migrans most common organism is that of *Ancylostoma braziliense* in North and South America.

Cyclophyllidean Cyclophyllidea is the order for the tapeworms (cyclophyllidean) that includes the most important cestode parasites of both humans and domesticated animals.

Cyclops Copecod that is implicated in the transmission of *D. medinensis* organism contracted by drinking water containing a copecod called a *Cyclops*.

Cyclosporiasis Infection with the protozoan *Cyclospora cayetanensis*, a pathogen transmitted by fecal matter or feces-contaminated fresh produce and water.

Cyst Also means "bladder" or open cyst; may also be a sack that encloses an organism during a dormant period, such as in the case of certain parasites that would be destroyed in the stomach acid if not encysted.

Cyst form A stage of a protozoan that is nonmotile and is surrounded by a protective wall; stage that is readily transmitted to new hosts; the trophozoite stage is motile but the organism may be transformed between these two stages (cyst and trophozoite) readily.

Cysticercus Refers to the larval form of a tapeworm, consisting of a single scolex that is enclosed in a bladder-like cyst which is also called a hydatid cyst.

Cysticercosis Infection with cysticerci in tissues of the body that include subcutaneous, muscle, or central nervous system tissues.

Cytoplasm The part of the cell not including the membrane and the nucleus; the cytoplasmic appearance may be smooth, rough, or with inclusions, etc.

Cytoplasmic granules Ingested cells and materials, organelles, secretory inclusions such as enzymes, proteins and acids, nutrient inclusions (glycogen, lipids), pigmented granules.

Cytostome Mouth-like opening of certain protozoa (the term *stoma* means "mouth."

Cytotoxicity Cellular immunity where natural killer (NK) cells attack invading organisms; certain chemicals are also cytotoxic, such as medications for eradicating parasites.

D

Daughter forms The process of mitosis produces two genetically identical cells to that of the parent cell, containing the same type and numbers of chromosomes.

Dead-end hosts Organisms termed as *dead-end hosts* are those from which infectious agents are not transmittable to other susceptible hosts (maybe accidental hosts).

Deer flies Genus for a biting fly that transmits parasitic diseases to humans and animals.

Deer fly fever Highly infectious disease of rodents, in particular squirrels and rabbits, that may be transmitted to humans by ticks or flies or by handling infected animals.

Deer tick Includes several ticks of the genus Ixodes that are parasitic for deer and other herd animals; ticks transmit infectious organisms of febrile diseases.

DEET Abbreviation for diethyltoluamide, an extremely effective insect repellent useful in protection from vectors of parasites.

Defecate Act of elimination of solid waste products from the body.

Definitive host This is the organism in which a parasite passes its adult and sexual stages of existence.

Dehydration A condition that occurs when a body contains less fluid than is adequate; can result from illness, weather conditions to which exposed, inadequate intake, and certain medications that cause loss of body fluids.

Dermacentor A genus of tick (*D. andersoni* and *D. variabilis*) belonging to the order Acarina and family Ixodidae.

Dermatitis Inflammatory skin rash usually accompanied by redness and itching.

Desiccated To dry out thoroughly; commonly used in laboratories as a freeze-dry process to preserve specimens and control samples.

Deworming Procedure for ridding an animal of worms.

Diagnostic stage The stage of development where an organism is most easily identified; (i.e., cyst or trophozoite), larvae or ova.

Diarrhea Extreme loss of fluids through frequent defecation of watery feces; often related to infectious process including certain parasitic infections.

Digenetic Reproductive functions include two stages of multiplication, one sexual in the mature forms and the other asexual in the larval stages.

Dioecious Presence of separate individuals that possess either male or female sexual characteristics relating to organisms.

Direct tests Procedure that tests for the actual organism or antigen, rather than antibodies formed against the particular organism.

Dissected The prefix *dis-* means to separate into parts and *-sect* means to separate and to cut. Quite often the word is mispronounced as di'sect, which would merely mean "to cut into only two parts, as in bisect" (dis·sect/, dĭ-sekt').

Disseminated Term meaning that a condition is spread over a large area of the body.

Dorsoventrally Refers to the back and the belly surfaces of the body and passing from the back to the belly surface.

Dracunculiasis Infection with a genus of nematode parasites, including *Dracunculus medinensis* (guinea worm), a threadlike worm, widely spread over India, Africa, and Arabia; burrows into subcutaneous and intermuscular tissues of humans and other animals, particularly the lower limbs, causing dramatic swelling (elephantiasis).

Duckworms Common term for intestinal trematodes common in a number of areas including coastal New Jersey where duck and other water fowl that are infected may contaminate the water and infect humans.

Duodenal fluid Both fresh liquid stool specimens and duodenal aspirates (fluid in the aspirates duodenum of the intestine) may yield trophozoites of *Giardia lamblia* or the antigens of the organism.

Duodenum First and shortest segment (approximately 1 foot long) of the small intestine originating from the pylorus of the stomach.

Dysentery Diarrhea that contains blood and mucus, and originates with extreme inflammation of the intestines.

E

Echinococcosis Infection with an *Echinococcus* organisms (tapeworm).

Ectoparasites Lice and mites that live outside the human body.

Ectoplasm The outermost layer of the protoplasm of animal cells.

Edema Swelling or accumulation of fluids in a region of the body; may be generalized.

EDTA Anticoagulant to prevent blood from clotting; preserves morphology of RBCs.

Ehrlichiosis Caused by a bacterium of the family called Rickettsiae, which causes significant numbers of serious diseases around the world. These diseases include Rocky Mountain spotted fever and typhus, and all are spread by the bites of ticks, mites, and fleas. There are two types in the United States called human monocytic ehrlichiosis (HME) and human granulocytic ehrlichiosis (HE).

Elephantiasis Grotesque swelling of lower limbs and genitals as a result of *D. medinensis* infection (guinea worm).

Ellipsoidal Elongated circle with three planes that are based on three coordinate axes.

Emaciation Term describes the substantial loss of fat and other tissue, causing the organism to appear extremely thin.

Embryonated eggs Female parasite deposits embryonated eggs as a prelarval stage, giving rise to microfilaria which grow into an infective stage that are generally passed to others through the bites of insects.

Embryos This is the term for the developing young of a living organism and is the young stage of development. From the moment of fertilization the zygote that will eventually become the offspring is undergoing a period of rapid growth.

Empyema Fluid gathered in the thoracic cavity between the lungs and the chest wall.

Encapsulated Confined in or surrounded by a capsule or a membranous sac.

Encapsulated zygote An encysted or encapsulate zygote of a sporozoan protozoan is called an oocyst protozoa, which develops into a sporozoite or a sporocyst that contains a number of sporozoites.

Encephalitis Inflammation of the lining of the central nervous system.

Encystation Transformation into a cyst from a trophozoite.

Endemic The term means that a specific illness occurs with predictable regularity in a specific geographic region or in a population group.

Endoparasites Group of parasites that inhabit the atria and organs inside the host's body.

Endoplasm The central cytoplasmic fluid of a cell as separate from the ectoplasm.

Endoplasmic reticulum Endoplasmic reticulum (ER) involves organelles that form a network of tubules, vesicles, and storage areas within the reticulum.

Endosome In a eukaryotic cell which has an organized nucleus, an endosome is a membrane-bound compartment in the cytoplasm.

Enterocytes These cells are simple columnar epithelial cells for absorption that are found within the small intestines and the colon.

Eosinophilia Condition of an increase above approximately 3 percent in the white blood cells called *eosinophils*; often related to immune reactions such as those found in allergic conditions and parasitic infections where the tissue is invaded by the parasitic organisms.

Eosinophilic enteritis Inflammation of the intestines, which includes colitis, **eosinophilic enteritis**, celiac disease, other malabsorptive disease, lactase deficiency, and obesity.

Epidemiological surveillance Often conducted by governmental agencies and universities, where gathering and analyzing data related to disease states, drawing inferences, and interpreting the data derived, its significance and the distribution of important epidemiologic.

Epigastric Upper central region of the abdomen just under the sternum.

Epsom salts May be used as a purgative to aid in eliminating toxins and parasites following administration of parasiticidal medications.

Erythema chronicum Expanding red rash found in acute infections with Lyme disease agents and is in migrans response to the actual skin infection with the Lyme bacteria.

Erythematous rash Redness and eruption of the skin caused by dilatation and congestion of the capillaries that are often a sign of inflammation or infection.

Esophagus Muscular tube that carries food and liquids from the mouth to the stomach.

Ether and formalin Used in the formalin-ethyl ether sedimentation procedure for the detection of parasites and their eggs.

Ethyl acetate Ethyl acetate for safety has replaced ether for some procedures as this compound is quite flammable and explosive. The procedure using this chemical is primarily for the routine recovery of protozoan cysts, helminth larvae, and ova (including operculate and schistosoma eggs) but is not as useful for other organisms.

Etiologic agent The organism or microorganism that is responsible for causing a disease.

Eukaryotic Condition where the nucleus is organized and enclosed within a membrane.

Excystation "Hatching" of a cyst, which becomes metacystic trophozoites.

F

Febrile A condition characterized by a clinically significant rise in the body temperature.

Fecal-oral route Refers to handling or coming in contact with objects or food materials that have become contaminated by feces and are transferred to the mouth by hand or some other mechanical means.

Feces Solid waste material.

Feline Refers to members of the cat family.

Fertilized An ovum is fertilized where there is a fusion of gametes to produce a new organism. In animals, the process involves a sperm fusing with an ovum.

Fibrils Threadlike fiber or filamentous appendages such as a myofibril or neurofibril as a component of a cell or a parasitic organism.

Filariasis Condition where a chronic disease is present due to filaria or microfilaria.

Filariform infective *Strongyloides stercoralis* is an example of the roundworm that stage larvae lives in soil. The larvae have two stages in their life cycle: a rod-shaped (rhabdoid) first stage, which is not infective; and in the second stage the threadlike (filariform) larvae can penetrate intact human skin and even internal organs.

Flagellates Protozoa with long hairlike tails (flagella) that provide locomotion.

Flame cell Specialized excretory cell that performs functions similar to a kidney; found in many freshwater invertebrates such as nematodes, flatworms, platyhelminthes, and rotifers.

Flatulence Excessive gases in the stomach and intestines.

Flatworm Belong to the phylum Platyhelminthes.

Fleas Ectoparasites that are wingless and have stout legs for jumping. Fleas are generally parasitic for warm-blooded animals, particularly those that have hair. Fleas are capable of transmitting parasitic infections such as tularemia, typhus, and brucellosis. Fleas that are swallowed by animals and humans may also be infected by cat and dog tapeworms and may infect other animals and humans.

Flotation method A common method used to recover the eggs of parasites and oocysts is that of a flotation technique. This procedure relies on the differences in the specific gravity of the eggs that are contained in fecal specimens, where the eggs float and the fecal material is found on the bottom of the tube used for the test.

Fluke Parasitic worm of the trematode class.

Fly disease of hunters Hunters may be exposed to ill animals with epizootic hemorrhagic disease or bluetongue virus that are spread by a small, biting midge fly.

Folic acid Used to treat certain types of anemias, including those as a result of parasitosis.

Fomites Equipment or substances to which organisms cling and are able to transmit disease to those in contact with these items.

Fork-tailed cercariae Dermatitis caused by schistosomes may be called "swimmer's itch" and occurs in water when the skin is penetrated by a free-swimming, fork-tailed infective cercaria, which originate in a snail host.

Formalin Preservative for biological specimens and may be combined with other chemicals to achieve a more desirable result.

Fossilized Preserved remains or traces of animals, plants, and other organisms; ancient specimens may have had organic material replaced by minerals such as silicon or calcium.

Free-living Term refers to an organism with the ability to act or function independently outside a host.

Fulminant colitis Rapid and sudden onset of inflammation of the colon.

G

Gametocytes Malarial stage in life cycle of the genus Plasmodium which reproduces in the blood of the *Anopheles* mosquito.

Gelatin capsule Device attached to a string which is swallowed into the gastrointestinal tract upon which parasites may adhere.

"Germ of laziness" Term applied to those suffering from the effects of hookworm infection, such as accompanying anemia and malnourishment.

Giardiasis Condition of a victim who suffers from an intestinal infection by *Giardia lamblia*.

Giemsa stain Hematologic stain useful in demonstrating morphology of blood parasites.

Glandular Generally used for diseases that relate to, affect, or resemble a gland.

Glycogen vacuole Glycogen is similar to starch and will stain with a variety of stains; this is a food storage vacuole found in certain amoebae; humans also store glycogen in tissues and organs to be used as energy sources.

Golgi apparatus Series of curved and parallel sacs that may concentrate products for the secretory cells; in other cells their function is not completely understood.

Golgi complex   Termed the "export complex" with unique proteins that seem specialized for information flow to and from ER (endoplasmic reticulum) and the Golgi complex.

Gomori stain   The stain provides for a permanent stained smear that enhances detection and identification of cysts and trophozoites where a permanent record of the protozoa is required.

Graft rejection   Immunologic destruction of transplanted organs or tissues that is based on both cellular and humoral (antibody-mediated) reactions.

Graft vs. host reaction   The T-lymphocytes of the donor's tissues or bone marrow may recognize the recipient's body tissues as non-self and when this occurs, the transplanted bone marrow cells attack the transplant recipient's body.

Gram negative bacteria   Stain that differentiates between two broad groups of bacteria. The Gram-positive organisms retain the crystal violet portion of the stain while the Gram-negative organisms retain the red-colored counter stain comprised of safranin.

Granular   Granular material is described as a conglomeration of discrete solid, macroscopic particles giving an inconsistency to the homogeneity of the material.

Granulocytes   White cells that arise from a myeloid stem cell, and include neutrophilic segmented or polymorphonuclear cells, eosiniphils and basophils; neutrophilic WBC's may engulf bacterial organisms and destroy them by lytic processes; eosinophils play a major role in the killing of parasites, particularly for enteric nematodes as their granules contain a unique, toxic basic protein and a cationic protein.

Granulomatous lesions   A group of inherited diseases where certain cells of the immune system have difficulty forming the reactive oxygen compounds through oxidative or "respiratory burst" activity required to kill certain ingested pathogens.

Gravid proglottids   Gravid proglottids from tapeworms encompass egg capsules and when they break free they pass out in the feces and then release the egg capsules.

Ground itch   An itching sensation caused by the penetrating and burrowing into the skin of larvae of hookworms *Ancylostoma duodenale* or *Necator americanus*.

Guillain-Barre syndrome   Neurological disease following acute infection with *Campylobacter jejuni*, cytomegalovirus or Epstein-Barr virus that is rare; ascending paralysis of the motor functions and progresses to the respiratory muscles; some residual damage may remain after disease is resolved.

Guinea worm   Refers to the filarial form of *Dracunculus medinensis*.

Gundi   Small, stocky rodents that live in rocky deserts across northern Africa as important reservoirs of leishmania.

H

Habitat   Geographic location where organisms may dwell.

Hard tick   The hard ticks are those that transmit the most pathogens; these ticks have a hard shield or scutum on the back and mouth parts that project from the head. The families of Ixodidae, Amblyomma, Bophilus, and Dermacentor, and several other less important vectors are all hard ticks.

Heartworms   A heartworm is a parasitic roundworm (*Dirofilaria immitis*) infecting dogs, but other canids particularly and rarely humans may be infected. The disease is spread from host to host through the bites of mosquitoes.

Helminthiases   Condition of being infected by flatworms (platyhelminthes).

Helminthology   Study of parasitic and other worms.

Helminths   A wormlike animal belonging to the phyla Platyhelminthes (flatworms).

Hemaphroditic   An animal or plant that possesses both male female reproductive organs.

Hematuria   Presence of blood in the urine.

Hemiptera   Several insects of the order Hemiptera possessing biting or sucking mouthparts and two pairs of wings. Hemipterans include the leafhoppers, treehoppers, cicadas, aphids, scales, and true bugs.

Hemoflagellates   A flagellated protozoan that inhabits the blood; most important hemoflagellates are the genera *Trypanosoma* (malaria) and *Leishmania*.

Hemorrhage   Literally means "bursting forth" as in the act of bleeding copious amounts.

Hemorrhagic pancreatitis   Pancreas inflamed to such an extent that bleeding occurs, possibly resulting in massive, difficult-to-control bleeding.

Hepatitis B   Liver infection caused by the hepatitis B virus (HBV) that may become chronic and lead to liver failure, cancer, and cirrhosis.

Hepatomegaly   Enlargement of the liver.

Herbivore   Grazing animals that predominantly eat grass and other vegetation.

Hippocratic Oath   Oath exacted of the students of Hippocrates for student physicians; historically one of the oldest documents outlining expectations of a professional. The oath basically requires treatment of the sick to the best of one's ability, preservation of patient privacy, and teaching of medicine to the next generation. The oath has been modified several times from the original document.

Hirudinea   Class of parasitic or predatory annelid (segmented) worms with 34 annelids or rings around them; the common name is *leech* and the organism uses terminal suckers for both attachment to its prey and for locomotion.

Hookworm larvae   The means of infectivity for hookworms is through the larvae found in the soil that are able to penetrate the skin; hookworm eggs are not infective.

Host   Organism from which nutrients are obtained for the parasite, and is part of the parasite's life cycle.

Human granulocytic ehrlichiosis (HGE)   Rare infectious disease caused by a genus of bacteria that belongs to the Ehrlichia family. The bacterium is carried and transmitted by certain ticks, namely the deer tick (*Ixodes dammini*) and the American dog tick (*Dermacentor variabilis*).

Human hydatid disease   The larval stage of the dog tapeworm *Echinococcus granulosus* is responsible for hydatid disease in humans; acquired from animals through ingestion of tapeworm eggs excreted in the feces of infected dogs.

Human Immuno-deficiency Virus (HIV)   A retrovirus that can cause acquired immunodeficiency syndrome (AIDS).

Human monocytic ehrlichiosis (HME) Three tick-borne diseases caused by the intracellular bacteria of the genus *Ehrlichia* have been described. Human monocytic ehrlichiosis (HME) was first identified in 1986 and is caused by *Ehrlichia chaffeensis*.

Hyaline shell Clear, translucent covering of a cyst.

Hydatid larva (cyst) Cyst in the tissues, especially the liver where development of the larvae of the dog tapeworm has been encysted; may grow for years to extremely large size.

Hydatid sand Term for the hydatid cyst caused by *Echinococcus granulosus*, where a floating membrane or cyst may contain possibly up to 400,000 protoscolices per milliliter of fluid.

Hydatiform Fluid-filled cyst that forms most often when an individual is infected by a tapeworm such as in the disease of echinococcosis.

Hypersensitivity reactions The term refers to an excessive reaction to an allergen (antigen), which includes parasitic organisms; severity ranges from a mild reaction to severe systemic reactions leading to anaphylactic shock and shut down or damage to systems of the body.

Hypostome Hardened and sharp harpoon-like structure found in the mouth area of some certain parasitic insects that includes ticks and mites. The structure enables the ectoparasite to maintain a firm grip while withdrawing blood from its victim. This mechanism is the reason for the difficulty in removing ticks, during which the head is often left attached when the body is removed.

I

IgE One of the immunoglobulin classes of antibodies is that of IgE (immunoglobulin E). These antibodies are found in high concentrations in various tissue spaces and are chiefly involved in ridding the body of intestinal parasites as well as reacting to allergic conditions.

Immunocompetent An immunocompetent individual possesses the ability for the body to react normally in an immune response to allergens.

Immunocompromised Refers to the inability to develop a normal and limited immune response, appropriate for the situation, which may be due to conditions of disease, malnutrition, age, or immunosuppressive medications.

Immunodeficient Being immunodeficient may relate to cellular (white blood cell reactions) or humoral (production of antibodies against the offending antigen) that results in an impaired immune response; a number of conditions predispose one to infections and certain malignancies.

Immunoglobulin Refers to five classes of immune globulins that are gamma globulin proteins found in the blood, body fluids, and tissues of vertebrates as antibodies. The immune system uses these antibodies to aid in identifications of and neutralization of foreign bodies such as parasites, bacteria, and viruses.

Immunosuppressive Drugs or other agents may be immunosuppressive that inhibit or prevent activity of the immune system. Steroidal use is a prime example of immunosuppressive drugs.

Incidental host Incidental hosts may also be referred to as accidental; this means that the food source may be the primary host that is infected, but then is ingested by the accidental host and therefore infected.

Incysting To enclose or become enclosed in a cyst.

Indirect test Testing for the evidence of an organism rather than for the organism itself, for example, antibodies toward a parasite is an indirect test in which the parasite itself was not found. Several of these are performed as indirect fluorescent antibody tests for parasitic diseases such as for toxoplasmosis and malarial infections.

Infection Growth of microorganisms inside the body.

Infectious jaundice Jaundice is caused by excessive destruction of RBCs. It occurs from infections by bacteria or viruses, and in particular the parasite responsible for malaria.

Infective stage Certain stages in a parasite's life cycle are infective; in some, the larval form is infective, in others the eggs may be infective, and for various others, spores are the infective stage. For some organisms, there is only one stage and that is the infective stage.

Infestation Growth of organisms on the body's surface.

Insect repellent Agent that discourages the presence of insects but does not kill them. DEET is the most well-known of these repellents.

Insects Any members of the six-legged class within the arthropods that have a hard exoskeleton, three-part body, compound eyes and two antennae that distinguish them from spiders and other arachnids.

Integument Commonly refers to a covering that may include various layers and their appendages or investment and most often refers to the covering of the body as the skin.

Intermediate host An organism in which a part of the life cycle of the parasite is spent while undergoing morphological changes, before it infects a definitive host.

Intestinal coccidian A common intestinal coccidian infecting humans is that of *I.belli*. This organism causes a self-limiting diarrhea in healthy individuals and a chronic disease in those who are immunocompromised due to underlying medical conditions or infectious diseases.

Intestinal fluke These organisms are transmitted by humans and pigs primarily in Asia. *Fasciolopsis buski* is the most common and is called the giant intestinal fluke.

Intestinal lumen A cavity or channel within a tube such as the intestines is the lumen. The lumen may become constricted in a variety of intestinal conditions.

Intracellular Refers to a condition within the cellular membrane of the cell.

Intra-erythrocytic Refers to a condition in which organisms or inclusions are contained within the membrane of the RBC. A common intra-erythrocytic parasite is that of the *Plasmodium* genus responsible for malaria.

Intraperitoneal Refers to the abdominal cavity and digestive organs of vertebrates.

Intrapleural In humans as well as other vertebrates, the pleural cavity refers to the body cavity that surrounds the lungs.

Intrauterine Refers to "within the uterus" or womb.

Iron deficiency Refers to a condition where insufficient iron in the correct form is available for the body's needs, particularly for hematopoiesis (manufacture of RBCs).

Iron supplements   Vitamins that contain iron in a form used by the body; often necessary for certain medical conditions where anemia is primary or is the result of another disease process.

Iron-hematoxylin stain   Type of stain used to differentiate the internal morphology of cells and organisms, to include parasites.

Itch mite   An extremely small parasitic arthropod (insect) which is most commonly. *Sarcoptes scabiei* burrows into the skin of humans and causes a condition called scabies or one type of mange in dogs or cats.

Ixodidae   This term refers to a family of ticks called "hard-bodied ticks" and are important vectors of many tick-borne diseases.

J

Jaundice   A yellowing condition of the skin caused by destruction of RBCs. This condition may originate from an infectious process by bacteria, viruses, or parasites such as those that may be intraerythrocytic.

Jejunum   Refers to the middle portion of the small intestine, between the duodenum and the ileum.

Jigger   The name given to any of several species of small red mites (includes *Tetranychus irritans* and *T. americanus*) which can penetrate beneath the skin of humans and a number of animals, and found mostly in the southern part of the United States.

Joint myalgia   Myalgia literally means "muscle pain" and is a symptom of many diseases and disorders, but is called "joint myalgia" when the pain is associated with a joint, where a muscle may be attached.

K

Karyosome   A body included in the chromatin of the nucleus that usually stains a darker color than the remainder of the nucleus; varying appearances useful in identifying some amoebae.

Katayama disease   The disease referred to *Schistosoma japonicum*.

Kinetoplast   Small mass that stains darkly and is the base of the flagellum; provides movement to the flagella.

Kleptoparasitism   Parasitism by theft in a literal sense. Kleptoparasites take over food sources from their hosts without providing any advantage to the host.

L

Laboratory diagnosis   Refers to the conducting of laboratory tests to diagnose or to confirm a diagnosis made by other means.

Larvae   Demonstrate a distinct juvenile form as a stage of metamorphosis into adults.

Leech   Refers mostly to a bloodsucking aquatic worm or sometimes a terrestrial worm (similar to an earthworm) of the class Hirudinea; certain freshwater species were once in wide use in medicine for bloodletting, supposedly to cure a variety of diseases.

Leishmaniasis   Infection caused by a flagellate protozoan of one of the infective species of the genus Leishmania, normally transmitted to humans or animals chiefly by flies; causes a disease with two distinctive ulcerative skin diseases.

Leukocytes   White blood cells.

Leukopenia   Low numbers of white blood cells.

Lice   Extremely small (1 mm or less) wingless insects of the order Anoplura; some of these are parasitic on humans and other mammals and some infest mostly birds; having sucking mouthparts; examples include the body or head louse, *Pediculus humanus*, and *Phthirius pubis*, which is commonly called the crab or pubic louse.

Lindane   One of the medications used to treat scabies, head lice, and crabs is lindane.

Liver abscesses   Ranges from bacterial infections with pus generated from the site, to hepatic amebiasis; the amebic liver abscess is a collection of pus in the liver caused by an intestinal parasite, often by *Entamoeba histolytica*, the same organism that causes amebiasis, an intestinal amoebal infection. The organism is transported through the circulatory system from the intestines to the liver.

Liver fluke   A trematode, *Faciola hepatica*, from the phylum Platyhelminthes. Liver fluke adults are found in human livers and various other mammals. They feed on blood and produce eggs which are passed into the intestine.

Loa loa   Also known as *Loa loa* filariasis and several regional and local names. Tropical swelling and African eyeworm is commonly heard for a skin and eye disease caused by the nematode worm. Humans contract the infection through the bite of deer or mango fly vectors after which the adult filarial worm migrates through the subcutaneous tissues of humans.

Loamy soil   Composed of a mixture of sand and silt, and is perhaps the best soil for agricultural uses; frequently contaminated by hookworm larvae.

Lone star tick   The *Amblyomma americanum*, or lone star tick, is widespread in the United States, covering an area from Texas north to Iowa in the Midwest east to the Atlantic, and as far north as Maine. The female tick has a white spot on its back resembling a star. As are most ticks, it is found mostly at the edge of wooded areas and especially in forests with thick underbrush. The lone star tick is a vector for several parasitic pathogens, but is best known as a transmitter of human granulocytic ehrlichiosis (HGE).

Louse   Singular form for lice.

Lugol's iodine   First made in 1829; is a solution of elemental iodine and potassium iodide dissolved in water. It has had a variety of uses since first being formulated, including treatment for hypothyroidism and for making dirty water potable. In parasitology and bacteriology, it is used primarily for staining starch structures in parasites and in bacteria, and is a component of the common Gram stain used for staining bacteria.

Lung fluke   Parasite known as the lung fluke; is a parasitic flatworm of the species *Paragonimus westermani*. It is prevalent throughout Africa, Asia, and Latin America, but rarely in North America.

Lyme disease   Caused by the spirochete bacterium *Borrelia burgdorferi*. A certain tick (of the genus *Ixodes* in the majority of cases in the United States) carry these organisms. The disease was originally identified in Old Lyme, CT, but is now found in most parts of the United States. There are three stages of Lyme disease, that of primary, secondary, and tertiary.

Lymph nodes   Small kidney-shaped enlargements of lymphoid tissue that lie along the lymphatic vessels; lymph nodes are linked by lymphatic vessels and are found throughout the body. They function as filters for foreign materials such as organisms and contain WBC's that use oxygen to destroy invasive organisms

Lymphadenopathy   Activation of lymphocytes and other phagocytic white blood cells may cause an engorgement of the lymph system, resulting in lymph nodes that are noticeably larger and perhaps harder. Many infectious diseases cause lymphadenopathy, but in addition rheumatoid arthritis, sarcoidosis, and a number of less common diseases may result in lymphadenopathy.

Lymphatic filariasis   Refers to infections by worms of *Wuchereria bancrofti*, *Brugia malayi*, and *Brugia timori*. These worms invade the lymphatic system, including the lymph nodes and sometimes result in a disease called *elephantiasis*, due to the grotesquely large limbs of its victims.

Lymphatic varices   Dilated submucosal veins that occur in various parts of the body such as the stomach and the exophagus, as well as in diseases of veins, lymphatic vessels and lymph nodes.

Lymphocytes   White blood cell that is responsible for much of the immune response. Lymphocytes are found primarily in the lymph system, with a small percentage found in the circulating blood. Lymphocytes are divided into T-cells, B-cells, and natural killer (NK) cells.

M

Macrogametes   In heterogamous reproduction, where both male and female gametes exist, the larger and usually female of a pair of conjugating gametes is called the macrogamete.

Macronucleus   Found in eukaryocytes where the nucleus is organized into one large structure and is surrounded by a nuclear membrane (prokaryocytes, as are most bacteria, lack the organized nucleus surrounded by a nucleus).

Macrophages   Refers to a white cell called a monocyte that has left the vascular system and has matured (becomes much larger) in tissues of the body such as the spleen, tonsils, alveoli of the lungs, lymph nodes, and the liver (Kuppfer cells) as well as many other tissue types, including that of the central nervous system (microglia).

Mad cow disease   Disease caused by a subviral particle (i.e., prion), and is known variously as mad cow disease (bovine spongiform encephalopathy or BSE), scrapie, or Creutzfeldt-Jakob disease.

Malaise   A nonspecific and generalized feeling of discomfort, illness, or lack of well-being. The symptom can occur with almost any major disease condition.

Malaria   A hemolytic disease characterized by periods of fever based on species of malaria infecting the victim; four species of the genus *Plasmodium* infect humans, with differing geographic locations, incubation times, fever cycles, symptoms, and manner of treatment.

Malarial stippling   This is a useful method for a rapid and presumptive identification of the species of malarial parasites.

Malignant disorders   Conditions are capable of invading into adjacent tissues, and are frequently capable of spreading to widespread tissues.

Malnutrition   General term for a medical condition resulting from insufficient diet but is caused by a number of malfunctions of the body as well as low intake of nutrients. Causes other than insufficient consumption relate to poor absorption or excessive loss of nutrients, which often occurs in parasitosis.

Maltese cross forms   When a stained blood film shows a Maltese cross form for an organism, this may be presumptively diagnostic of babesiosis and will differentiate between babesiosis and malaria.

Mammillated   Refers to a structure, organism, or cell that has relatively small protrusions from the exterior that occur primarily on the surface.

Mandibles   Lower jaw of a vertebrate animal is the most common use, but biting insect mandibles are a pair of appendages near the insect's mouth.

Mange   Term for a persistent and contagious skin disease caused chiefly by sarcoptic mites for some types of the disease. They generally infect domestic animals including dogs but are capable of affecting humans.

Maturation   Process of reaching full development and size as a growth process.

Mature proglottids   Segments of the tapeworm, those closest to the scolex, that have matured to the point that they are capable of producing eggs.

Meningitis   Inflammation of the membranes (arachnoid, pia, and dura mater) of the central nervous system; may be as result of bacterial, viral, amoebal, mycobacterial (TB or associated organisms), or fungal infection, and in some cases from chemical irritation and from toxins.

Measles   Infection of the respiratory system by a virus seldom seen due to childhood immunizations. It is caused by a virus of the genus Morbillivirus.

Meningoencephalitis   Medical condition that concurrently resembles meningitis, an infection or inflammation of the meninges surrounding the brain, and encephalitis which is an actual infection or inflammation of the brain.

Mecuric chloride   Chemical used as a fixative when the preservatives that include polyvinyl alcohol (PVA) are used.

Merozoites   In infections by *Plasmodium* spp., chiefly, a breaking up of schizonts in the asexual reproductive process, merozoites are freed and invade other red blood cells, where they again undergo schizogony or develop into gametocytes (for sexual reproduction by union of two gametocytes).

Mesenteric veins   Blood vessel that drains blood from the small intestine (jejunum and ileum).

Metacercaria   Encysted stage of the life cycle of a trematode (flatworm) which occurs in an intermediate host and then infects the definitive host.

Metastasis   Change in location of a disease by movement of bacteria or diseased body cells to another location.

Metazoan   This form of life is multicellular, in comparison with the protozoan, a one-celled organism.

Methylene blue   This dye is used in a variety of staining procedures for bacteria, cells, and parasites.

Microcrustacean copecods   Copepods are a group of small crustaceans found in the sea and nearly every freshwater habitat. These organisms are the hosts for certain stages of parasitic development, and when eaten by fish are able to transmit the organisms to others.

Microfilaria   Immature form of the filarial worm.

Microgametes   The male version of the gamete for conjugation in the protozoa, specifically in the *Plasmodium* spp. reproductive process.

Microgametocytes   The gametocytes for the male reproductive structure is the microgametocyte and the larger, the female macrogametocyte, are ingested by an *Anopheles* mosquito during a blood meal.

Microsporidia   Once thought to be protists, the microsporidia are now known to be fungi and constitute a phylum of spore-forming unicellular parasites.

Microvilli   Refers to an increase in the exposed surface of a living organism or cell by the presence of hair, pilli, or folds that increase surface area.

Miracidia   Larvae that are free-swimming and that arise from a digenetic fluke (undergoes either sexual and asexual reproduction alternately). After leaving the egg, it infects a particular species of snail and becomes a sprorocyst.

Mites   Small arachnid, some of which are parasitic, and cause or aggravate conditions such as allergies, asthma, mange, and scabies; occasionally are intermediate hosts for certain cestodes.

Mitochondrion   A rod-shaped or oval-shaped organelle of a cell; participate in aerobic respiration of the cell.

Mode of transmission   Refers to the manner in which transmission takes place (e.g., eating poorly cooked beef containing larvae).

Mollusks   Invertebrate animals of the phylum Mollusca; found mostly in water and most often have a hard and protective outer shell. They have a muscular foot for locomotion and a well-defined circulatory and nervous system. Mollusks include gastropods that are important in parasite transmission as an intermediate host.

Molt   Term used to describe an activity related to growth or change of season, and means to cast or shed the feathers, scales, and skin.

Monogenea   Type of flatworm that lives on the outside of their host. They are not free-living and always need another creature to which to live.

Mononuclear cells   Cells that have only one nucleus, or a nonsegmented nucleus.

Mononucleosis   Acute infectious disease caused most frequently by the Epstein-Barr virus of the herpes virus group; characterized by swollen lymph nodes and elevated and abnormal presence of lymphocytes.

Morbidity   Pertains to disease states as a statistical value of the number of cases in a certain population group (often accompanied by mortality rates or the number of deaths for a given disease).

Morphology   Structure and shape of an element, such as a cell or organism.

Mortality   The condition of being mortal means a susceptibility to experience death.

Motility   Ability to move from one location to another.

Mucocutaneous   Area of the skin which contains mucus membranes.

Multicellular   This term refers to the opposite of unicellular, meaning that an organism is composed of more than one cell.

Multivesicular   The term refers to numerous small vesicles or blisters.

Mutualism   Parasitic relationship where both organisms benefit from association.

Myalgia   Refers to muscle pain.

Myeloproliferative disorders   Refers to atypical proliferation of the stem cells that provide blood production.

N

Nagana   A disease caused by *Trypanosoma brucei*, and which may affect humans, horses, and other animals; transmitted by the tsetse fly.

Nemanthelminthes   Refers to roundworms, organisms of the phylum Nemanthelminthes.

Nematodes   Refers to the parasites that are roundworms.

Neorickettsia   This strain includes species that are coccoid or pleomorphic cells found in cytoplasmic vacuoles within monocytes and macrophages of dogs, horses, bats, and humans.

Nephrosis   The condition is also called nephrotic syndrome or nephropathy, and is a kidney disease characterized by degenerative lesions of the renal tubules.

Neurocysticercosis   Cysticercosis, which is also called neurocysticercosis, is the most common parasitic infestation of the central nervous system worldwide.

Neutrophils   White blood cell with a segmented nucleus; responds primarily to bacterial infections.

NHANES   National Health and Nutrition Examination Survey.

Nit   The egg of a louse or other parasitic insect; often visible when head or body lice lay eggs on a hair shaft.

Norwegian scabies   A strain of scabies; a contagious ectoparasite skin infection characterized by superficial burrows and intense pruritus (itching), that is characterized by larger number of organisms than for other strains of the mite.

Nucleus or nuclei   Structure(s) normally at the center of a cell that contains the chromosomes with DNA and RNA and is/are responsible for the cellular metabolism, growth, excretion, and production.

Nymphs Stage of development for a variety of insects; the nymph is an immature form of some invertebrates, particularly insects, which undergoes gradual metamorphosis (hemimetabolism) before reaching maturity.

Nymphal tick stage Immature stage of the tick, where the organism are small; for some species the nymphal stage may also be an infective stage.

O

O & P examination Procedure for determining the presence of either the ova (eggs) of a parasite or the parasite itself.

Obligate Term for an absolute need or necessity for a material or condition.

Occult filariasis An infection in which microfilariae are not observed in the blood, although they may be found in other body fluids.

Ocular micrometer The device enables the measurement of the size of magnified objects. Has a ruled scale etched into a glass disk that fits in a microscope eyepiece.

Oculoglandular Enlargement of the lymph node around the eye and in many cases is accompanied by conjunctivitis.

Ohara's fever The disease is also known as or related to deerfly fever or tularemia and is caused by infection by the bacterium *Francisella tularensis*.

Onchocerciasis Infection by the organism *Onchocerca volvulus*, known to cause river blindness; a parasitic worm that is capable of migrating to the skin and into the eyes.

Oncosphere Tapeworm embryo with six hooks and is the earliest differentiated stage of a cyclophyllidean tapeworm also called a hexacanth embryo larval stage; the oncosphere burrows through the gut wall to reach various tissues of the host, where they develop into encysted cysticerci or bladder worms.

Oocyst Cystic form of a sporozoan (protozoan) that might or might not have a hard, resistant membrane for protection.

Oocytes Refers to a female gametocyte, cell which develops into an egg or ovum by meiosis.

Ookinete The fertilized form of the malarial parasite in a mosquito's body, formed by fertilization of a macrogamete by a microgamete.

Operculum Something resembling a lid or cover; a lid or covering is found in eggs of a pseudophyllidean tapeworm but the cyclophyllidean species do not have an operculated ovum.

Opisthorchiasis Condition in which an infection or disease has occurred due to liver flukes of the genus *Opisthorchis*.

Opportunistic Refers to a microorganism that is able to avoid immune reactions only under certain predisposing disease conditions, for example, when a person's immune system is impaired due to a variety of reasons.

Orgnelles Literally means "small organs" and refers to intracellular structures in the cytoplasm of a cell or a one-celled organism.

Oriental sore Known by a number of other names and is the most common form of leishmaniasis. It is a skin infection caused by a single-celled parasite of which there are approximately 20 different species that is transmitted by sandfly bites.

Oropharyngeal Part of the pharynx between the soft palate and the epiglottis.

Osteitis deformans Chronic bone disorder caused by an increase in the breakdown and re-growth of bone tissue.

Ovum An alternate term for egg.

P

Paget's disease Osteomalacia, or softening and bowing of the long bones; also called osteitis deformans; disease occurring chiefly in the elderly in which the bones may become enlarged and weakened in structure, often leading to a fracture or deformity.

Palaeoparasitology Study of evidence from fossils of long ago, showing evidence of parasitic infections.

Pallor Paleness and lack of normal color.

Palpitations An unusually rapid or somewhat violent beating of the heart; perhaps with ineffective pumping of blood.

Papillae Refers to small nipple-shaped projections or elevations such as those on the tongue or the small elevations at the root of a developing tooth, hair, feather projection, or elevation.

Paragonimiasis A food-borne parasitic infection caused by the lung fluke which is most frequently *Paragonimus westermani*. Human infection occurs mainly via ingestion of raw or undercooked freshwater crabs or crayfishes.

Parasitism Condition of being infected with a parasite or parasites.

Parthenogenetic A form of reproduction in which an unfertilized egg develops into a new organism; found frequently among insects and several other arthropods.

Pathogenesis The development or the source of a diseased condition.

Pathogenic Disease organisms that are capable of producing disease (i.e., bacteria, viruses, or parasites).

Pathognomonic Term often used in medicine that indicates characteristics for a particular disease.

Pediculosis Refers to an infestation of lice, the blood-feeding ectoparasitic insects.

Pelvic veins Associated with the venous system in the pelvis, the lower abdomen, and groin.

Pemphigus Any of a variety of several acute or chronic autoimmune skin diseases resulting in clusters of itching blisters, particularly on the mucus membranes.

Perianal Condition occurring in, or around, the tissues surrounding the anus.

Periodontitis Infective disease process of the gums characterized by inflammation of the tissues caused by bacteria that infect the roots of the teeth and surrounding gum crevices, sometimes by an amoebic gingivitis; produces bleeding, pus formation, gradual loss of bone and tissues that support the teeth.

Peripheral chromatin Includes genetic material of DNA and proteins that condense to form chromosomes for cell division. This chromatin is located in the nucleus of a cell.

Periportal   Near the portal vein and branches of this vein.

Peristalsis   Refers to the symmetrical contraction of smooth muscles, particularly in the intestine, which propagates in a wave down the muscular tube.

Peritoneal   The abdominal cavity and folds whose linings are composed of serous membranes.

Peritonitis   Inflammation of the layer of a membrane called *peritoneum* that lines the inside of the abdominal cavity.

Permethrin   A topical insecticide used to treat for body and head lice, their nits, scabies, and to protect against various species of ticks in the outdoors.

Petroleum jelly   Commonly called by the brand name Vaseline, petroleum jelly is a colorless-to-amber semisolid mixture of hydrocarbons obtained from petroleum and is used as a lubricant and in medicinal ointments.

Phagocytosis   Literally means "eating by cells" such as white blood cells that engulf pathogens as an immune function.

Phylogenetic   A map of the development or evolution of a organisms belonging to a particular group; studies similarities and possible common origins.

Pica   Abnormal craving for unnatural materials as part of the diet, such as white dirt or clay.

Pinocytosis   Refers to the ingestion of dissolved materials by taking in liquids through the cell membrane; also called *endocytosis*. The cytoplasmic membrane invaginates and pinches off small droplets of fluid that are retained in vesicles formed by this process.

Pinworms   Threadworms that infect mostly children; scientific name for this organism is *Enterobius vermicularis*.

Plasmodium   Genus of organism causing malaria in humans, birds, and animals.

Platyhelminths   Flatworms.

Plerocercoid   Worm-like larval forms of certain tapeworm that develop in secondary hosts.

Pneumocystosis   Infection with the *Pneumocystis carinii* (*P. jirovecii*) organism.

Pneumocystis carinii   Opportunistic organism that frequently infect those who are immunocompromised, leading to pneumonia; often a condition found in AIDS victims.

Pneumonia   An inflammation of the lungs, most often caused by infection. Bacteria, viruses, fungi, parasites, and even some chemicals can cause pneumonia.

Pneumonic form   The pneumonic form of both the plague, caused by *Yersinia pestis*, and that of anthrax, caused by *Bacillus anthracis*, have pneumonic forms of the infections, and are gravely serious conditions.

Polymerase chain reaction   Technique to amplify or increase the numbers of a single or few copies of a strand of DNA greatly, generating thousands of copies that can be used for testing and for incorporating into other organisms.

Polymorphic nucleus   Indicates a nucleus that may appear as segments such as in the polymorphonuclear leukocyte or the segmented neutrophil.

Polyvinyl alcohol (PVA)   Used in a number of applications including a broad-use adhesive and as a water-absorbent substrate which when incorporated with mercuric chloride is used as a fixative for cell and parasite preparations for microscopic examination.

Pores   Refers to small channels or tiny openings that may be microscopic, as in plant leaves, skin and the cell membranes, and walls of other organisms such as parasites and bacteria, through which fluids may be absorbed or eliminated.

Pork tapeworm   *Taenia solium* infects the intestine and is contracted through eating raw or poorly cooked and contaminated pork, and less often from beef or freshwater fish.

Portal of entry   Break in the natural immunity such as the protective skin, giving organism an avenue into the tissues of the body.

Precystic form   A trophozoite (motile form) stage often found just before complete encystations.

Prions   A microscopic protein particle that is subviral (less than a virus) and lacking nucleic acid from which DNA is built, is thought to be an infectious agent for mad-cow disease as well as perhaps for certain other diseases.

Procercoid   Refers to the first stage in the aquatic life cycle of certain tapeworms where the elongate larval stage of some tapeworms develop in the body of a freshwater crustacean called the copepod.

Proglottids   Segments of the cestode (tapeworm) that are capable of forming eggs and breaking off to infect other areas.

Progressive pernicious anemia   Seriously grave blood disease resulting in a continuing, devastating decrease in the number of erythrocytes and accompanying fatty degeneration of the various tissues; commonly the victim exhibits a lemon-yellowish discoloration of the skin.

Promastigotes   Amistigotes undergo changes to become flagellated forms called promastigotes, an infective stage.

Prophylactic   Preventive measure to avoid infection primarily.

Prostatic secretions   Prostatic secretions are expressed from the glands of males and the secretions are tested for evidence of inflammation or infection by various microorganisms.

Protein deficiency   Often related to hookworm infections, where poor nutrition as well as loss of nutrition to the parasites lead to anemia and protein deficiency states, which results in emaciation and wasting.

Protista   This is a division under Kingdom Protoctista and Protoctista; eukaryotic one-celled living organisms as differentiated from multicellular plants and animals that includes many of the parasitic protozoa.

Protoscolices   One large cyst resulting from *E. granulosus* infection may contain tens of thousands of protoscolices which, after ingestion, the protoscolices attach to the intestinal mucosa where they develop into adult stages.

Protozoa   Member of Kingdom Protoctista and Protoctista, Division of Protista; includes unicellular animal-like organisms.

Pruritis   Itching, burning, and sometimes tingling of the skin.

Pseudomembranous colitis   Term used for diarrheal disease that often occurs in hospitalized patients with extensive antibiotic therapy has enabled overgrowth of the bacterium *Clostridium difficile*, which is identified by a toxin it produces.

Pseudophyllidean Relates to tapeworms (cestodes), order Pseudophyllidae.

Pseudopod Means "false foot" and is a temporary extension or protrusion of an amoeba that is used for locomotion and for phagocytosis (surrounding and feeding).

Pseudopodia Plural form of pseudopod, indicating more than one false foot.

Pulmonary trichomoniasis Trichomoniasis is usually found as the common sexually transmitted form, but are also known to cause bronchopulmonary infections in patients with preexisting pulmonary conditions that weaken the immune system.

Pupa The pupa is one of the life stages of some insects undergoing transformation from the egg through the pupa, larva, nymph and adult stages (found only in holometabolous insects).

Q

Q fever Acute infection caused by the rickettsia *Coxiella burnetii*, that is found intracellularly; transmitted through milk, inhaling dust, or handling stock animals.

R

Rabbit fever Term used for tularemia, along with Pahvant Valley plague, deerfly fever, and Ohara's fever. Rabbit fever is a serious infectious disease caused by the bacterium *Francisella tularensis*.

Redbugs Also called chiggers, jiggers, and harvest mites, of the family Trombiculidae; a larval mite that that is parasitic on land vertebrates, and sucks the blood of vertebrates including human beings causing extreme irritation.

Redia A larva of certain trematodes that during its life cycle is produced within the sporocyst; redia are formed within this sporocyst and develop into additional rediae or to cercariae.

Reduviid bug Member of the order Hemiptera; produces the genus of the true bugs, some of which prey on man; their bite may transmit *Trypanosoma cruzi*, better known as Chagas's disease.

Relapsing fever Illness that is characterized by a recurring high fever; disease is transmitted through the bites of both infected lice and ticks; disease produces episodic stages of high fever accompanied by chills, headache, muscle pain, and nausea; these signs and symptoms may recur every week or 10 days for up to several months.

Repellent The term generally refers to a substance applied to skin, clothing, or other surfaces to discourage insects and other arthropods from remaining in a given area or landing on the body.

Reservoir host A reservoir host serves as a source of infection and potential reinfection of hosts such as humans by sustaining a parasite when no suitable host is available.

Rhabditiform larva Rhabditiform larvae are passed in the stool and can either molt twice and become infective filariform larvae (direct development) or undergo four separate moltings and become free living adult males and females that mate and produce fertilized ova from which rhabditiform larvae hatch.

Rhinitis Inflammation of the nose.

Rice paddy itch Cercarial dermatitis is the technical name for a malady that is known invarious geographic locations by different names. In developing countries, swimmer's itch has been called rice paddy itch, clam diggers itch, and duck fleas. Several different parasites can cause reactions after swimming, but these itch infections usually refer to infestation with trematode parasites.

Rickettsial organisms Rickettsial diseases and other similar diseases are caused by a group of gram-negative, obligatively intracellular coccobacilli include ehrlichiosis, Q fever, Rocky Mountain spotted fever, and Lyme disease.

Ring form Trophozoite form of *Plasmodium* sp., which cause malaria.

River blindness (onchocerciasis) Onchocerciasis is one of the leading causes of blindness in the world and is caused by *Onchocerca volvulus*, a nematode that can live for up to 15 years in the human body but can also live in other mammals. Transmission to humans is through the bite of a blackfly.

Rocky Mountain spotted fever Acute infectious disease of the causative agent called *Rickettsia rickettsii*; transmitted by ticks of the family *Ixodidae*, most often by *Dermacenter* sp. or *D. variabilis*; manifested by a skin rash (bull's eye rash), muscular pains, high fever, and skin eruptions, and is endemic throughout North America.

Rodents Rodentia is an order of mammals known as rodents and is characterized by two continuously growing incisors in the upper and lower jaws which must be kept short by gnawing materials that will grind away the tips of these prominent teeth. Rats, beavers, squirrels, and many other animal species are rodents.

Romanowski(y) Stain used for determination of malaria, using thick and thin blood films stained with Giemsa or Romanowski dyes for diagnosis; developed in 1891 by Ernst Malachowski and Dmitri Leonidovich Romanowsky by combining the stains eosin Y and oxidated methylene blue.

Rostellum Structure protruding from the leading end of the scolex of a tapeworm; possesses spines or hooks for attachment in the intestines.

Roundworm Nematodes parasitic to humans as well as other organisms. Several different species of these worms cause infections in the intestines.

S

SAF Sodium acetate, acetic acid, formalin.

Sand gnats Known by various names depending on location. A number of species or genera of flying, biting, blood-sucking dipterans found in sandy areas. In the United States, the sandfly may refer to certain horse flies known as *greenheads*.

Sandflies Flies are dipterans, meaning two-winged; the genus Phlebotomus is known in Africa to transmit onchocerciasis, caused by a filarial worm *Onchocerca volvulus*.

Sarcoptidae The family of the order Acarina, this mite is responsible for scabies (itch) in humans and mange in other animals. The species most often responsible for these conditions is *Sarcoptes scabiei*.

Scabies   Scabies is an itchy skin condition caused by a tiny, eight-legged burrowing mite, an arachnid called *Sarcoptes scabiei*. The condition is known as the "itch," and is the contagious ectoparasite that causes a skin infection characterized by superficial burrows and intense pruritus (itching).

Scavengers   Term is used for any animal, including both birds and insects, that gains its nourishment from dead or decaying matter.

Schistosomiasis   A condition of being infected with one of the blood flukes of the genus of *Schistosoma*.

Schistosomula   The cercariae of *Schistosoma* burrow through the skin of the host and develop into schistosomula that migrate through the body until they reach their final position in the blood vessels where they mature.

Schizogony   Term used for asexual reproduction by multiple fission, a reproductive process for many sporozoan protozoans; fission refers to a division of the cell into two more or less equal parts.

Schizont   In the infection of malaria, sporozoites migrate to the liver where the parasite matures in the hepatocyte to a schizont containing many merozoites in it. After this hepatic stage, the erythrocytic stage begins following the formation of merosomes that contain thousands of merozoites, which bud off the hepatocytes. Within the erythrocytes the merozoite grow first to a ring-shaped form and then to a larger trophozoite form.

Scolex   The head portion of the cestode; the anterior, first segment of a tapeworm that possesses organs such as suckers, muscular jaws, or hooks for attachment.

Scotch tape prep   Use of cellophane tape to obtain the eggs laid in the anal region during the night by the female pinworm called *Enterobius vermicularis*.

Scutum   Hard shield-shaped chitinous plate covering the upper dorsal surface of hard-bodied ticks, a feature that distinguishes them from the wrinkled appearance of soft-bodied ticks.

Sebaceous glands   Glands of the skin that produce a secretion of fat; an oily solution that resembles fatty materials, the sebaceous secretions of some plants, or the sebaceous humor of animals.

Secretory IgA   Secretory IgA is a dimer of the immunoglobulin A and is the primary molecule of the mucosal surfaces and is one of the first lines of defense against invasion and colonization by potentially harmful microorganisms.

Sedimentation method   One of the two major techniques available for parasite assays and identification in separating eggs and even cysts from fecal material and concentrating the organisms or their ova.

Seed ticks   Nymphal form of some ticks that may be capable of transmitting infection.

Segmented neutrophils   A phagocytic leukocyte also called a *seg* or *poly*; when mature has a segmentednucleus (it is called a seg or poly). The immature neutrophil has a horseshoe-shaped nucleus called a band.

Semisulcospira   Species of freshwater snail with an operculum (lid-shaped cover) that is an aquatic gastropod (stomach-foot) mollusk capable of acting as the intermediate host for a number of parasites.

Seroprevalence   Refers to the frequency or probability of individuals in a population group that have a particular type of antibodies to a certain organism in the blood serum.

Sexually transmitted diseases (STDs)   Any of a variety of bacterial, viral, fungal, or protozoal organisms that are transmitted primarily by copulation (sexual intercourse).

Sheather sugar   Sheather's flotation method is a method for examining fecal samples for the presence of worm eggs or larvae using a saturated solution of sugar or saline.

Siberian liver fluke   A freshwater parasite called the *human liver fluke* is found in areas of Thailand, Japan, and Siberia where the species was first identified and studied. This parasite may trigger cancer in humans by creating harmful cell mutations, encouraging tumor formation in the liver.

Sigmoidoscopic   Most frequently a flexible tube connected to a fiber-optic camera is used in which a physician examines the large intestine.

Sleeping sickness   A parasitic disease found primarily in sub-Saharan African, trypanosomiasis is a parasitic disease in people and other animals that is transmitted by the tsetse fly, and is caused by several species of the genus Trypanosoma.

Slime molds   Originally classified as a fungus and no longer considered as such, *slime mold* is a general term for identifying fungi-like organisms that reproduce by spores.

Snails   Mollusks that have a muscular foot (Gastropoda) and that are capable of being parasitic vectors or intermediate hosts.

Soft tick   Any tick of the Argasidae family that lacks a dorsal shield, or scutum, and has the mouthparts on the underside of the head.

Southern Tick-associated Rash Illness   Also called STARI; emerging infectious disease related to Lyme disease that occurs in southeastern and south-central United States. The disease is spread by the bites of the tick called the lone star tick, *Amblyomma americanum*. The causative organism has not been definitively identified.

Spirochetes   Slender, motile organism with spiral shape; such as *Treponema pallidum*, the pathogen that causes syphilis.

Splenomegaly   Enlargement of the spleen located in the abdominal region.

Spontaneous generation   An obsolete assertion that life can spontaneously occur from nonliving matter. The appearance of maggots in meat sealed in a lidded container was used as "proof" that this occurred initially.

Sporocyst   A protective case or cyst where sporozoites develop and are then transferred to different hosts; also a bladder or saclike larval stage in many trematode worms.

Sporozoans   Class of parasitic protozoa that includes *Plasmodium, Cryptosporidium*.

Sporozoites   Undeveloped sporozoans that are produced by multiple division of a zygote or spore; stage where it may infect a new host cell.

Sputum   Thick, mucopurulent material from the air passages of the respiratory system that is coughed up and frequently expelled from mouth; mucus or mucopurulent matter expectorated due to various infectious diseases, including certain parasites, of the air passages.

St. Louis encephalitis   The disease caused by the mosquito is a form of encephalitis virus is related to Japanese encephalitis virus. This disease mainly affects the United States and less frequently Canada and Mexico.

Stoma   Mouth-like opening of certain protozoa (the term –*stoma* means "mouth").

Stramenopiles   Kingdom for protists of this group have flagella with fine hairlike projections and motile reproductive cells are flagellated. The organism is neither a yeast nor a protozoan and is now found in a new kingdom known as the Stramenopiles, which include algae, mildew, diatoms; was responsible for the Irish potato famine and the organism responsible for sudden oak death disease.

Stratum corneum   Outermost horny and keratin-rich layer of the epidermis.

Stratum germinativum   Layer of epidermis in which division of cells occurs leading to the formation of new skin.

Striated skeletal muscle   Muscles with fibers that are divided by transverse bands into striations; such muscles are voluntary and serve primarily to make gross motor movements of the body.

Strobila   Proglottids or segmented main body part of the adult tapeworm.

Strongyloidiasis   Infection with the roundworm called *Strongyloides stercoralis*.

Subcutaneous   Layer of skin lying beneath the horny, outer layer of skin called the *epidermis*.

Subcutaneous filariasis   The condition of filariasis is divided into three groups according to the organs occupied (i.e., lymphatic, subcutaneous, and serous cavity filariasis). Subcutaneous filariasis is caused by *Loa loa* (the African eye worm), *Mansonella streptocerca*, *Onchocerca volvulus*, and *Drancuculus medinensis* (guinea worm). These worms occupy the subcutaneous layer of the skin or the fatty layer.

Subphylum   A taxonomic category that occurs between a phylum and a class.

Suckers   Anatomic structure on the mouthparts of parasites that enable stronger attachment to a host.

Sudden oak death disease   Caused by organisms of the kingdom Stramenopiles.

Supernatant   The term for the liquid portion lying above a layer of precipitated and insoluble material.

Surra   A condition affecting mostly camels and horses and is caused by *Trypanosoma evansi* through the bites of flies.

Swimmer's itch   A number of organisms may be responsible for the condition as an itchy rash or dermatitis caused whose hosts are waterfowl and freshwater snails. Names ascribed to this condition are duck itch, cercarial dermatitis, and schistosome cercarial dermatitis, which is usually a short-lived immune reaction of the human skin.

Symbiosis   A parasitic relationship between two or more different organisms that may but do not always benefit each of the members.

Syndrome   Refers to the association of a number of clinically identifiable features such as signs observed by medical professionals and symptoms (subjective) that are reported by an individual.

T

Tabanid flies   The bloodsucking dipterous flies of the family Tabanidae, including horseflies, that are involved in transmission of several bloodborne parasites.

Tachycardia   Rapid cardiac rate of well over 100 beats per minute.

Taenia tapeworms   *Taenia* is a genus of tapeworm including medical and economically important parasites of humans and livestock. The most important representatives from the genus *Taenia* are *T. solium* (pig tapeworm) and *T. saginata* (beef tapeworm).

Talmud   Record of Jewish law, ethics, history, and customs which outline rabbinic laws restricting certain practices, such as eating certain meats.

Tapeworm   Narrow, segmented worm of the class *Cestoda*.

Taxonomy   Science of classification according to morphology and ecological niches occupied by specific organisms.

Tenesmus   The term describes the constant feeling of the need to defecate along with pain and cramping that may accompany inflammatory diseases of the intestinal tract.

Teres   Term related to muscle shapes, such as the anatomical feature of being round and long.

Tetracycline   Bacteriostatic antibiotic used for several parasitic species, including *C. trachomatis*.

Tetrachloroehtylene   Liquid used some exclusively years ago as an anthelmintic medication has now been replaced safer and more effective drugs.

Tetrad   Term most commonly identifies a group or set of four; in biology often refers to division within a spore mother cell during meiosis as in *Babesia* sp. reproduction.

Tetraethylene   Refers to a molecular arrangement of four functional groups.

Thin smear   For laboratory diagnosis of malaria, both thin and thick blood smears are stained for microscopic examination.

Thoracic   The thoracic cavity is the chest cavity of the human body containing the lungs and the heart.

Threadworms   The filaria of *Strongyloides stercoralis* are called threadworms, but less often and not exclusively, the worms of *Enterobius vermicularis* are also called *threadworms* or *seatworms*.

Thready pulse   Arterial pulse, that when palpated, is fine and barely perceptible.

Thrombocytopenia   Decrease in the absolute platelet (thrombocyte) count in the blood.

Thymol   Synthetic or natural thyme oil useful in antibacterial and antifungal treatments that is also used as an over-the-counter preparations for treatment of hemorrhoids, acne, and tinea pedis (athlete's foot). It may be used as a stabilizer preservative in some preparations.

Tick typhus   Any of several tick-borne rickettsial diseases identified as the typhus group (vs. spotted group) of *R. prowazekii*, *R. typhi*, and *R. Canada*.

Tissue flukes   Refers to a number of flukes that are identified by the anatomic portion or organ of the body that the various species primarily infect.

Toe itch   Old term for sores between the toes from the burrowing of hookworm larvae.

Toxocariasis   This term refers to an infection caused by the dog or cat roundworm, *Toxocara canis* or *Toxocara cati*, respectively. Ingestion of these worms may lead to visceral larval migrans and ocular larvae migrans.

Toxoplasmosis   Infection with the organism, a protozoan, called *Toxoplasma gondii*. At least 1/3 of the population of the United States has been exposed.

Trachea   Portion of the respiratory system that carries air from the mouth and nose through the neck and into the upper lungs.

Trachoma   Chronic and contagious type of conjunctivitis caused by the *Chlamydia trachomatis* organism, and is a leading cause of blindness in the world.

Translactational   Ability of toxins and pathogens that may be transmitted through the milk of a lactating mother.

Transplacental   Term that refers to toxins or pathogens capable of crossing the membranes of the placenta separating the mother from the fetus, to whom such substances may be dangerous

Treatment   Course of action designed to alleviate a medical condition.

Triatomid   This term refers to some blood-sucking species, particularly the *Triatoma* spp. spp. and are also known as kissing bugs due to their habit of biting sleeping humans on the lips and eyes; a number of these insects are found in Central and South America, and are capable of transmitting Chagas's disease, which is also called *American trypanosomiasis*.

Trichina   Genus of parasitic roundworms of the phylum Nematoda that cause trichinosis. Other names frequently used for this genus are trichinella or trichina worms.

Trichinellosis   Another term for "trichinosis"; is a parasitic disease that occurs from eating raw or undercooked pork and sometimes wild game meat that is infected with the larvae of one of the species of the roundworm *Trichinella spiralis*. A few cases occur annually in the United States as a result of eating undercooked game meat or home reared pigs that were fed uncooked garbage contaminated with the larvae. This is a common condition found in the developing areas of the world where pigs are mostly fed raw garbage.

Trichrome stains   The stain refers to a method utilizing a combination of three different dyes to identify organisms, cells, and tissue elements.

Trophozoite   This is the motile form of many protozoa during which time the organism feeds, multiplies, and grows within the host it has infected; other names for this form are "vegetative" and "trophic" forms.

Trypanosomes   The most notable trypanosomal diseases is trypanosomiasis (African sleeping sickness and South American Chagas's disease); these are caused by species of the genus *Trypanosoma*.

Trypanosomiasis   Condition of being infected with one of the organisms of the *Trypanosoma* genus.

Tsetse belt   An area that stretches from West to East Africa and is the geographic location where most tsetse flies abound.

Tsetse fly   The tsetse fly is found only in Africa and is known for transmitting trypanosomes as disease agents causing human sleeping sickness and animal trypanosomosis.

Tularemia   Infectious disease caused by the bacterium *Francisella tularensis* that chiefly affects rodents but can also be transmitted to humans through bites of various insects or contact with infected animals.

Turkey ticks   Larval forms of *Amblyomma americanum*; is a tick known somewhat incorrectly as "turkey mites."

Typhoidal   The term refers to an infectious disease caused by the bacterium *Francisella tularensis* that chiefly affects rodents but can also be transmitted to humans.

Typhus   Forms of infectious disease caused by rickettsia, especially those transmitted by fleas, lice, or mites.

U

Ulcerations   Condition where ulcers have occurred and have caused a breakdown of the tissue.

Ulcerative colitis   The condition is an inflammatory bowel disease with infectious and psychological impact, and causes chronic inflammation of the digestive tract. The disease primarily causes abdominal pain and diarrhea.

Ulceroglandular   The condition is usually manifested in ulceroglandular tularemia as the most common form of the disease. Signs and symptoms are characterized by a skin ulcer that forms at the site of infection, most often in the area of an insect bite.

Ulcers   Often associated with the stomach, but an ulcer is a lesion of the skin or a mucous membrane often accompanied by pus (discharge containing WBCs) and necrosis of adjacent tissues.

Undernourished   The condition may result from consuming too little food over a period of time or the lack of certain nutrients but may occur due to infections by parasites that rob the body of essential nourishment.

Uncinariasis   Genus *Uncinaria* relates to hookworm infection; Latin for hook-shaped.

Undulating membrane   Occurs in flagellated forms of some organisms such as that of *Trypanosoma*, which has a fin-like ridge along the dorsal area of the organism. A flagellum may be buried in this ridge, with the end extending as a flagellum for locomotion; movement of this structure causes the body of the organism to engage in wavelike repetitive movements of the cell membrane.

Unembryonated eggs   Embryonated eggs containing larval worms can be seen while an unembryonated eggs is absent in larval form.

Unilocular   The term means having but one cavity or compartment.

United Nations   Although multiple roles and functions are occupied by the organization, it is an international organization whose stated aims are facilitating cooperation in international law.

Urethral occlusion   Characterized by the failure to pass urine, the urethra may be blocked by edema, renal stones, or parasite eggs such as in schistosomiasis.

Urethritis   Urethritis refers to inflammation of the urethra, usually as a result of infection.

Uterine pore   Small opening through which eggs of certain tapeworms are discharged.

V

Vacuolar   Structure or organism with small cavities called *vacuoles* spread through the cytoplasm of cells.

Vacuole   Small cavity in the cytoplasm of a cell, bound by a single membrane and containing water, food, or metabolic waste.

Vascular system   Veins, arteries, and heart of an organism such as a mammal.

Vector   Organism that carries and perhaps transports parasites from one host to another; snails, other mollusks, and insects often serve as vectors for parasites as well as viruses and bacteria.

Vincent's angina   An acute communicable infection of the respiratory tract and mouth marked by ulceration of the mucous membrane.

Visceral larva migrans   Caused by parasitic worms that infect the intestines of dogs and cats. The dog parasite is called *Toxocara canis* and the cat parasite is called *Toxocara cati*. The disease is contracted where eggs in the feces of infected animals enter soil and allow the infection to spread to humans.

Vitamin B$_{12}$ Used to treat pernicious anemia.

Volutin   Granular, phosphoric substance that stains with basic dyes and is found in the cytoplasm of some bacterial and fungal cells.

W

West Nile virus   Mosquito-borne virus that can cause encephalitis or meningitis (inflammation of the membranes surrounding the brain).

Western blacklegged tick   This tick is a three-host tick that primarily feeds on lizards or small rodents before adulthood and on large mammals, commonly deer, canids, and dusky-footed woodrats. This organism is the principal vector for Lyme disease in the western United States, as it readily bites humans.

Wet mount   In order to allow light to pass through a microscopic preparation more effectively, a wet mount of water or normal physiological saline may be used for microscopic examination under a high-power objective.

Wheatley modification   Wheatley's modification of Gomori's trichrome technique is useful in examining stained fecal film for the presence of parasites.

Whipworms   A slender, whip-shaped, parasitic nematode worm (*Trichuris trichiura*) that often infects the intestine of humans.

WHO   World Health Organization.

Wolbachia   The term refers to a genus of bacteria that infect a wide variety of invertebrates that includes insects, spiders, crustaceans, and nematodes.

Worms   Used as a general description of a variety of parasites other than protozoa.

Wright stain   Hematology stain for staining blood cells for differentiation, morphology.

Wright's-Giemsa   Combination hematological stain useful for identifying intracellular parasites.

Wyle's disease   Caused by spirochetes that are also responsible for relapsing fever, infectious jaundice, Lyme disease, sores, ulcers, and Vincent angina.

Y

Yellow dog tick   The American dog tick is from a genus of hard-bodied ticks of which most species are important vectors of disease. It has a decorative white or yellow outer dorsal covering called the *scutum*.

Yellow fever   This disease is an acute viral hemorrhagic disease resulting in jaundice due to the destruction of RBCs. *Aedes aegypti* mosquitoes primarily but along with some other species are capable of transmitting the virus which is prevalent in tropical and subtropical areas in South America and Africa.

Z

Zinc sulfate   The specific gravity of zinc sulfate is adjusted to a particular level and is used as a fecal flotation medium for finding the ova and some cysts of parasites.

Zoonosis   Diseases of animals, such as rabies, that can be transmitted to humans.

Zygote   This term is used for the union of two gametes resulting in a complete cell that may develop into a mature organism.

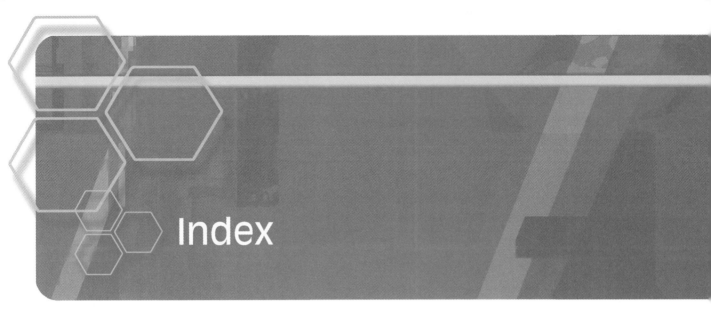

Index